DIFFERENCES IN MEDICINE

D0757499

BODY, COMMODITY, TEXT

Studies of Objectifying Practice

A series edited by

Arjun Appadurai,

Jean Comaroff, and

Judith Farquhar

DIFFERENCES IN MEDICINE

Unraveling Practices, Techniques, and Bodies

Marc Berg and Annemarie Mol,

editors

▼

Duke University Press   Durham and London 1998

© 1998 Duke University Press
All rights reserved
Printed in the United States of America on acid-free paper ∞
Typeset in Minion by Tseng Information Systems, Inc.
Library of Congress Cataloging-in-Publication Data appear
on the last printed page of this book.

CONTENTS

ACKNOWLEDGMENTS

We would like to thank Els Goorman, Maura High, Jean Brady, Hellen Heutz, Richard Morrison, and Ken Wissoker for their help and support in getting this book in print.

Parts of Marc Berg's chapter have appeared in Marc Berg, *Rationalizing Medical Work* (Cambridge, Mass.: MIT Press, 1997). Parts of Monica Casper's chapter have appeared in Monica J. Casper, *The Making of the Unborn Patient: A Social Anatomy of Fetal Surgery* (New Brunswick, N.J.: Rutgers University Press, 1998). An earlier version of Charis Cussins's chapter was published in *Social Studies of Science* 26 (1996): 575–610.

DIFFERENCES IN MEDICINE

DIFFERENCES IN MEDICINE:
AN INTRODUCTION

Annemarie Mol & Marc Berg

▼

In 1981 Barbara Smith published an article under the title *Black Lung: The Social Production of Disease*. She stressed that not just anybody risks developing the disease "black lung." What turns it into a reality for some—miners—and not for others—for instance, the shareholders of the mining companies—is social relations. Moreover, the often early and severe development of black lung that Smith encountered in the region she reports on, West Virginia, is not an inevitable consequence of mining. The onset and course of the disease depend on the specific working conditions in the mines: on the amounts of coal dust and on the levels of oxygen miners get to breathe. And, related to that, on the extent to which miners are or are not granted control over the way they work.

But what happens to the lungs of miners is not all that is socially produced. Social relations also shape the *categories* used in discussing health conditions. Smith, for example, examines which specific miners were judged to be ill enough to be entitled to a financial compensation from the mining company they worked for or, later on, from the government. She shows that there is not just one set of terms with which to discuss this question but *two*. Initially, one might note that it is possible to make an *X ray* of a miner's lungs: the whiter the picture, the blacker the lungs. Above a certain threshold the miner can then be said to be ill enough to deserve compensation. This, in fact, is how company doctors proceeded. They wanted an objectified image to point at, a picture that could be measured against a standard, to avoid the complexities of further discussing the rights and wrongs done to people in specific cases.

But the miners didn't agree. Such objectified images had little to do with their suffering. Standardized judgments of X-ray images led to what they saw as completely arbitrary decisions: one worker might get compensation while his neighbor, who was worse off, got none. The miners felt that they deserved financial compensation, not if their X rays were bad, but if they *suffered:* if, say, they were no longer capable of working in their garden, or climbing the stairs. Doctors who did not work for the mining companies often supported the miners in their challenge of X rays as a diagnostic criterion. These doctors thought that the severity of black lung deserved to be assessed in terms of *respiratory disability*, something that does not correlate neatly with X ray images.

Smith argues that medical categories are intertwined with their social background and usage and that, therefore, these categories come in pairs of two, one on each side of the class struggle. There is black lung that translates the interests of the companies and black lung that reflects the position of the miners. And there is a fight between them: which of these two wins out as the "real" black lung when compensation is decided upon? Smith describes how this fight about reality figured in the strikes of West Virginia miners in 1968. She warns health advocates involved in other struggles elsewhere: they, too, may have to challenge the definitions of the diseases they try to eradicate by changing the social relations that produce them.

Smith's article appeared in the *International Journal of Health Services*. But it was never routinely cited in other articles in this or other journals. Its argument was that social struggle does not stop when it encounters the boundary of medicine but simply crosses it. Class conflict does not respect the boundary of what, in medicine, is called scientific: the struggle continues right into the "heart" of biomedicine. Smith's text shows this convincingly and in detail for the case at hand. Even so, it seems to never have convinced — or even reached — many readers. Maybe this is due to the overtly activist tone, to the polarization between Marxists and anti-Marxists of that time. Or maybe it is due to the way Smith's radical moves thwarted the more careful strategies of contemporary philosophers and social scientists. Smith took the way patients interpret their condition as something relevant to debates *inside* biomedicine. The dominant strategy of these theorists, on the contrary, was one of *addition*: biomedical knowledge was seen as "too limited," as requiring a psychosocial supplement. But they left its content unchallenged. They believed that attending to people's personal interpretations, to their "illness," had to be done as something on top of, or next to, attending to "disease."

Smith's challenging article was almost forgotten: for quite a while, the unity of medicine was a favorite trope amongst medicine's investigators — until, slowly, creaks and cleavages began to show. Medicine's social diversity, its regional variations, its embeddedness in different contexts, were gradually dissected. Marxist, feminists, and antiracist researchers did their bit in topicalizing "difference" — until "difference" became a theme that went beyond their primary concerns and reached everywhere. This book is a product of that process. This is our point of departure: medicine is not a coherent whole. It is not a unity. It is, rather, an amalgam of thoughts, a mixture of habits, an assemblage of techniques. Medicine is a heterogeneous coalition of ways of handling bodies, studying pictures, making numbers, conducting conversations. Wherever you look, in hospitals, in clinics, in laboratories, in general practitioners' offices — there is multiplicity. There is multiplicity even inside medicine's biomedical "core."

A few years ago Donna Haraway wrote: "But if there has been recognition of the many non-, para-, anti-, or extrascientific languages in company with biomedicine that structure the embodied semiosis of mortality in the industrialized world, it is much less common to find emphasis on the multiple language *within* the territory that is so often glibly marked scientific."[1] We have accepted the challenge: it is this territory — "so often glibly marked scientific" — that we venture to explore. In one way or another, all our chapters investigate the *contents* of medical diagnosis and intervention: the way people's bodies and lives are shaped by the activities of doctors, nurses, technicians, and technologies, and the work involved in making textbooks come true. So this is the first commonality that links the various chapters: they explore differences in the shape accorded to the physical body and its diseases. They open up the so-called hard core of medicine, the business of medical judgments, decision making, intervention. They focus on the very biomedical facts that for such a long time seemed beyond the grasp of philosophers and social scientists.

There is another commonality. We proceed not just by exploring the ideals and ideas of medicine. We also investigate its practices and performances: the manipulation of fluids and numbers in the laboratory, the physical examination of suffering patients, and the filling out of forms. We have studied the interactions of doctors and patients, and the meetings where professionals make plans or draw conclusions — pointing their fingers at pictures or graphs. Of course each of us has studied these practices in a slightly different way. Between our chapters, there are divergences, overlaps, disputes, and resonances: partial connections.[2]

UNITIES AND DISAGGREGATION

If medicine is not a unity, then other unities implicated with it dissolve, too. The traditions in which these "unities" were created form a part of our intellectual backgrounds. But the process of their dissolution has been going on for some time now. It is that process in which we are caught up, and to which we

ence was the place of unity par excellence, a place where coherence was not incidental, but essential. The idea was that in the realm of science each logical contradiction would be explored and resolved, with all the work of investigating and arguing this implied. It might take some time, but in the end this work would yield consensus. A global picture. For science was taken to refer to a reality beyond itself. A final arbiter that, even if it could only be asymptotically approached, was undoubtedly singular in nature.

The social study of science, however, has loosened the link between science and its objects. It shifts the attention to the relation between scientific stories and the places from where they are told. Studies focus on labeling and accounting practices, on the manipulation of petri dishes and calculators, on the rhetorics of writing, on publication and citation practices, on interests and ambitions: practices that hang together through a complicated set of rules and their transgressions. If the objects of study matters to the outcome of all this, it is as one element among many, an element that no longer holds the power to draw divergences together. If unification is ever reached, this no longer seems to follow from the objects: it is, rather, a sociomaterial accomplishment, an in-situ achievement, a construction that necessarily remains local and rare. That science might be unified, then, becomes more and more difficult to conceive. The idea that the combined efforts of everything and everyone involved in thousands of highly divergent, scientific practices could ever merge into a unity seems like a far-fetched fantasy.[14]

We have touched upon four failing coherences. And we're not there yet. A fifth unity to be disrupted is the *patient*. At first glance, this might seem odd: hasn't the complaint against medicine for a long time been that it *disrupts* the unity of the patient? That it dehumanizes persons, takes their bodies apart, reduces them to organs and functions?[15] But in the process of framing this criticism, the "patient as a whole" was erected as a normative standard—as a philosophical dream against which actual practices could be measured and discarded. "The patient" was something undividable, an in-dividual: the true foundation for the normative requirement to be humane.

Some scholars have started to work in a different way. Instead of departing from preestablished truths or norms, they wonder how truths and norms get established. Instead of attempting philosophical judgments from an outside vantage point, they try to dissect from the inside, and by empirical means. At that point, both truth and norms start to look like parts of ongoing practices, mobilized in specific situations by some participants and not others. And their multiplicity appears to be overwhelming. The idea that there is a single body preceding knowledge and treatment is no longer self-evident. Instead, many bodies shaped in medical practices are displayed. In the light of the many possible existing reductions, it sounds, paradoxically, more and more empty to say that the person "is reduced." Instead, these authors begin to attribute advantages and disadvantages to various reductions. Analyzing and confronting those seems a richer, more powerful, and yet less imperialistic strategy than using a single standard — always and everywhere. Thus, the single human being that forms the heart of humanism gives way to a composite picture involving many measurements, numbers, intuitions, habits, humans — not to mention dead ends and (often unresolvable) contradictions.[16]

The image of a unified medicine gives way to one that overflows with diversity. But how is this diversity to be understood? Is it not a mere artifact, an effect of coming ever closer to the messiness of practice? What is its relevance?

First, diversity is sometimes taken to be a *problem*, something to fight against — as it is, for example, by those who complain about so-called medical practice variations.[17] They take unity to be the norm against which variety must be measured and discarded. They take diversity to be a temporary state that may be overcome through such things as evaluation studies, protocols, and the standardization of terminology. Our authors, however, do not believe that diversity is a temporary state of affairs. Instead, several of us argue that diversity, problem or no problem, good or bad, is here to stay. Even if it is countered by massive means, diversity will remain a feature of any complex practice, medical practice included. Instead of countering it, it would therefore be better to find more creative ways to handle it.

A second way to conceive of diversity is to imagine that however impressive it may look on the surface, a deeper unity hides behind it,[18] a unity that is all the stronger because of its disguise. For as long as the battles on the surface attract a lot of attention, nobody delves beneath them. Thus the underlying unity is left untouched. Again, this is not the way the authors of this book conceive of diversity. Neither do we subscribe to the opposite image, in which the existence of diversity signals the triumph of liberal pluralism and proves the freedom of all. But if diversity neither hides a fundamental unity nor signals a freedom that deserves celebration then what does it do? That question, we think, is precisely what requires investigation. Our studies show both unifying and disruptive forces; both continuities and discontinuities. They point at *tensions* among shaping practices, bodies, and lives in various diverging ways: tensions between making the world run in this, rather than in some other way.

diagnostic, research, and treatment practices in and around a Dutch university hospital. She shows the effort involved in linking the object "atherosclerosis" of the pathology department or the hematology lab with that of the outpatient clinic or radiological imaging. There is no single object waiting in the body that guarantees the possibility of such links. Links only exist if they can be practically performed. Thus some links are missing.

Charis Cussins takes us to a Californian infertility clinic in an attempt to move beyond Enlightenment notions of agency. She argues that the various *objectifications* to which women are subjected in this clinic are not antithetical to their agency or subjectivity. Instead, they are used by the women as a means of pursuing agency and becoming a self. Cussins analyzes how the (self-) attribution of agency fluctuates and shifts throughout the process of in-vitro fertilization and relates this to its failure, success, or as-yet-open outcome.

Stefan Timmermans, Geoffrey Bowker, and Susan Leigh Star discuss the creation of the Nursing Interventions Classification, a nursing classification scheme originating in Illinois, meant to be widely used in the United States and elsewhere. They claim that making a successful classification scheme depends on the balancing of a *series of demands that can never be met simultaneously.* They show how the designers deal with the tensions among these demands. Making things visible and comparable, creating intimacy, and allowing for manageability may all be desirable but trade off against one another.

Marc Berg discusses decision support tools developed to replace the "messiness" of ordinary medical practice with the "order" of a deliberate, agreed-upon strategy. With examples from the introduction of a breast cancer protocol, he shows that a protocol may indeed alter local diagnosis and treatment. Instead of obliterating messiness, however, it complexifies the relation between "order" and "disorder." Protocols, Berg argues, do not create homogeneity, but introduce *new kinds of diversity* in medical practices. They may help to manage differences, but they produce new ones in the process.

None of us tries to say that medicine lacks something, the coherence it would surely have if only it were scientific. Quite the contrary. "Incoherences" as we describe them here can be found in all practices informed by, and in their turn informing, scientific knowledge. Medicine doesn't fail to meet the standards: the standards fail to meet reality. Whoever wants to study scientific practices outside the research laboratory may go as we did to the hospitals and other sites we studied, to find science there, as well as divergences.

Do these divergences have their origins elsewhere—in society? Are they a product of some social difference or influence that doesn't stop short at the boundary of medicine but crosses it? Sometimes this may be the case. But it isn't always easy to project the differences we describe onto a preexisting social relation that generates and explains them. Social relations do not necessarily precede medicine. They also follow from it — and they can be found inside it. Whoever wants to study society may go, too, to the sites we studied, for there it is — in all its ambiguity, ambivalence, shifts and balances, efforts at coordination, conflicts, and compromises.

NOTES

1 Haraway 1991: 204.

2 For an insightful study on "difference" and "comparability," introducing the term "partial connections," see Strathern 1991.

3 From Freidson 1970 until Abbott 1988. For a broad overview of the tradition of medical sociology from the fifties to the eighties, see Gerhardt 1989.

4 Good examples of this are Fox and Swazey 1978; Bosk 1979; Strong 1979; Strauss et al. 1985; and Atkinson 1995.

5 For national differences, see, e.g., Vos 1991; for a combination of national and socioprofessional differences, McCrea and Markle 1984; for professional differences that coincide with political ones, Smith 1981; for differences between nurses and physicians, Anspach 1993; for different conceptions of general practitioners' tasks, Singleton and Michael 1993; for differences between different groups of physicians, Baszanger 1992; 1995.

6 See for a recent example of a study in which Western medicine is severely criticized as so much poorer than the healing practices of "the others": Gordon 1988. See, for a more subtle depiction of the difference between "cosmopolitan" and other — in this case various Asiatic — medicines Leslie and Young 1992. Interestingly enough, most authors contributing to the latter book describe the various Asiatic medicines they studied as containing the kind of differences we attribute to cosmopolitan medicine — which they take to be united.

7 The titles of these studies suggest the move was daring: *Physicians of Western Medicine; American Medicine as Culture; Anthropologie de la maladie*, etc. See Hahn and Gaines 1985; Stein 1990; Laplantine 1986.

8 See, e.g., Kleinman 1980; Good and Good 1980; Helman 1978; Young 1981; contributions to Lock and Gordon 1988; Willems 1992; Martin 1994; O'Neill 1994; Good 1995. See also Payer 1989.

9 For some examples, see Hohlfeld 1978; Dodier 1993b; 1994; Hirschauer 1991; 1993; Lindenbaum and Lock 1993; Haraway 1991; Frankenberg 1992; Mol and Law 1994.

10 For highly divergent examples, see Ehrenreich and English 1978; Reiser 1978; Starr 1982; and for a tradition of focusing on ruptures in the contents of medical knowledge, Canguilhem 1966; Foucault 1963. And see the critical Foucauldian studies of,

e.g., Armstrong 1983 and Arney and Bergen 1984. Or, in a different vein again, Rothshuh 1978 and Böhme 1980.

11   An important text here is Fleck 1935, rediscovered in the late seventies.

12   See, e.g., Marks 1988; Pasveer 1992. And see, e.g., Warner's seminal work 1986.

13   For examples of histories that show no breaking points, but shifts, inclusions, juxtapositions, etc., see Mol and van Lieshout 1989; for one that analyzes the creation of "time" along with history: Latour 1984. On different times in medical practices see, e.g., Roth 1979; Frankenberg 1992; Star and Bowker 1997.

14   For some crucial examples, see Latour and Woolgar 1986; Knorr-Cetina 1981; Collins 1985; Star 1989b; Traweek 1988. For studies especially attending to "difference," Goodman 1978; Haraway 1991; Jordan and Lynch 1992; Lynch 1993. An early application of some of these perspectives to medicine was Wright and Treacher 1982; see also Bloor 1978. For studies on medical work drawing on social studies of science perspectives, see Fujimura and Chou 1994; Casper 1998; Berg and Casper 1995; Timmermans 1995; Berg 1997.

15   For some examples, see Clavreul 1978; Cassel 1982; Wulff, Pedersen, and Rosenberg 1986.

16   See, e.g., Treichler 1990; Duden 1991; Haraway 1991; Strathern 1992; Rapp 1993; Heath and Rabinow 1993.

17   See, e.g., Andersen and Mooney 1990.

18   The work of Foucault has often been read in this way. For although Foucault explicitly states that there are cleavages in the present as well as in history, his studies always regard the latter, not the former. See Foucault 1963 and, as examples of unifying readings, Armstrong 1983 and Arney and Bergen 1984.

19   See, e.g., Haraway 1991.

PERFORMING SEXES AND GENDERS
IN MEDICAL PRACTICES

Stefan Hirschauer

▼

To talk of differences in medicine is to evoke the vast array of heterogeneous discourses and practices among different medical disciplines, settings, and groups, and the various diseases and bodies incorporated in these discourses and practices. This chapter contributes to this discussion by showing how three medical disciplines involved in a sex change determine the sex of an individual and how they define the meaning of "sex" by various differentiating practices: practices that set apart, divide, distinguish, categorize, classify, segregate, dissect, discriminate, and separate.

The specific case of sex change also raises the question of how a difference already made in everyday life (the sex difference) is drawn into, reproduced, and changed in medicine. This question of "differences in medicine" concerns the way in which medical disciplines reconstruct, protect, and mould the life-world distinction between men and women. And by looking at how medical practice is embedded in a wider cultural context, we are also able to see how the disunity of medicine can be induced and reduced by this context.

Some of the practices that construct "sexes"[1] in everyday life are well known through ethnomethodological and interactionist research. Participants in public and private interactions maintain ongoing processes of gender presentation and gender attribution in order to display and categorize each other as members of a specific sex category (Garfinkel 1967; Goffman 1976; Kessler and McKenna 1978; West and Zimmerman 1987). In current feminist contributions on the performance of gender (Butler 1990), these phenomena have given rise to theories of the contingency and esthetic multitude of gender. Unfortunately, poststructural discourse analysis has not taken into account *empirical* explorations of the performative dimension of sex membership. In fact, it has highlighted the contingency of gender by implicitly contrasting it with a biomedical notion of sex as a monolithic, ontological entity. Since outside of identity politics there is no need to oppose ontologies, I will try, instead, in this essay to *reconstruct* the ontologies inherent in different medical practices.

From the biographical perspective, the process of sexing an individual starts in a medical setting: in the deciphering of the gray shadows of ultrasound pictures or—more important for the legal fixing of gender—at birth. Knowing that the strange creature emerging there must be either a "boy" or a "girl," a doctor or a midwife takes certain anatomical features as a good reason to apply one or other gender category to the baby.

To understand transsexuality as a social phenomenon, it is useful to think of it as a delayed revocation of that first attribution: "No, I'm not a girl. I'm a boy." Such a revocation leads to uncertain social situations with opposing categorizations, that is, to a micropolitical conflict between, on the one hand, a person making a verbal claim to being one gender and, on the other hand, people in his/her environment who believe him/her to be the other gender because of his/her public appearance or their past knowledge of this person. Two parties emerge here: the first is the majority of people, embarrassed by this severe interruption of the routine workings of their classificatory practices; the second is that tiny minority who develop a modest rhetoric of self-determination as a consequence of their political weakness. They don't aggressively claim to be the other gender or simply live as such, but they subjectively *feel* it "inside."

In the history of the medicalization of this social conflict, such clashes have been reconstructed as divides between "body" and "soul," "sex" and "gender" (Stoller 1968)—divisions that reflect territories of different medical disciplines. These divides have given rise to the well-known formula of a person with a "female (or male) soul being captured in a wrong body." The formula has a life-world predecessor. In nineteenth-century Germany it was framed in *moral* language that implied that gender deviants (called *Urninge*) had the wrong body, given their sexual preferences: "What we do is not false, what is false is our body." At the end of the nineteenth century this sense of wrongness acquired *theoretical* meaning, with the development of a biological etiology and symptomatology for homosexuals. Finally, since the 1920s, the wrongness has acquired *pragmatic* meaning with the development of genital surgery. A body now can be experienced as "wrong" because it can be corrected.[2]

The delegation of the problem to medicine has also shifted its controversial character into medicine. The disunity of people in families and at places of work over the gender of an individual became a profound disunity within medicine, which was expressed in heated ethical debates about the legitimacy of genital surgery.[3] The micropolitical conflict about whose gender definition must adapt itself was transformed into a question of medical treatment: whether one should adapt the soul to the body psychiatrically or the body to the soul surgically. And social conflicts about the validity of gender migrants' claims were transformed into theoretical controversies about nosological classification: labeling transsexuality a psychotic condition, a neuroendocrinopathy, a borderline syndrome, or a creative defense mechanism — each implied a political position with regard to the social conflict.

The debates were largely settled in the 1960s with the formation of interdisciplinary treatment programs for transsexuals, where careful selection of candidates was designed to guarantee a successful sex change under medical management (Green and Money 1969). Professionals participating in such programs included psychiatrists, urologists, gynecologists, plastic surgeons, endocrinologists, medical practitioners, voice therapists, cosmeticians, social workers, and legal experts.

In what follows, I will describe some aspects of this treatment program, which I studied in a two-year ethnographic project in Germany.[4] I will concentrate on the three most important medical disciplines, ignoring other professions and some of the local differences.[5] I make use of an ideal-typical description of practices that enables the contrasts and comparisons required for my argument—which can also be spelled out in a myriad of situated events and conversational details (see Hirschauer 1993). My analysis will not focus on the differences between medical *actors* in, for example, their education, ethos, theoretical views, and prejudices. Instead, my guiding questions are: What are the different praxeontologies of sex and gender that are incorporated in different medical *practices* of psychiatry, endocrinology, and surgery? And how are these disparate practices linked?

PSYCHIATRY: RECIPROCAL GENDER ATTRIBUTION

Psychiatry's task in the medical management of a sex change is to diagnose transsexuality—not so much for its own therapeutic approach but as a service for endocrinologists, surgeons, and judges. In the case of transsexuality, compared to other syndromes, psychiatrists do not have much to rely on in their diagnosis: the electroencephalograms of gender changers are not noticeably different, psychological testing mostly reveals nothing interesting, and their behavior isn't sufficiently "mad" to be called psychotic.

The diagnostic procedure that was designed to cope with this embarrassing situation consists of a one-year period in which the patients have to live as the other gender—the so-called everyday test—to prove their claim. This is combined with a series of interviews intended to rule out other syndromes and to understand the biographical development of the patients' "personal conflict."

The psychiatrists I studied were fairly nominalist in their attitude to the label

"transsexual." They either viewed the decision to label someone as a transsexual as "crucial but simple" — a matter of adding symptoms together — or
they were not concerned at all in whether "transsexual" was the right label for
a patient. Those who took the latter view were interested in understanding the
person's life and focused on the problem of the right treatment for a patient.

Psychiatrists' decisions about whether someone is a transsexual or not are
informed by heterogeneous factors, including their experience with different
types of gender changers, their detailed knowledge of a patient's personality,
or even by their wish to get rid of a difficult patient. But the most important
factor influencing their decision is what psychiatrists call their personal conviction that someone is a certain gender. Evidence for this is sought in three
ways: through biographical data, through whether the patients pass the "everyday test," and by interactive experience in the therapeutic situation.

First, patients are asked to tell biographical stories that show their long-
standing conviction that they are the other gender and have behaved like someone of that gender. Second, patients are called on to solve the problems that
come up in their everyday life as they actually live in their new gender; they are
urged to show that they "are" the other gender.

The problem with these two approaches is that psychiatrists know very
well that gender changers extensively reconstruct their biographies: they create
matching stories, conceal much and gloss over problems in their life as the new
gender when talking about their experience in the everyday test.[6] In a therapeutic context, doctors can only hope to observe the gradual adaptation of the
patients' public appearance to their verbal claims, that is, an increasingly routine gender presentation. But even so there is an additional complexity for —
in contrast to everyday relevances in gender diagnosis — a perfect presentation
may not convince the psychiatrist. Instead, it may lead to new questions about
whether the patient is suffering too little pain for the gender presentation to be
a proper proof that he (for example) is really a man. So sometimes psychiatrists
are more interested in efforts than in successes as signs of the patient's conviction.

Interaction thus becomes the most important factor for psychiatric diagnosis. To understand what happens it is not enough to look at the presentation
and attribution of gender separately. Distinguishing the production of gender
signals from their cognitive processing (Kessler and McKenna 1978) will not do.
Rather, one has to ask how the participants are able to recognize how they are
perceived by their coparticipants: the social reality of gender attribution lies in
the gender presentation of the other. This is a bodily account of what the other
sees when looking at an individual: his/her own gender, or the other one. This

applies both to patients and to psychiatrists: transsexual patients read from the psychiatrist's reactions how they are perceived. And the more convincing the transsexual's gender presentation becomes, the more psychiatrists are drawn into a different perception of their own gender.

If a male psychiatrist, for instance, sits casually and talks with a patient about women (as an absent gender), everyone understands that the patient is a man. If the same psychiatrist starts to flirt and use more polite forms of greeting and choice of words (especially in connection with sexual matters), everyone understands that the patient is a woman. Psychiatrists interactively realize the patients' gender together with their own, and vice versa. This coproduction of two interactive genders remains problematic for a long time. Transsexuals manage to convey their conviction by a permanent and refined imputation that they *are* convincing. And psychiatrists are constantly trying out the transsexuals' gender in their own behavior. They test whether patients can still be addressed in their old gender or if the imputation of their new gender is strong enough to support the psychiatrists' gender as well. The interaction of transsexual and psychiatrist often leads to situations of great uncertainty and suspicion. These may culminate in situations like the encounter of people unsure of whether they know each other, who communicate with their eyes about what can be seen.

If one puts this subtle interaction into the mechanics of a classification process, the subject and object of classification become blurred. The distinction of sexes in psychiatry, and in any interaction, is a case of classification as self-classification.[7] There are two sides to this: first, the object to be diagnosed suggests how it should be classified. It is not passive, simply receiving judgments, but acts as an active and powerful agent in its own classification: it provides a public appearance and arguments, it begs and urges in endless talk, it works and fights for its acknowledgment.

Second, when classifying a patient as a certain gender, the diagnosing psychiatrists also classify themselves: as belonging to the patient's gender or as being different from it. Treating a patient as a woman, for example, is at the same time a move to distinguish oneself from the patient or to join the patient in a fellowship of gender. Gender diagnosis draws or withdraws a distinction between those who interact.[8]

When they finally diagnose transsexuality in a patient, psychiatrists reconstruct the interactive accomplishment of two genders and the efforts of the object at self-classification as a psychological identity that this individual is supposed to possess — as it is revealed by psychiatric expertise. With this "glossing" diagnosis, patients are referred to endocrinology.

ENDOCRINOLOGY: SEXING FIGURES

Endocrinologists cannot diagnose transsexuality. No test exists to determine the syndrome in patients' bodies. There is nothing measurable. Rather, the only diagnostic task left to endocrinology is to rule out the possibility that transsexuals have any organic pathologies that could make them believe themselves to be the other gender. For example, a patient should neither have a tumor of the adrenal cortex, which leads to abnormal levels of sex hormones, nor an underdeveloped hypophysis with reduced hormone production. In other words, gender change patients should be endocrinologically sound.

This results in a paradoxical position for endocrinologists: in order to turn someone into a woman, the doctors need to know from her hormone level that she is a real man; and they need to know from the psychiatric diagnosis that the same person is really a woman in order to treat her as a woman, that is, with female hormones.

Like the midwife who knows that in order to determine the sex of a baby one must look between its legs, an endocrinologist knows that to determine the sex of a person one must first take some blood. The blood sample has then to be sent to a laboratory, accompanied by a form requesting measurements of the estrogen and testosterone levels.

At the observed laboratory, the incoming sample is placed alongside hundreds of other samples that are to be measured in the same way. They are all centrifuged for approximately fifteen minutes and then a radio immune assay is done. The basic reagents of this biochemical method are supplied by industrial manufacturers of so-called kits. A kit consists of three elements: monoclonal antibodies with a specific binding point; a tracer (a radioactivity-marked hormone); and so-called standards with a known concentration of hormone.

Two further "reagents" of a radio immune assay are supplied by the laboratory itself: they are the prepared blood sample and the laboratory assistants. The latter are each assigned one hormone to test each day. Members of the laboratory believe that this human "reagency" has to be as neutral as possible. In order not to disturb the natural reaction of the chemical substances, the assistants have to follow strict instructions: not to confuse blood samples, to be precise when they pipette, not to overlook hemolytic samples, to make sure that their timing is right, and so on.

The next steps in determining the sex of a patient are as follows: assistants dissolve standards and tracer in distilled water and they pipette fifty microliters of the standard and five hundred microliters of the blood sample into different test tubes. To reduce errors in pipetting, two tubes are filled per sample and the pipetting tip is changed for every sample. The whole set, with its chemical reagents, is then placed on a shaking grate to perform its incubation by itself.

Next, the laboratory staff locate the most important activity within the test tubes. They say that during incubation a competition takes place between the hormone molecules of the blood sample and the radioactively traced hormone molecules. These compete to bind to the antibodies as fast as possible. The more hormone in the blood sample, the more successful it will be in seizing binding points.

After a certain time, the assistants stop this action in the test tubes by placing them in a bath of ice water. Then the test tubes are centrifuged again, the superfluous tracer is decanted, and the test tube is put into a beta counter. The counter sends four-digit figures onto a screen, and a computer converts these into further figures and prints them out in long columns.

Having made figures out of blood, the next problem in endocrinological sex determination is how to make meaningful data out of these figures. There are three steps in their interpretation. First, all reagents in an assay are checked internally by looking at each measurement. The standard curve should be smooth, and the two figures for each sample should show only slight variation. If this is the case, then the figures are taken to be values of sample hormone concentration. However, measurements often have to be repeated the next day to get sufficiently similar figures for a sample.

Making values relevant for the sexing of patients is the second step in this interpretation. Listen to how an assistant sees two sexes in a column of figures:

> I would say *this* is a woman—*that* could be a woman—*that* is a man—*that* is a man *or* it is an abnormal woman—we've had women with a testo of 10 even. . . . *this* is a woman. 0.8 would be slightly pathological, if we presume that, let's say, 3 would be a man and has a testo of 0.8—then he would be highly pathological. . . . *This* is a man. Well, 8 is okay, it's a man, but it does not happen so often—here, most are around 6 or 7.

Of course, the sex attribution to figures is not left to the arbitrary decisions of laboratory assistants. They use reference frames for normal maleness and femaleness. The threshold values of these frames vary between both industrial manufacturers of kits and laboratories, which develop their own specific normality frames. In addition, there is some competition between laboratories as to which one will define the reference frames of radio immune assays. The more sex determinations a laboratory does, the better its chances of determining the reference frames for other laboratories as well.

The third step of interpretation returns us to the practice of the endocrinologist. The figures, which are now sexually meaningful, have to be turned into "reasonable values" a doctor can act upon. The doctors who determined the starting sex of a transsexual now have to decide the significance of the hormone values for the patients' treatment with hormones of the opposite sex: what dose the figures indicate in order to construe the new sex of the patients. This is a decision that has to find a middle way between wanted and unwanted effects in the bodies of the patients.[9] Some doctors start cautiously with a low dosage and later switch to a higher level; others start with a high dosage in order to reduce the patients' own production of sex hormones, and then look at the changes in the resulting values. There is continual alternation between measuring and administering hormones.

It is difficult to determine the right dosage because every patient decomposes doses at a different rate. Moreover, many transsexuals are not compliant: they manipulate their sex by consuming additional hormones on their own. For them, hormone values have less to do with scientific data than with their presentation of self.

Endocrinologists, however, aim to adjust their patients gradually toward an endocrinologically normal woman, for example—someone with a female hormone level. It is this measurable level that has the pleasant side-effect for the patients of developing breasts (or, for men, growing a beard), where they had none in their starting sex.[10]

Sex determination in endocrinology is a reflexive process. It does not happen between actors at a single location, as with psychiatry. Rather, it takes place between actors and reagents[11] in quite different locations: the sex of a person is classified in the careful pipetting at a workbench; in a computer program that calculates figures; in their sceptical interpretation by assistants; in the competition between reagents in a test tube and of laboratories in a scientific community; and finally in the decisions of doctors about levels of dose, which in turn are regulated by the production and interpretation of new values. At the center of all these loops, the role of figures as symbols of sex is established.

The reclassification of transsexuals up to this point entails a shift in contradictions. In the everyday test, the gender presentation of transsexuals is adapted to their verbal claims. This causes a contradiction between their public appearance and bodily symbols of sex such as breasts or the pitch of the voice. But as soon as hormone treatment has resolved this contradiction, it produces another one, between these features and the genitals. So transsexuals are referred from hormone treatment to surgeons in a hermaphroditic state of ambiguity.

SURGERY: REARRANGING FLESHY MATERIALS

Surgeons start their sex determination with a urological or gynecological examination of patients to determine the feasibility of a sex change, given the anatomical starting sex of the body in question. This examination is an inspection of the materials of skin, fat, and vessels, which might be more or less useful for the shaping of a new organ. If the conditions seem satisfactory, the surgeons can go ahead.

In the operating room the patient is turned into a body by anesthesia. Then the body is further reduced to the operating area. Blue fabric is spread over it, covering it completely, except for the "private parts," which are thereby rendered public. In other words, surgical sex determination continues by the optical dissection of a piece of body as relevant to the sex change operation.

In physical dissection, layers of skin and tissue that obstruct the view of the anatomical structures the surgeons are aiming at are cut through and spread apart. Operating can be regarded as a sequence of looking and cutting, of manipulations that provide visibility for further manipulations. Surgeons know that in order to classify something, one has to cut something else. The flesh is dense and compact, cohesive, and resistant to penetration, and one has to carve the relevant material out of a crevice that opens up in the depth of a wound. Dissection seeks to present anatomical structures in the clear, discriminating style of an anatomical atlas. There, the drawings display neatly separated organs; in the patient's body, this state must first be produced by isolating them with the scalpel and other instruments. The surgeons make local use of anatomical pictures in the terrain of the patient's body.[12]

In sex change operations this sculptural practice carves out materials that are used as follows: the skin of the penis is used for a vagina and the skin of the vagina for the urethra of a penis. The scrotum is used for labia, and vice versa. Parts of the labia may become nipples, preparations from the intestines may be used for a vagina, skin and vessels from the back of the foot and forearm as well as costal cartilage may be taken for a penis.

In the standard technique of constructing a vagina, surgeons first open up the scrotum along its middle line, remove the testicles and the spermatic cord from surrounding tissue and amputate them. The scrotum vanishes into a bloody trapezoid measuring about 10 by 20 centimeters. Then, with scalpel and fingers, the surgeons create a cavity, so that instruments normally used in dealing with a vagina can be used. The penis is then turned inside out, without cutting, thereby dividing skin from shaft. The surgeons examine whether the valuable skin has withstood this operation. Then the shaft is split into urethra and spongy bodies, and both are amputated. Only a piece of the glans is saved to later form a clitoris. The former genitals are now transformed into an apparently structureless bloody surface. The skin of the penis is then folded into the created cavity and fixed with threads. The trapezoid of the former scrotum is spread into two triangles, which are shortened and arranged in the form of labia. The surgeons spend a lot of time and effort to achieve as much similarity to female genitals as possible and to distinguish them from the appearance of male genitals.

Transsexuals often regard the operation as a second birth. To them it is an opportunity to reconstruct their biographical tale in a phase before and after an event that "really" turned them from one sex into the other. From an observer's standpoint there is also a close link between the sex determination at birth and in the operating room. The surgical construction of sex consists of the creation of artificial genitals. The social construction of sex in surgery, instead, consists in looking for bodily features that are relevant for social categorization, and in viewing certain features as being crucial for locating individuals within those categories. That is, it consists of the repetitive use of a perceptual scheme already used at birth: making a boy out of a penis — or a vagina; taking a penis as a good reason for calling a baby a boy — or as good material out of which to make a vagina. Both acts give meaning to pieces of the body that are indifferent toward any possible classification. But a sex change operation makes the process of meaning attribution observable because it *starts* by denying that genitals are signs of a sex, by destroying them, before reaffirming that very assertion.

THE COHERENCE OF PRACTICES OF SEX/GENDER

Different sexes are incorporated in the medical practices described above: sex as personal conviction, as the level of substances in the blood, or as an anatomical structure between the legs. The analysis of the differentiating methods behind all these facts of sex, reveals them to be contingent accomplishments. The meaning of a so-called gender identity emerges in interactional gender presentation; the meaning of figures as symbols of sex in hormonal sex determination depends on the methods used, on the competition of laboratories and on dosage decisions by doctors; the meaning of flesh as the insignia of sex is constructed by relating it to anatomical pictures of proper organs and to one of two social categories.

If one asks what each of these sexes *really* consists of, the answers will refer to interactive accomplishments, to loops in which meanings are constructed, and to differentially arranged materials of skin, tissue, and vessels. Each method composes its sex by mobilizing the specific internal environment of its own procedure. So the differentiating methods are relatively independent of one another.

They need, then, to be linked in multiple ways. There are coordinating mechanisms such as organizations (such as clinics, medical associations), persons (who combine different competences in a personal union), time schedules within a division of labor (that is, the sequence psychiatry-endocrinology-surgery), or communicative exchanges (either in the form of interdisciplinary publications and conferences or in the mundane form of referrals and mutual consultations by phone).

But all these intramedical linkages are not very specific to the case of transsexuality: this is a case of an *extra*medical unification of medicine. The coherence from the outside is brought about in two ways: by two classes of actors and by the relevances of the cultural context, which assume that a social conflict should be settled.

The first class of actors are the lawyers, judges, and politicians. In the construction of laws for transsexuals (which by no means allow a simple choice of sex) and in the authoritative decisions about transsexuals' personal statuses and names, they construct medicine as the *other* profession, responsible for expert judgments and coordinated services. Doctors should guarantee that "those people" have a medical condition instead of sexual-political claims.[13]

The second group of actors are those persons who strive to change their sex as part of their gender and who thus declare themselves patients in order to secure a strong ally in the conflicts around their style of living. Transsexuals are not embarrassed victims of the disunity of medicine (cf. Willems, this volume), but highly informed actors who skillfully play medical disciplines off each other. They take the initiative in bringing doctors into contact with one another; they create disorder (cf. Berg, this volume) within the schedules of their treatment and make their own sequences. By buying hormones on the black market, for example, they oblige endocrinologists to agree with their treatment in order to prevent overdosage; by persuading a cosmetic surgeon to construct breasts they force psychiatrists to certify a stage in the process of gender change, which then simply seems to need completion by further operations and name adjustment. This instrumental use of medical incoherence has been and still is the main reason for the creation of treatment programs that respond to such strategies by forming professional alliances.

With respect to the cultural context of medical practices, the outcome of treatment can be regarded as a displacement of contradiction. The treatment of transsexuals never loses the features of the social conflicts that arise if the sex given at birth is revoked. These conflicts are translated into theoretical controversies and into the psychiatric assumption that transsexuals suffer from an *inner* conflict. But by the end, the conflicting parties are presented with a settlement. The genital operations on transsexuals confirm "them" in their assertion that they now really are the other sex. But they do so by establishing that there has been a so-called sex *change,* and so prove to "us" that they were *not* the other sex before. For transsexuals, the new pieces of body are objective proof of their gender, not only because they are visibly there but because anyone who denied their objectivity would have to bear the (moral) costs of their removal, that is, would have to argue for a repetition of medical intervention. So the burden of proof has shifted.

On the other hand, medical treatment ties transsexuals to staying in their new gender: in the beginning a "gendered soul" wasn't much more than rhetoric suggested by their small chances in a social conflict. At the end of a course of treatment, which constantly lets them experience being the other gender, they are forced to *have* a gendered soul because there is no alternative to living with the effects of medical treatments: first with the stories and convictions uttered in psychiatry, then with the habitus gained in the everyday test, and finally with the sexual features produced by endocrinology and surgery. The treatment of transsexuals inscribes and "buries" their claim very deep within them, because after the irreversible alteration of their bodies regret is not an option that could be lived. In other words, the treatment materially constructs a gender identity as *part* of a person's sex. *Both* sex and gender identity belong to the deep structure of the practices of gender.

Therefore it would be misleading in the exploration of gender practices to follow the sex/gender distinction developed by medical discourses. This medical distinction yields strange contradictions: in the first instance, psychiatric theories of transsexuality have developed a notion of a constant, never-changing and early-determined gender identity from precisely those persons who actually change their sex and gender. Furthermore, psychiatrists have developed a procedure of sceptically testing the stability of gender identity as if they distrusted their own theoretical assumption that the "true" sex of an individual is simply revealed in what it determines itself to be. And surgery, which seemed to push the anatomical boundary between the sexes aside in a radical manner, only confirms with its genital transformations that anatomy remains crucial.

These contradictions are caused by the fundamental links between medical and everyday ways of defining the sexes. The methods of medical differentiation have a deep life-world bias, presupposing certain axiomatic features of sexes. They take into account two preconstructed categories, whether these are regarded as poles of a hormonal continuum, or whether surgical techniques allow genitals to be switched between them, or psychiatric sensibility and wit make it possible to accomplish and experience changes between same-sex and cross-sex interactions. All these medical modes of performing the difference between sexes reassure everyone involved in a sex change of the duality, distinctiveness, and constancy of the sexes.

So medical reclassification works to settle and normalize "gender troubles" in everyday life. Genital surgery has been successful in reducing the culturally hegemonic form of gender migration to a single event instead of a pattern of constant shifting, which could constitute a continuous subculture. But other forms of gender migration can and do articulate themselves when sex change is reclaimed from medicine: sex determination by hormone consumption is a routine cosmetic alteration of the body for some posttranssexual (Stone 1991) groups; the notion of gender identity and the ways of constructing its existence starts to become a tolerable version of being a sex in urban environments prepared for greater gender plurality; and transsexuality itself could be incorporated into the ongoing processes of gender attribution if this category were routinely applied to passers-by in the street in the same way as we identify men and women.

NOTES

1   The distinction between "sex" and "gender" in English poses a problem which does not exist in other European languages, such as Dutch, German, or Turkish. This problem will not be solved here. For the purpose of this article I shall use "gender" as an encompassing category, including "sex," i.e., the body shaped materially and experienced from "within." Nevertheless, sometimes I avoid the term "gender" because it has been semantically spoiled as mere "software" in the construction of two sexes.

2   I have described the history of transsexuality in detail in Hirschauer 1993: 66–115.

3   For the United States see Billings and Urban 1982; for Germany see the contributions in *Psyche* 1950/51.

4   Essential elements of the treatment program for transsexuals developed in the United States have also been implemented in Germany. One of the differences is that the German programs—like those in Britain (King 1987)—are less centralized in "gender identity clinics." I have done participant observation of psychiatric work in a sexology department, of endocrinological work in the practice of several gynecologists and in an endocrinological laboratory, and of surgical practices in four different clinics.

5   Medical disciplines are simply the unit of analysis chosen in this chapter. Another
    investigation might be made of the clashes within medical professions. For ex-
    ample, many surgeons and endocrinologists in Germany still refuse to treat trans-
    sexuals for ethical reasons. And in psychiatry there are conflicts between more
    permissive and more restrictive stances toward transsexuals. There is a maximalist
    position, which says that a psychic problem has to be resolved by psychotherapeu-
    tical means; a minimalist position, which refers the patients at their own discretion
    to surgery; and a middle position, which is dominant in specialist medical de-
    partments, protects some patients from the mutilating surgeries while supporting
    most seeking change. My description of psychiatric gender determination methods
    refers to this last case.

6   In their overadaptation to "normalcy" transsexuals have obstinately disappointed
    sexual revolutionary hopes. In the words of Sandy Stone: "The essence of trans-
    sexualism is the act of passing" (1991: 299).

7   This is not the only pragmatic meaning of the label "transsexual" in psychiatry. For
    a more detailed analysis see Hirschauer 1992.

8   This calls to mind Bourdieu (1979), who analyzed how the classification of aes-
    thetic objects at the same time distinguishes the classifier on a vertical dimension of
    social class. Instead, I would stress the unavoidable reciprocity of sex classification,
    which implies that participants *cannot* assume a position of distance from those
    with whom they interact. In psychiatric gender diagnoses this reciprocity is, of
    course, asymmetrical for several reasons: one of the participants is going to decide
    on the other's gender authoritatively, and s/he is equipped for that with a trained
    competence in interactive attributions and with a simple knowledge capable of in-
    validating the other's gender presentation — the fact that it does not "fit" the bodily
    constitution.

9   It should be noted that the "wanted effects" — e.g., chemical castration and breast
    development in transsexual women and amenorrhea and growth of beard in trans-
    sexual men — are "unwanted effects" from the point of view of the pharmaceutical
    industry. The drugs used are designed for many diseases (e.g., menopausal prob-
    lems), but not for sex change, and in the information for patients they include
    warnings about the very "side-effects" transsexuals are seeking.

10 In general, transsexual men (born women) — and their doctors — are more satisfied
    by hormonal effects than transsexual women. While beard and low voice mostly
    make a person an inconspicuous man in interaction, breasts often turn a trans-
    sexual woman into only a dubious man. This is due not only to the androcentric
    construction of bodily signifiers of sex (Kessler/McKenna 1978), but also to the fact
    that having a beard is regarded as more contingent than having breasts and there-
    fore can be better used to communicate a claim on sex membership.

11 In my description I was not looking for a general agency of things or for a primor-
    dial agency of humans — both of which could be argued philosophically (Latour
    and Callon 1993; Collins and Yearley 1993). Instead, I try to treat agency as a situ-

ated variable. Compare blood cells and laboratory assistants: if the latter attributed agency and competitive spirit to the former, I found it adequate to describe their mechanic functioning in turn as mere "reagency." On the other hand, I cannot imagine how the "activities" of scallops (for example) could ever be intelligibly described in the same way, for instance, as the fight of transsexuals who refuse to be treated as mere reagents on their "psychic conflicts." Thus I regard it as an empirical finding—to be contested—that humans are classificatory objects who engage in self-classification with an obstinacy not to be found in the objects of the natural sciences.

12 Again, the unity of the surgeons could be broken down much further into the participants actually involved in a surgery: gynecologists, urologists, assistants, anesthetists, and (different kinds of) nurses. For a more detailed description of the sculptural practice of surgery see Hirschauer 1991.

13 For the cooperation of psychiatrists and politicians in the formulation of the German law for transsexuals see Hirschauer 1993: 293–311.

WORKING ON AND AROUND
HUMAN FETUSES: THE CONTESTED
DOMAIN OF FETAL SURGERY

Monica J. Casper

▼

A special problem arises with interventional fetal procedures, especially those that require the expertise of specialists from very different fields. . . . Because no single specialty training provides the total spectrum of skills and experience, this is an area in
which "turf" battles between medical specialties and "ego" battles among team members may sabotage the fetal treatment enterprise. It is also an area in which cooperative
efforts and teamwork can be productive. M. R. Harrison, *The Unborn Patient*

At its core, sociology is about "doing things together" (Becker 1986), how
groups of people collectively weave and maintain the fabric of social life. Just
as society itself is a collective enterprise, so too are its many institutional and
cultural components, such as medicine and science. Biomedical and scientific
work are not only collective but are also heterogeneous, as explored in the rich
vein within medical sociology, which examines the manifold contributions of
medical work. Different sets of people with diverse skills, resources, and power
do things together within particular institutional contexts, such as hospitals
and laboratories. They use a variety of technologies in their work and draw on
a wide range of general and specialized knowledges. The objects and goals of
their work may be quite diverse, and the cultural meanings they attach to their
work may also vary considerably. As the editors of this volume point out in
their introduction, biomedicine in the late twentieth century is heterogeneous
along many dimensions. This has important implications for medical work and
how it unfolds in local settings.

Drawing on interview and ethnographic data, the empirical study presented
in this chapter focuses on experimental fetal surgery as one such setting.[1] In
fetal surgery, a fetus is partially removed from a pregnant woman's uterus via
hysterotomy (similar to a cesarean section), operated on surgically, and, if it
survives the operation, replaced within its mother's body for continued development and subsequent delivery by cesarean section. Fetal surgery is currently

limited to terminal conditions, such as congenital diaphragmatic hernia and urinary tract obstructions.[2] The objective of fetal surgery is to repair damage *in utero* to save the fetus or to prevent life-threatening conditions from developing at birth. Approximately half of the fetuses that undergo treatment die, while those who live are unlikely ever to be fully healthy and *always* require postnatal treatment of some kind. As one informant, a hospital social worker, told me, "This is a very rigorous sort of deal for a fetus, a newborn, make no mistake about it. This baby comes out, it's already been operated on, its guts are hanging out its side, it's on a respirator. . . . If you talk to the people on the team it's like a walk in the park for them. But you know I watch the moms watch these babies, and I watch these babies myself. It's a lot for a tiny immature person to go through."

Maternal mortality statistics are somewhat better; as one surgeon assured me, "We haven't lost a mom yet."[3] Yet in terms of morbidity, the pregnant women's health, after two cesarean sections and often several weeks of intensive clinical management, may be severely compromised (Harrison and Longaker 1991). Because fetal surgery is highly invasive, both pregnant women and their fetuses must be monitored extensively throughout the remainder of pregnancy and often beyond. Every woman, without exception, must take medications called tocolytics to prevent preterm labor and many must also remain in bed constantly, often for up to two or three months. This often takes a considerable toll on the women. One patient remarked that "it was a very hard thing physically," and another stated, "I had no idea it would be like this." Fetal surgery thus has significant implications for the health and well-being of pregnant women as well as for their fetuses and, after birth, for their babies.

Fetal surgery is characteristic of other medical specialties where diversity and heterogeneity are omnipresent. Contemporary fetal surgery requires the participation of a broad array of medical workers and technologies. It is an enormously complex undertaking, in part because fetuses, located *inside* pregnant female bodies, are notoriously difficult to access. Finding and operating on the fetal patient and attempting to safeguard maternal health during these procedures requires multiple skills and tools.[4] There is a clear and necessary division of labor, which forms the institutional contours of this new specialty and is constantly reinforced through professional interaction. Yet fetal surgery is complex for other reasons as well. Because it is an emergent specialty, currently in what Bucher (1988) calls the "consolidation phase" of formation, its territory is not yet defined and staked out. Of the many different medical specialties involved in fetal surgery today, which set of workers will ultimately control fetal surgery remains to be established. Consequently, there is continual jockeying for position among the various groups in this domain.

Fetal surgery is thus a contested domain, an intersection of multiple practitioners with a range of skills, interests, and commitments. Differences abound here and shape this specialty in multiple ways. Yet the most significant interactions, as the prefatory quote illustrates, are but two sides of the same coin: *cooperation,* which makes the achievement of fetal surgery possible, and *conflict,* which threatens this achievement at every turn. Participants are well aware of their need to cooperate with one another to make the fetal surgery enterprise successful even while they may disagree vociferously about exactly how to accomplish this. Fetal surgery is not a static, stable construction, but rather is continually changing shape as its practitioners negotiate and attempt to work things out. This chapter explores key aspects of the interactional scaffolding of fetal surgery, focusing both on the "cooperative efforts" and on the "turf battles" that Harrison (1991: 9) describes. Throughout, it attends closely to the implications of these differences for work practices, for the medical practitioners involved, for pregnant women and their fetuses, and for the emergent enterprise of fetal surgery.

SOME THEORETICAL TOOLS

Within social studies of technoscience, there has been considerable interest in the practices through which science and increasingly medicine are accomplished.[5] Interactionist perspectives in particular have focused on diverse aspects of science and medicine closely related to work, such as organizational arrangements, tasks, tools, and research materials.[6] This body of scholarship reflects a long-standing interactionist tradition in which *work as collective action* is taken as a central unit of analysis.[7] These perspectives situate work as a set of important social actions located at the intersection of social processes and orders. The social organization of work is seen both as a product of specific work activities and as something that constrains and shapes broader arenas of collective action.

Two interactionist concepts are pivotal to this chapter, the first of which relates to Mead's (1934) notion of *social objects.* People are seen as living and working within contexts of meaningful objects, which are conceptualized as human constructs rather than as "self-existing entities with intrinsic natures. Their nature is dependent on the orientation and action of people toward them" (Blumer 1969: 68). In this view, an object — including its classification as either human or nonhuman[8] — is defined according to the meanings it has for the actor(s) for whom it is an object. These meanings derive from the ways in which a person acts toward an object, rather than from any inherent nature or quality of objects. Objects are conceptualized as social products in that "they are formed and transformed by the defining process that takes place in social interaction" (ibid.). As Blumer points out, "to identify and understand the life of a group it is necessary to identify its world of objects; this identification has to be in terms of the meanings objects have for the members of the group" (ibid.).

Building on Mead's definition of social objects, I have developed the concept of *work objects* to more fully grasp the concrete, hands-on, and contextual dimensions of work and its place in social organization. I define work objects as the material entities (human, nonhuman, technical, or hybrid) around which actors construct meanings and organize their work practices. In sociological research on work, little attention has been paid to the objects of work.[9] The analytical significance of focusing on work objects is in examining how the "nature" of the object, or its material and symbolic characteristics and properties, shapes work practices and how the object itself is simultaneously and mutually shaped by the work and its social contexts. In this framing, analytical emphasis remains focused on human action and meaning (Strauss 1993), yet incorporates an understanding of how work objects may constrain, enable, or otherwise influence these processes.

The second concept of relevance here is *negotiated order,* developed by Strauss and his colleagues (1964: 176) to characterize structure and social order as artifacts of interaction. Based on research in a psychiatric hospital, they argued that the structured life of the institution is constituted by "continual negotiative activity." Negotiations may be patterned, as for example within a web of institutional relationships, but must be continually reconstituted as the basis for social order. Negotiations are conceptualized as emergent, contingent, constrained, and fluid—hallmarks of interactionist approaches. Strauss and his colleagues argue that these negotiations are integral to the coordination of work: the shapes of wards, clinical and administrative arrangements, and institutional rules are all products of negotiation.[10]

Both the concepts *social object* and *negotiated order* are important for the purposes at hand. This chapter links these concepts to show how negotiations occur around particular *work objects* in the shaping of work in a new specialty. Like other medical practices, many of which are discussed in this volume, fetal surgery is characterized by the intersection of heterogeneous elements. Yet fetal surgery is emergent, experimental, and focused on a particularly contested object in American culture and technoscience—the human fetus.[11] Not only are fetuses contested at the level of cultural politics, but they are also highly contested within local domains as well. One important site at which fetuses are socially and culturally constructed is the actual work done on and around them. This might include, for example, pregnant women's emotional and physical work prior to birth, the work of scientists who use fetal tissue in their research, the work done within abortion clinics, and the work of physicians who treat fetuses prenatally. Examining the construction of fetal work objects in experimental fetal surgery thus provides a lens through which the different meanings attributed to pregnant women and their fetuses may be analyzed. The shape of fetal surgery is, in an interactionist sense, a negotiated order.

"A SPIRIT OF COOPERATION": MAKING THINGS WORK

IN A FETAL TREATMENT UNIT

The rich diversity of participants in fetal surgery demands that practitioners cooperate in order to make things work. Yet while cooperation may be a necessary building block for "doing things together" in fetal surgery, it is by no means a naturally occurring phenomenon. Rather, cooperation, like all human interactions, must be achieved. The production of fetal surgery as a cooperative enterprise is characterized by numerous institutional activities, such as regular staff meetings designed to enable actors in this domain to work together. However, cooperation is not only the means to achieve certain ends, such as a reasonably healthy fetus, but may also be seen as an end in itself to satisfy certain institutional requirements related to fetal surgery. For example, in attempting to secure funding for experimental surgery or the approval of institutional review boards, it is more expedient for fetal surgeons to portray the fetal surgery enterprise as cooperative rather than as riddled with conflict. What follows is an elaboration of the cooperative components of fetal surgery which make this nascent specialty possible.

The Fetal Treatment Unit (FTU) at Capital Hospital began in the early 1980s when a pediatric surgeon, a sonographer, and an obstetrician began working together on experimental fetal surgery. Prior to this time, these physicians often attempted unsuccessfully to save newborns whose diseases were too advanced for treatment. Their resulting frustration at not being able to save these neonates, coupled with important historical precedents in fetal treatment, prompted the three colleagues to consider operating on fetuses *prenatally* in order to repair defects and/or to prevent life-threatening conditions from developing at birth. In the 1960s, extensive animal research and limited human experimentation in Puerto Rico and New Zealand had laid crucial groundwork for both noninvasive and surgical fetal treatments.[12] This early work served as an important influence on subsequent practices; indeed, William Liley, a pediatric neuroendocrinologist from New Zealand who pioneered prenatal treatment for maternal/fetal Rh incompatibility, has been called the "patron saint" of fetal medicine (Koop 1986).

Contemporary fetal surgery became possible, however, only with the advent of prenatal diagnostic technologies such as ultrasound, which is capable of visualizing defects for subsequent treatment. Importantly, this key technological development necessitated that experimental fetal surgery would require the input of a sonographic team. Further, because pediatric surgeons had little understanding of maternal health and the physiological intricacies of pregnancy, it was considered crucial that obstetricians be involved in the early phases of the program. Sonographers and obstetricians at the institution I studied had already been treating fetuses *nonsurgically* for many years, beginning with intraperitoneal transfusions for Rh incompatibility based on Liley's work in the 1960s. Open fetal surgery was deemed necessary only when a fetal catheter inserted nonsurgically to treat a blocked urinary tract refused to stay in place; replacing the catheter required surgically opening a pregnant woman's abdomen to access her fetus. Once a new catheter was developed it proved to be less recalcitrant than the old model, rendering open surgery unnecessary for this condition.[13] By that time, however, the door to fetal surgery had itself been reopened and contemporary physicians had begun to consider applying this "new" technique to other diseases and conditions. A combination of technological innovation, professional goals, and institutional conditions resulted in renewed interest in open fetal surgery two decades after Liley's pioneering efforts in fetal treatment.

Since its inception, the Fetal Treatment Unit has been multidisciplinary. The feasibility of experimental fetal surgery and the likelihood that it will become a routine medical practice are seen by participants as resting on cooperative interaction among its diverse practitioners. According to some participants, "the institutional setting, organization, and *coordination* of the FTU are elements critical to its success" (Howell, Adzick, and Harrison 1993: 143; emphasis added). From the initial triad of pediatric surgeon, sonographer, and obstetrician, the fetal surgery team has grown to include a range of practitioners with diverse skills, perspectives, and backgrounds. These include perinatologists skilled in fetal diagnosis, fetal blood sampling, and intrauterine transfusion; neonatologists, who must often intensively manage newborns after birth and during subsequent postnatal treatment; social workers who address psychosocial (including emotional, financial, employment, and social support) issues faced by pregnant women, their partners, and families; pediatric and obstetric anesthesiologists; nurses representing different specialties; geneticists; medical ethicists; and fetal physiologists knowledgeable in basic fetal biology. A successful fetal treatment center is, according to a prominent fetal surgeon, a "blend of skills and expertise" (Harrison 1991).

Practitioners within this domain are acutely aware of the diversity of requisite skills and knowledges. In addition to its attention in the published literature, every informant spoke at length about the necessity for cooperation. One fetal surgeon remarked, "It has to be a team approach. . . . The team approach is key." Another surgeon stated, "This is the most complex undertaking in surgery. . . . We've got to enlist the aid of every person who's involved in every stage of this." An obstetrician, speaking at a professional meeting, stressed that "it's important to have a well-rounded unit for fetal surgery, including neonatologists, pediatric surgeons, and so on." A sonographer agreed that there is a great degree of cooperation and remarked that "considering some of the problems we've had, generally I would say it's a reasonably orderly group of people." And a social worker remarked, "I think the days of territorialism are long gone. . . . Because there's so much to be done for these families, everybody sort of pitches in. And I think there is a spirit of cooperation on this team that makes it reasonable to work on."

The significance of the "team" metaphor to describe working arrangements in the Fetal Treatment Unit cannot be overstated. According to practitioners, a number of general principles have evolved since the inception of contemporary fetal surgery to guide its development. Chief among these is that "fetal surgery is a team effort requiring varying amounts of input from all team members" (Harrison 1991: 9). As well as specifying all the requisite members of the team (e.g., obstetrician, perinatologist, geneticist, surgeon), these principles also lay out additional rules underlying the organization of fetal surgery. For example, "[A]lthough all members of the team can contribute to any particular procedure, there must be a team leader" (ibid.). Who is selected as team leader may be a source of conflict, spurring negotiation, despite the rule that "the procedure is done by the team member who is most likely to produce the best outcome" (ibid.). Further, just as experimental fetal surgery is a proving ground for developing and implementing new procedures, it also provides "an invaluable opportunity to work out . . . the professional relationships that will enable the team to function smoothly. The lines of responsibility must be drawn clearly among team members before the choice of doing a procedure is offered to a patient" (ibid.).

Certain organizational conventions within the FTU also indicate that cooperative teamwork is extremely important. At ongoing fetal treatment staff meetings, a range of practitioners come together to discuss specific cases and strategies for treatment, evaluating past activities as well as planning for the future. Also, regular "consensus meetings" are held among clinicians and researchers to discuss current basic scientific research as it relates to clinical practices. It is here that new fetal technologies, developed in a fetal treatment lab using animal models, are first introduced into a clinical setting. In addition, fetal surgeons, obstetricians, genetics counselors, and social workers routinely meet with potential patients, often coordinating their schedules and agendas to coincide with a family's visit to the hospital. Further, there are ad hoc meetings on particular issues, such as a discussion of fetal and maternal management following a rash of postoperative maternal health problems and fetal deaths. In introducing the topic of this ad hoc meeting, a fetal surgeon referred to those present as a "working group" to address the issue of maternal safety.

An illustration of the continual quest for cooperation was provided in a talk presented by Dr. Graham for other practitioners at Capital Hospital. The presentation was given during grand rounds for obstetrics and gynecology, with most of the audience representing these two specialties. Entitled "Prenatal/Perinatal Management of Anomalies," the talk was clearly designed to "enroll" (Latour 1987; Latour and Woolgar 1986) obstetricians as allies, or members of the team, in the enterprise of fetal surgery. Not only are many obstetricians vocal critics of open fetal surgery (for reasons discussed below), but they also possess the skills and expertise in maternal health issues that fetal surgeons may be lacking. For example, preterm labor is a major problem in fetal surgery, and obstetricians traditionally have been viewed as best equipped to resolve it. Graham strategically emphasized throughout his talk that his team is very concerned about maternal safety. Significantly, in terms of establishing cooperative working relationships, he invited the obstetricians to "talk about [fetal surgery] together, both its limitations and new approaches." He remarked that surgeons are "looking to forge a new partnership." Graham closed his talk by emphasizing that the success of the Fetal Treatment Unit at Capital Hospital "depends on people rubbing shoulders in the hall, talking informally, and working together." In short, the presentation was a strategically delivered invitation to obstetricians to participate in the fetal surgery enterprise as a cooperative venture.

In sum, then, there seems to be an ongoing commitment to cooperation and teamwork among the practitioners who work in the fetal surgery domain. To some degree, any cooperation that is achieved is based in part on shared understandings of the work of fetal surgery. Yet, however each medical worker may conceptualize fetuses and pregnant women, the institutional shape of this domain situates the fetus as a primary locus of practice. Simply stated, the chief reason that people work together in fetal surgery is because a pregnant woman has been admitted with a fetus requiring treatment. There may be ancillary reasons for the collective nature of fetal surgery, but these are shadowed by the broad aim of "saving babies." As one might expect, however, the picture of cooperative harmony painted by fetal surgeons and others in this domain seems too good to be true. While there is certainly a great deal of cooperation, as displayed in staff meetings and in operating rooms, this is often achieved despite deep and profound differences between medical workers in this specialty. As any chemist (or sociologist) knows, affinity is only one possible reaction to mixing different elements; sometimes the end result is a volatile compound.

"FOLKS ARE ALWAYS RUBBING SHOULDERS":
WORKING AROUND DIFFERENCES THAT MATTER

Although cooperation is necessary for open fetal surgery to work, conflict among practitioners is pervasive in this domain. There are both minor disagreements and major fights about how both fetuses and pregnant women are talked about and worked on; about proper treatment plans; about postoperative procedures; about who is responsible for which work tasks; and so on. There is a seemingly infinite number of possible reasons why participants in fetal surgery do not always "get along" with each other, some of which they themselves recognize and articulate.[14] A fetal surgeon had this to say about conflict in the program: "Well, I think that any time you have a group of people, sort of management by committee, there are going to be problems. People just have different views, particularly when you have groups of people from different backgrounds." Another surgeon remarked: "But that's just because things are new, and things aren't worked out, folks are always rubbing shoulders. . . . Sure, we've had terrible conflicts, arguments, and things that were strictly differences of opinion medically."[15]

Yet is it entirely a case of different professional training, or are the differences between social actors in this domain more complex? A social worker describes this diversity in more detail: "It was a baptism by fire. . . . Meaning that I was surprised at how, in some ways, unprepared I was for the politics of the program. . . . We all have a slightly different vantage and orientation and perspective and cultural agenda. There are so many subtle ways in which we are different from one another, both because of our professional training and because of who we are as human beings." These profound differences between actors in this domain affect the shape and trajectory of this practice in often highly consequential ways, both locally and downstream. Yet how actors organize their work practices on and around fetuses in turn shapes differences between actors by impacting access to work objects. There are three significant areas of difference at the local level of work arrangements, to which I now turn, focusing on the ways in which these differences are made meaningful.

Different Definitions of Work Objects: Negotiating the "What" of Fetal Surgery

A major site at which differences emerge and coalesce in fetal surgery is in definitions of work objects. The fetal patient is positioned as the primary work object within this domain (Casper 1994a). For example, every fetal operation is videotaped for research and recording purposes. Taping begins after full anesthesia of the pregnant woman has occurred and surgeons have opened her uterus, and it ends when they are finished working on the fetus, illustrating graphically what/whom is considered the important work object in fetal surgery. In addition, the Fetal Treatment Unit recently instituted a descriptive toll-free number for referring physicians and potential patients who desire information about the practice: 1-800-RxFETAL. Further, surgeons have proposed a Fetal Intensive Care Unit (FICU) where fetuses (and presumably "moms") may be monitored postoperatively. The name of the unit — FICU — gives no indication that a fetus is still inside its mother's body during this postoperative period.

Yet as ubiquitous as the fetal patient is in this domain, not all of the actors define fetuses as their primary work objects. Different actors attribute diverse, sometimes conflicting meanings to fetuses, and this is related to how work activities are organized differently. This often leads to considerable strain between fetal surgeons, who define fetuses as central work objects, and other practitioners with different tasks and agendas. For example, most obstetricians generally consider pregnant women to be their primary work objects and are concerned with fetal health secondarily or only in relation to maternal health. Indeed, relations between fetal surgeons and obstetricians have become increasingly difficult in recent years, with the latter group being, in one obstetrician's view, slowly "pushed out" by the fetal surgeons.[16] An obstetrician, dissatisfied with the direction of the FTU, stated: "[We] are having trouble with [fetal surgery] because we're seeing lots of complications in women. . . . The obstetricians of course take care of the maternal patient." He later remarked, "[Fetal surgeons] don't take care of the woman afterward. We've had women who've not been able to leave the hospital, who've been in and out of labor for the rest of their pregnancies. Those are the successes!"

Another informant, a social worker, confirmed these sentiments and described difficult relations between fetal surgeons and obstetricians: "The OBS are used to managing [maternal] patients. . . . A lot of angry stuff between the OBS, who is going to be in attendance at these deliveries, you know, people who really didn't want to do it or believe in it. They think it's bad medicine, bad to take a pregnant woman and cut her open." Note that this is the same informant who remarked earlier that the days of territorialism in fetal surgery were over!

Comments of fetal surgeons are especially revealing about conflict between "baby doctors" and "mom doctors." For example, the FICU described above has proven somewhat controversial. According to one fetal surgeon, "Anytime you have new concepts like [the FICU], you're bound to encounter some resistance. . . . That was a new concept for many people and it led to friction." When pressed about the source of resistance, he remarked "Well, you know, it's just a different way of dealing with things. I'm used to doing big operations and having patients in the ICU, and some of the obstetricians and OB nurses are not used to that. . . . They view the postoperative period as the preterm labor problem. . . . But it was clear that patient management went far beyond just management of preterm labor, and we couldn't *not* be responsible outside of monitoring. That led to friction." Of course, monitoring means that the pregnant woman must remain in the hospital after surgery, often for up to several weeks.

Another fetal surgeon described, in somewhat more critical terms, key differences between patients as work objects: "The unfortunate part is that the obstetricians have been taking care of the fetal/maternal pair for so long it's driven into them. . . . But *our* patients aren't like their patients. *Our* patients are mid-gestation fetuses, *our* mom has just undergone a major operation, *our* fetus has just undergone a major operation, there's been prolonged anesthesia, and now there's problems with pain control, volume fluctuations, and all the normal perioperative things. . . . Obstetricians don't understand anything about perioperative management; they don't understand anything about management of a patient in the perioperative period."[17] Note the carefully articulated distinctions here between *fetal* patients/work objects as clearly constituting the territory of fetal surgeons, and *maternal* patients/work objects as part of the proprietary but increasingly shifting terrain of obstetricians. Fetal surgeons are more and more advancing on obstetrical territory and claiming authority for mothers as well as fetuses.

This same surgeon ascribes such differences to professional training and background: "Basically every group of physicians have their own personality. Surgeons tend to be a little more aggressive, we tend to push harder, get things done. It's just a personality thing. . . . The obstetricians now have seen enough problems with fetal surgery that they're absolutely opposed to it. They don't like it. They don't want it to happen. They're against it. The only reason they're going through the moves right now . . . is because it's protocol driven." A fetal physiologist echoes these points: "Well, I think it's again a turf issue. Obstetricians feel that they should be responsible for all prenatal care—care of the fetus *and* mother. And surgeons feel that the fetus is their patient and have therefore assumed some responsibility for the mother." Although professional training may be significant, it is the implementation of such training in local work arrangements that both shape and reinforce crucial distinctions between different actors in this domain.

The availability of direct access to fetuses is an important constraint on how, by whom, and under what conditions fetuses are defined as meaningful work objects. This is illustrated in Harrison's (1991: 10) discussion of which specialist should perform fetal surgery, or rather, which specialist should be the team leader. He begins by stating that the most politically expedient solution would be to have each specialist do his or her part of the overall procedure. This would mean that obstetricians open and close the uterus, and the pediatric surgeon operates on the fetus. This easy solution is, according to Harrison, "likely to keep team members comfortable in their accustomed roles." Yet he goes on to state that this practice is not likely to yield the best outcomes because "it assumes that traditional skills will suffice; that is, that obstetricians can close the uterus as they do in the case of an empty uterus and that the pediatric surgeon can do with a fetus what he learned in a neonate. Neither is true." He argues that "tag-team surgery is never ideal," particularly where exposure and closure of the fetus by hysterotomy is complicated by preterm labor problems. Thus, despite the rhetoric of teamwork, it seems that a division of labor by extant specialties may not work or be construed as ideal. In terms of defining fetal work objects as the province of one set of specialists, Harrison claims that "fetal surgery cannot develop and will not succeed unless a few surgeons are willing to devote considerable time and effort to developing, practicing, and perfecting all aspects of this new procedure."

Further complicating matters, social workers in the FTU define their work objects quite differently from both the fetal surgeons and the obstetricians. One social worker is "troubled" by fetal surgery because, in her words, "every baby was dying. Every step of the way, we've been thwarted . . . by consequences of surgery that have high morbidity and high mortality for these babies." Because negative outcomes often seem to create or intensify conflict,[18] this social worker decided that she would be "an advocate for the parent." Yet differences in status within the FTU between social workers and physicians often make this difficult. The social workers are frustrated in their attempts to advocate for the pregnant woman by surgeons more intently focused on fetuses. For example, women who are prime surgical candidates clinically may not be good candidates psychosocially (discussed more fully below). One social worker's judgment about a particular patient was challenged, leading her to remark: "I was incensed about it. . . . At that point, my confidence was shaken, and I felt that if I'm going to be the psychosocial person on this team, I'm going to have to have the support of the members of the team." While her recommendation was ultimately supported by an outside psychiatrist, she felt that the incident "forced [her] to look again at [her] role and [her] interactions with the team."

As these examples illustrate, there are a number of divergent positions on who or what are, and are not, work objects in fetal surgery: different actors ascribe different meanings to work objects in this domain. For fetal surgeons, fetuses are first and foremost patients and objects of treatment-based work practices such as surgery. For obstetricians, pregnant women are (usually) the first and most important patients and objects of maternity care, while fetuses are secondary work objects. Most obstetricians do not completely reject the notion of a fetal patient; indeed, one of the striking developments in medicine in recent years is the emergence of maternal-fetal medicine as a replacement for standard obstetrics (Creasy and Resnick 1994). However, conflicts between obstetricians and fetal surgeons tend to center on other aspects of treatment, such as how to keep pregnant women healthy while operating on them *solely* for the benefit of their fetuses. For social workers, fetuses are only direct work objects in a tertiary sense; for example, the social worker quoted above was concerned that too many fetuses were dying. For social workers, the pregnant woman and her family are the primary work objects and are defined in terms of psychosocial care rather than surgical treatment, even while outcomes may be of great concern.

In sum, a fluid relationship exists between how work practices are organized and the meanings that each work object has for different actors. There is a certain medical "logic" at work here in terms of identifying what to do next in the clinical setting (Berg 1992). That is, if the fetus is seen as a patient, then it must be treated. If the pregnant woman is seen as a patient, then she (and secondarily her fetus) must be cared for. If a pregnant woman and her partner are viewed as needing psychosocial care, it will likely be provided by the appropriate person, generally one of the social workers. This is one site where differences matter in terms of clinical decision making and patients' trajectories. Yet despite these tensions surrounding different work objects and practices, the Fetal Treatment Unit *qua* organization is collectively geared toward "saving fetuses," which continue to be *institutionally* defined as the most significant work objects. Who, then, decides what are primary work objects? Under what conditions? With what consequences? How do institutional hierarchies shape this process?

In the examples below, additional dimensions of difference are explored, both of which are related to definitions of work objects and their "sitings" within particular locales. Each of these examples represents a possible consequence flowing from diverse meanings attributed to work objects in fetal surgery.

Different Criteria for Patient Selection:
Negotiating the "Who" of Fetal Surgery

Based on their definitions of work objects, different actors in fetal surgery use different criteria for patient selection, or who is considered a good candidate for treatment.[19] There is an ongoing debate in fetal surgery over what constitutes valid criteria for selecting patients, with some actors advocating strictly "clinical" criteria and others emphasizing "nonclinical" factors. Clearly, if there is disagreement over who/what a patient is, then there are likely to be substantial differences over how to select for patients.

Fetal surgeons generally define selection in terms of fetuses (Harrison 1991), while obstetricians consider maternal health a priority; both groups tend to rely primarily on what they define as "clinical" criteria. In the clinical literature,[20] guidelines for patient selection suggest that a fetus should be a singleton (i.e., not a twin, triplet, etc.) prenatally diagnosed and found to have abnormalities. The family should be fully counseled about the risks and benefits of surgery. Further, a multidisciplinary team should be used during treatment, and high-risk obstetrical and intensive care units should be available. Last, bioethical and psychosocial consultation should be made available for both practitioners and patients. In local practices, however, these global guidelines are not necessarily followed; depending on circumstances and conditions, some factors may take precedence over others in the selection process, revealing that "clinical" decisions are rooted in nonclinical priorities.

For example, one fetal surgeon described selection and treatment considerations for congenital cystic adenomatoid malformations (c-CAM). This is a condition in which a benign lung tumor takes up too much space in the chest and can cause fetal hydrops, or excessive accumulation of fluids in the body's tissues and cavities leading to heart failure. The disease is particularly dangerous because fetal hydrops can cause pregnant women to become quite sick, and possibly die, through the mechanism of placental transfer. As fluids are released from the placenta into the woman's bloodstream, she may develop severe preeclampsia (hypertension) or pulmonary edema (accumulation of fluid in the lungs). A fetal surgeon stated, "this is called the *maternal mirror syndrome* because the mom's condition begins to mirror that of the fetus." After several fetuses died either during or after C-CAM surgeries, the fetal treatment team determined that the bigger the tumor, the less likely a fetus (and possibly the pregnant woman) is to survive surgery. As one fetal surgeon pointed out regarding the initial fetal deaths, "Along the way, you actually learn more from things that are not successful than from things that are successful." Laboratory research in fetal lambs subsequently generated a technique for resecting lung tissue, deflating the chest, and "curing" the hydrops. According to this surgeon, patient selection for C-CAMS currently rests on a clinical evaluation of fetuses that includes assessment of lung tumor size, gestational age, and the degree of advancement of fetal hydrops.

Yet as the above surgeon's comments indicate, this "clinical" evaluation is also related to the broader scientific research goals of experimental fetal surgery. As one fetal surgeon pointed out, there have been "a number of biologic spin-offs from this work." These include, for example, wound-healing research in which scientists investigate why fetuses heal without scars;[21] the "preterm labor problem," including introduction of new drugs and technologies to prevent it;[22] and a host of other questions. Not everybody involved with the Fetal Treatment Unit is enthusiastic about these scientific "advances." An obstetrician remarked: "The [fetal] surgical group constantly wants to introduce new things that have not been thoroughly tried.... There's a very different approach to how experimental things should be introduced." In response to probing about the ethics of experimentation, this same informant sharply stated, "Are you asking me whether I think the human pregnant woman and fetus should be used as an experimental animal? . . . I think that is what's happening."

The contradiction between what are defined as "clinical" and "nonclinical" factors in selection is particularly evident in conflicts between fetal surgeons and others, such as social workers, over criteria for surgery. Consider the situation in which a social worker's evaluation was dismissed in favor of "narrow" clinical criteria, with particularly unsettling consequences. April Saunders, a nineteen-year-old white, single woman with one child and on public aid, whose fetus was diagnosed with a congenital diaphragmatic hernia, was referred to the FTU for treatment. Below are excerpts from field notes taken at a meeting at which Saunders's treatment was discussed:

The meeting began with a description of the patient to be operated on. Ultrasound had been abnormal, indicating a possible diaphragmatic hernia. The woman smokes (mentioned by Graham as a health status indicator) and is on public aid, at which point Graham commented that the only thing that means for the Fetal Treatment Unit is they won't be paid. Social worker Barbara Greenwood responded to Graham's and Siegel's questions about Saunders' background and social situation. Greenwood commented that April is smart, "has religion," knows that her baby might die, and is "quite remarkable for a 19-year old," which garnered several grunts of agreement from the others present. According to Greenwood, the bottom line is that April knows the risks and wants the surgery. Based in part on Greenwood's assessment of April's emotional condition and Siegel's and Graham's medical assessments, the decision was made to go ahead with the surgery. They decided to schedule it for 8:00 A.M. on Thursday. April would be admitted to the hospital on Wednesday evening.

It is interesting to contrast this record of the decision-making process with the social worker's recollection and interpretation of it. According to the social worker, April Saunders "had been a product of foster homes. . . . She had a little kid, she was in a second relationship, new partner, *but she was like a perfect physical specimen.* She was young, she was strong, the baby had the right liver. And it was one of the real successes of the program. But in the end she took him home and shook him, shook her baby, and he was taken away." [23] Here the social worker points out that even when a case seems ideal from a clinical point of view, unknown and unanticipated factors may influence the outcome. Her narrative suggests that fetal surgery may be a traumatic experience for pregnant women, and consequently for their families downstream, particularly when a pregnant woman's life circumstances and social support networks are less than optimal, as in this case. Here "nonclinical" factors bleed into "clinical" decision making, with disturbing implications.

While social workers do not dismiss clinical criteria or outcomes, which are often quite serious, they are most interested in whether a pregnant woman will be able to psychologically withstand the rigors of fetal surgery and has adequate social support in place. These are issues that fetal surgeons and obstetricians, focused on clinical factors, consider only peripherally in practice. Thus, emphasis on treating fetal patients/work objects draws attention away from other participants and considerations in fetal surgery, such as the physical and emotional health of pregnant women and their families. The social workers in the Fetal Treatment Unit strive to provide adequate psychosocial care to their constituency, but are constrained in how much they can actually do by clinical practices aimed at "saving" fetuses and by institutionalized hierarchies of hospital care in which social workers typically have little say. Simultaneously, although surgeons and obstetricians consider psychological and social factors, these criteria often seem to play second fiddle to clinical criteria. Thus, "patient selection" is one set of work practices that in part shapes the conditions under which work objects are defined in this domain, while definitions of work objects in turn influence patient selection.

Different Views of a Disease and Its Treatment:
Negotiating the "How" of Fetal Surgery

The third area of difference concerns fetal disease or, more specifically, what should or should not be done about particular diseases. I focus on congenital diaphragmatic hernia (CDH), a particularly problematic and contested defect. CDH is a condition, diagnosable by ultrasound, in which fetal abdominal organs migrate upward into the chest through a hole in the diaphragm. The disease is often fatal because normal, healthy lung development is impaired and fetuses die in utero of respiratory failure. Sometimes an infant born with CDH can be operated on successfully, and many CDH cases are treated after birth. Fetal surgeons pursue *prenatal* surgery for CDH with the hope and expectation that early treatment will prevent the condition from worsening. Their prevailing clinical logic is that prenatal treatment will enable an adequate growth period in utero for fetal lungs following surgery. However, fetal mortality for CDH cases is near 60 percent (Harrison, Adzick, and Flake 1993), and even fetuses who survive are not completely healthy; *all* surviving fetuses require some additional postnatal surgery and follow-up. For these reasons, CDH has become a sort of rallying cry around which critics of fetal surgery organize their resistance, while fetal surgeons struggle to meet the challenges posed by this difficult-to-treat disease. Not all fetal surgical treatments are as controversial as CDH, and what makes CDH particularly contested is the very high fetal mortality rates. Other procedures have been far more "successful" than open surgery for CDH in terms of fetal mortality. For example, repairing blocked urinary tracts is seen as somewhat "routine" in the overall fetal surgery enterprise.

Fetal surgeons are very enthusiastic about prenatal treatment for CDH, even while recognizing that their lack of success makes the procedure controversial. For example, the FTU received a large grant from the National Institutes of Health to conduct a controlled clinical trial of CDH cases. According to one fetal surgeon, there is a great deal at stake in the study: "We've just begun this NIH trial, and we've been in starts and stops, moratoriums, you name the process, we've been through it. It's been extremely frustrating, and it's hard to know if formal diaphragmatic hernia repairs will be possible before birth. We're hoping that this trial will have the answer, so we can tell the rest of the world that yes this is worth doing, or no, stop doing it, and you have to just take your chances after birth." So far, outcomes have been discouraging to surgeons because many fetuses have died. Yet the fetal surgeons keep trying and hoping. As one points out, "Most of the mistakes, or most of the things we've learned, have been the result of frustrations doing the first few clinical diaphragmatic hernia repairs. And things that you couldn't have predicted no matter how many fetal animals you've done. So that's a very controversial area of treatment." When confronted with negative grumblings about CDH cases from other practitioners, this surgeon remarked: "But that's fine, that's good, at least now we can sort of put it to the test and see once and for all, after incredible painstaking review by the NIH. That's the way it gets sorted out."

While fetal surgeons continue to investigate surgery for CDH, other actors have become increasingly outspoken in their criticisms of the practice. One obstetrician remarked, "I think now you'll get divergent opinions—they are still enthusiastic about [CDH], we are definitely not and I'm willing to go on the record saying that . . . I would not recommend that any of my patients have open CDH surgery. The chance of survival is much greater to not have surgery and deliver in a tertiary center than the surgical survival is right now. There are just problems that have never been solved." When asked if he thought the conflict had to do with different professional training, he replied angrily, "It's not a disciplinary split! Get the actual numbers of how many CDH cases have been done and what the success rate is, and how many of those kids are living. Then compare that to the fact that if you come in here and have a CDH that we diagnose prenatally, and you deliver in a tertiary center, there's very good evidence that you will have a 40 percent survival rate. And you will draw your own conclusion as to whether you would ever have such surgery or whether you would ever suggest to a patient that they have it." With respect to *postnatal* surgery for CDH, he went on to say that "[the pediatric surgeon] still gets to operate on them, but it's a less sexy thing and it's something everybody's doing."

Social workers and obstetricians, who often disagree about criteria for treatment, often find themselves on the same side of the CDH debate. One social worker is deeply disturbed by these cases; in her words, "I found myself feeling like maybe this wasn't the best thing we were doing . . . it would be a relief to me if they weren't doing fetal surgery for the diaphragmatic hernia." Her reasons are similar to the obstetricians' and have to do with the mortality rates. She points out, "I can't recall very many healthy survivors of the fetal surgery program [for CDH]." And like the obstetricians, this social worker feels a certain amount of distrust for the fetal surgeons: "I was wondering about the presentation and whether we hadn't been manipulating statistics in a way to make it sound like this was an alternative to these kids going to term. . . . I really felt although they were trying to be honest, it was very hard to really paint an accurate picture and expect that anybody would actually do a thing like this, put themselves through this." As we spoke about the CDH cases, she grew visibly upset and finally remarked, "I don't know how many more moms and babies we can bring up to the altar of fetal surgery with the outcomes that we're having. . . . It's not as though you go through this and you're gonna have a healthy kid at the end!"

Both the obstetricians and social workers represent the CDH cases as in part motivated by professional interests of fetal surgeons. For example, fetal surgery is often referred to as the "final frontier" in reproductive medicine, and has certainly been a career-making enterprise for the surgeons in the FTU. In response to questions about why fetal surgeons continue to do CDH surgery in the face of high mortality rates, one obstetrician replied bitingly, "Well, they believe in themselves. They believe they're going to stamp out disease and save babies. . . . And I think what they're doing at this point is unfair and it borders on being immoral. Therefore our group is no longer part of it." And a social worker remarked, "There are kids who have hernias the size of the Grand Canyon. . . . And Dr. Graham is the kind of guy who really likes to take on something like diaphragmatic hernia, it's one of the most vexing problems. Sometimes I look at the surgeons, and I think, Can't they see that this isn't really going very well? When are we going to say, Gee, this isn't really working? Maybe we need to move on to something else. But the further along they get, the more dogged they get in their determination to meet every problem with a solution."

In sum, conceptualizations of fetal disease relate to definitions of work objects in ways similar to criteria for patient selection. The meanings that actors attribute to work objects order their work practices, just as work arrangements simultaneously shape the meanings given to fetuses and pregnant women. Fetal surgeons, for whom fetuses are central objects of work, are ostensibly dedicated to "saving" their patients, though they may well have other commitments and goals. Thus a central meaning ascribed to fetal work objects by surgeons is that the fetal patient *qua* work object must be repaired. Within this framework of meaning, attempting to surgically correct a terminal fetal disease is seen as the most logical action taken by surgeons. In turn, acting on this meaning by operating on a diseased fetus contributes to a social definition of the fetus as both patient and work object.

Neither obstetricians nor social workers consider the fetus to be a primary work object despite the Fetal Treatment Unit's collective institutional definition. For these actors, work practices center not on "saving" the fetus clinically, but rather on saving fetuses from fetal surgeons through activities that promote maternal and fetal health and well-being. These may well include criticizing fetal surgeons for treatment plans and outcomes that seem inconsistent with overall goals of healthier babies and "moms." In their view, the outcomes of surgery for congenital diaphragmatic hernia are not sufficiently positive to risk the physical and emotional health of pregnant women. Thus CDH, which has so far proven remarkably resistant to prenatal treatment, occupies different positions in the system of meanings held by each set of actors in the fetal surgery domain about their work. Despite both obstetricians' and social workers' concerns about maternal health and less than satisfactory fetal outcomes, fetal surgeons continue to advocate prenatal surgical repair of diaphragmatic hernias.

THE POLITICS OF DIFFERENCE:
SHAPING THE PRACTICE OF FETAL SURGERY

This chapter has shown that fetal surgery is a negotiated yet fluid order, given institutional and practical shape through the interactions and work practices of its participants. As a diverse enterprise, fetal surgery is characterized by cooperation, conflict, and a range of other interactional dynamics. Actors coalesce around fetuses and pregnant women in different ways, and there is both agreement and discord surrounding who or what is the work object in fetal surgery. These interactional dynamics shape such aspects of fetal surgery as patient selection and definitions of diseases and their treatment. Differences between practitioners are thus mobilized in certain ways to produce a negotiated order, a cooperative outcome that supports the overall institutional goals of the Fetal Treatment Unit while conflict may continue to rage internally. The politics of difference, then, refers to how diversity is mobilized and articulated in different ways and for different purposes.

The politics of difference also means that while there are many participants in this domain, some are heard and seen more clearly than others. Focusing on how different actors define work objects and organize their work practices highlights the many alliances and cleavages formed in this domain. Fetal surgery may well be a negotiated order, but it is continually evolving in response to other factors shaping negotiation. A context in which fetuses are defined as primary work objects leaves little room for the practical differences among actors to filter up to the institutional level. Most significantly, fetal surgeons have been successful in framing fetal surgery in line with their own commitments and interests. As one fetal surgeon remarked, "None of [the other practitioners] would be needed, it would be down to a single group of physicians, if we could just make them realize the goal is to get the fetus to survive the operation. We need a czar. . . . We need to *be* the czar." My point here is not to demonize fetal surgeons or to impugn their commitments to healthier babies, but rather to show how negotiations are patterned within and by institutional hierarchies, access to work objects, and investments in human fetuses.

Focusing on the politics of difference also means carefully considering the broader implications of experimental fetal surgery and how local work practices might seep out of the operating room and into other spheres of social life. For example, surgeons' emphasis on fetal work objects constructs pregnant women as barriers that must be passed through in order to reach the primary patient. Although there are actors in this domain who advocate for pregnant women, such as social workers, the interactional fabric of fetal surgery is woven in such a way that being an advocate for anybody other than a fetus is *very hard work*. The social workers, self-proclaimed "handmaidens" to the clinicians, are often unable to address psychosocial concerns of pregnant women because clinical criteria applied to fetuses take precedence and because social work is positioned low within the medical hierarchy. While obstetricians also attempt to advocate for pregnant women, their more circumscribed clinical orientation often precludes attention to important psychosocial and emotional issues. These dynamics have a number of implications for the specific practices of fetal surgery, including possible compromised fetal and maternal health and well-being. This is not to suggest that if social workers were more powerful and able to advocate for pregnant women, fetal surgery would be unproblematic. The issues here are much more complex than simply replacing "clinical" concerns with "nonclinical" ones. Rather, an important analytical task is to determine how these categories are constructed in the first place and where they overlap to impact the health of pregnant women and their fetuses.

How might the differences discussed here affect the future of experimental fetal surgery? As an emergent and contested specialty, it is in an uncertain position. The longevity of fetal surgery may well be shaped by the local factors presented here, as well as by broader developments in the U.S. health care system and the cultural politics of reproduction. The salient differences related to definitions of work objects will likely continue to occupy participants in this field, even while they strive cooperatively to meet the Fetal Treatment Unit's institutional aims of "saving fetuses" from certain death. Yet how, and if, these differences will be resolved is contingent upon an array of factors. There is little reason to believe that contestation will simply cease should fetal surgery become a routine medical specialty. The differences pointed to in this chapter will undoubtedly reshape both global and local definitions of fetuses, definitions of the work involved in operating on them for life-threatening diseases, and the health care of pregnant women. Current practices in this contested domain are indeed shaping the future of fetal surgery.

NOTES

Special thanks to Marc Berg, Annemarie Mol, Adele Clarke, Vicky Singleton, Lynn Morgan, Mike Curtis, Lisa Jean Moore, Sharon Kaufman, and Peter Taylor for helpful criticism and comments. Thanks also to my informants for agreeing to be interviewed and observed for this research. An earlier version of this paper was presented at the 1993 meetings of the Society for Social Studies of Science, Lafayette, Ind., where I received valuable feedback.

1 Data were collected through interviews and ethnography in a fetal treatment unit (FTU) at a major urban teaching facility that I call Capital Hospital. In order to protect the anonymity of my informants, I use pseudonyms or simply describe people by their occupations. While there are a multitude of different participants in this domain, this chapter focuses primarily on fetal surgeons, obstetricians, sonographers, and social workers. I selected these groups because they are key figures in fetal surgery, they work together closely but not always cooperatively, and they represent different professional backgrounds. Because work objects are the focus of analysis, examining the perspectives of those who work most closely on and with fetuses seems logical. Although not discussed here, pregnant women are also quite active in constructing fetuses as work objects, with implications for defining fetal surgery as a women's health issue.

2 Congenital diaphragmatic hernia (CDH) is a condition in which there is a hole in the diaphragm, causing fetal organs to migrate upward into the chest cavity and to impair lung development. Fetal surgery for CDH is designed to repair the diaphragm *in utero* and reposition the organs in the fetal abdominal cavity, thereby making room for subsequent lung development. Many fetuses with CDH die at birth; those who live and undergo surgery after birth generally have respiratory and other problems for the rest of their lives. Urinary tract obstructions, which may be caused by a number of factors, generally result in an excess build-up of fluid in the kidneys, leading to severe kidney damage and/or renal failure. See Harrison, Golbus, and Filly 1991 for a discussion of other conditions for which fetal treatment has been proposed or is being used.

3 A number of people I interviewed indicated that if a maternal death were to occur, it would have significant repercussions, including "maybe even shutting down the program."

4 Harrison (1991: 9) states that "the fetus with an anomaly requires the attention of a team of specialists working together. . . . Whether the patient is inside or outside the womb, its care is a continuum that requires the expertise of physicians trained in the care of mothers and babies. It is hard to imagine how one specialist, no mat-

ter how broadly trained, could take sole responsibility for the treatment of a fetus with a complex malformation."

5   Pickering 1992; Berg and Casper 1995.

6   See, e.g., Clarke 1987; 1990b; Clarke and Casper 1992; Fujimura 1987; 1988; 1992; and Star 1983; 1989b; 1991c; 1994, among others.

7   See Hughes 1971; Bucher and Strauss 1961; Strauss et al. 1964; Strauss 1978b; Strauss et al. 1985; and Bucher 1988.

8   See Shapin and Schaffer 1985; Ashmore, Wooffitt, and Harding 1994; Casper 1994a; 1994b; 1995; and others for an elaboration of the social construction and attribution of human and nonhuman within technoscience and biomedicine.

9   In a roundabout way, medical sociology has moved in this direction by focusing intently on patients as work objects, although this has not been articulated theoretically or explicitly.

10   In subsequent research, Strauss (1978b; Strauss et al. 1985) elaborated the concept of negotiated order in different ways, both by broadening the definition to include different dimensions of social order and types of negotiations, such as those constrained by coercion, as well as by linking negotiated orders to work activities more explicitly. More recently, Strauss (1993), building upon his earlier concept, proposed *processual ordering* to reflect that negotiation is but one type of ordering process. Strauss (1993: 253–54) writes, "A quick review of the original usage of [negotiated order] will show that it referred to the overall order of mental hospitals, and perhaps of most hospitals in general. . . . My use of a verb—ordering—instead of the usual noun is meant to emphasize the creative or constructive aspect of interaction, the 'working at' and 'working out of' ordering in the face of inevitable contingencies, small and large. . . . It is still my belief that though negotiation is only one of the interactional processes, it must be a major contributor to any social ordering." Although Strauss's newer concept is provocative, I have used "negotiated order" in this chapter because it resonates more clearly with the data.

11   Human fetuses are highly contested entities in the late twentieth century, particularly in the United States where opposition to abortion is often increasingly violent. Fetuses are situated culturally and physiologically at the margins of humanity and are thus imbued with diverse and often contradictory meanings (Casper 1994a). In the United States, where individuality is ideologically and politically significant, the ontological status of fetuses is especially controversial because they are not autonomous organisms. Fetuses exist within and are dependent upon the bodies of pregnant women. Yet in all domains in which pregnancy and fetuses are salient, the reigning conceptual paradigm is that of maternal-fetal *conflict,* in which the fetus is symbolically excerpted from a pregnant woman's body and represented as a separate entity with its own needs and concerns. Within these ubiquitous representations, the fetus is positioned as an individual social actor imbued with human agency while the pregnant woman is often conceptually erased as an active participant (Casper 1994b). For example, emergent fetal rights frameworks in ethics

and law often assert fetal interests and relegate pregnant women to the status of containers (Purdy 1990). This dynamic forms the broader cultural and political context of work on fetuses in the United States and other countries where human reproduction is a highly charged public issue.

12   Liley 1963; Adamsons et al. 1965.

13   The new technology was called a Rocket catheter and is still used widely in fetal treatment practices.

14   They may also recognize other reasons but choose not to discuss these publicly.

15   This informant's usage of "rubbing shoulders" differs slightly from Dr. Graham's, indicating conflict where Graham's usage invoked interaction. Vicky Singleton (personal communication) has suggested that this term also captures how the FTU is a place where practitioners work closely together and engage in ongoing interaction, which may include both cooperation and conflict.

16   The Fetal Treatment Unit at Capital Hospital is often approached by other hospitals interested in starting fetal surgery units. One fetal surgeon told me that the FTU has advised a major East Coast hospital "*not* to include obstetricians from day one." In other words, if obstetricians are not invited in as cofounders of this program, then some of the problems "plaguing" the FTU discussed here might be avoided at other institutions.

17   Emphasis added. This is a somewhat ironic criticism, as obstetricians have historically, and routinely, performed cesarean sections and must have at least a passing knowledge of "major operations."

18   One informant, a fetal surgeon, told me that if everything "worked right," everybody would "get along fine." A sonographer remarked, "If everything was red, white, and blue banners flying all the time about the successes, then believe me, there would be no conflict. Everybody would be so happy. The only conflicts would be who got to stand first in line for the laurels. We're more likely to have conflict when we have failures."

19   Not all patients referred to the FTU end up having fetal surgery, which is only one, albeit the most invasive, of several available treatment options. Other options include nonsurgical interventions such as drug therapy, aborting the fetus, and/or not treating at all.

20   E.g., Harrison 1991.

21   There is considerable excitement about fetal wound-healing research. As one fetal surgeon put it, "Ten years ago no one would have predicted a huge investigative effort now in trying to figure out how the fetus can heal without scarring. . . . If the fetus can teach us how he or she can heal without scarring, we can use that same blueprint to treat problems after birth. That would be incredible." Possible applications may include, for example, cosmetic surgeries (both reconstructive and elective) and use in the cosmetics industry.

22   A fetal surgeon stated that "the preterm labor problem is to fetal therapy what rejection is to transplantation. And we're working like crazy to come up with the

medication, like cyclosporin was for transplantation, to treat the preterm labor problem. If folks here can do it, then that would have implications beyond our little tiny fetal therapy enterprise. That would have implications for a huge health problem."

23 Emphasis added.

CLINICAL PRACTICE AND PROCEDURES
IN OCCUPATIONAL MEDICINE: A STUDY
OF THE FRAMING OF INDIVIDUALS

Nicolas Dodier

▼

In this chapter, I show how doctors, when asked for an expert appraisal, use codified rules to deliver judgments on specific individuals. I propose to demonstrate that the use of these rules by medical experts depends on the manner in which they "frame" the individuals with whom they are dealing. What is meant here by "frame"? Extending recent studies, I propose the general hypothesis that a person adjusts to a situation not by using discrete resources, but through arrangements of resources (words, rules, objects) in which past experiences are inscribed, that is, through frames. When a person mobilizes a rule, a word, or an object, he or she must at the same time take note of all the other elements associated with it in this arrangement or complex. For example, in a medical consultation, the doctor initiates with his or her stethoscope the whole of the clinical approach, which gives the noises heard through the stethoscope a diagnostic meaning (Dodier 1993b). The technical object only becomes operative in an activity if all the connections are made to ensure its integration into a network (Latour 1987; Akrich 1993). The word is only integrated into a concrete situation through a language game that encompasses it in the web of ordinary language (Wittgenstein 1961). When we wish to make use of one element, the whole fabric comes into view. The area of personal involvement illustrates this process very clearly: once people seek to establish some sort of connection with others within a certain relationship, they are automatically involved in the web of associations already woven by past events. They are faced not only with the stethoscope, the actual technical object, or the word, but with medical practice, a sociotechnical network, or a language game.

Several scholars have identified such complexes of resources and their role in action. Boltanski and Thévenot have identified "forms of coordination": vast assemblies of resources integrated by doctrines stemming from political philosophy, through which people manifest their sense of justice in everyday life

(1991). In his work on frames of experience, Goffman (1974) looks at the co-ordination of actions at lower levels of integration. Coordination with others is assured by gestures, objects, or behavior, but especially by interior shifts in the way of seeing things. Goffman makes a vast inventory of possible frames, illustrated by a host of examples. He notes the large number of possible ways of dealing with adjustments. He indicates the many rifts between frames, as manifested by awkwardness, difficulties, uncertainties, hesitations. Frames can thus harmonize with each other or conflict with each other. The architecture of frames takes form as much in the web of interior experience as in sequences of interaction with other beings. Goffman defines the articulation of several re-sources as a frame and leaves open the possibility of combinations occurring between frames. His form of classification is very similar to Austin's pragmat-ics (1970). Recent research on the work of doctors shows that contemporary medicine is a place where resources coexist between frames: the establishment of "medical-decision making" formats, based on a conversational analysis of consultations (Silverman 1987); the distinction between "modes of decipher-ing pain" through a meticulous comparison of actual medical consultations in specialized centers (Baszanger 1995); the articulation of several "frames" of re-lationships with dying persons (Perakyla 1989).

This research suggests that several frames are generally available for each situation. Therefore, people must manipulate a multiplicity of frames, as well as the eventual ruptures that emerge in the course of the interactions. Different frames can therefore succeed each other, conflict, or mix in a given situation. The analysis of frames is a tool for developing a *sociological pragmatics* (Dodier 1993a). According to this approach, making a judgment on a human being ne-cessitates a choice among different "frames" of this person or a combination of several. Focusing on medical judgments, I will develop this point by showing that the same rule can be mobilized differently depending on the framing of the situation adopted by the doctor.

A number of sociological works have illustrated the web of interpreta-tion that doctors use to apply rules to concrete situations. It is principally in the domain of ethnomethodology (Garfinkel 1967), of conversational analy-sis (Atkinson and Heath 1981; Heath 1988), of cognitive sociology (Cicourel 1975; 1985), or of artificial intelligence (Schnaffner 1985) that this work has been pushed the farthest. The introduction of frame analysis offers a supplementary element: "following a rule" is an activity that can have diverse meanings de-pending on the status that one accords to this rule with regard to action. It is in exploring the different statuses of rules that the concept of frames is useful. The way in which doctors frame the situation affects their attitude toward codi-fied rules.

I will address the relationship between two frames: the *administrative frame*, in which all people of the same category are treated in the same way, and the *clinical frame*, in which the doctor follows a course that leaves room for the individual's unpredictable particularities. At the center of this analysis are the relationships established by doctors between rules and particularities. The doctor encounters the following questions: How much should I take into consideration individuals' particularities? Should I systematically refer to codified rules? To what extent is a rule a guide for a decision? The heterogeneity of contemporary medicine, which interests us here, must be understood not only as a difference between places of medical care but also as internal tensions in action.

I use the example of occupational medicine in France as the point of departure. Occupational physicians are responsible for the fitness report that has to be drafted for each employee on recruitment and once a year thereafter. This report is transmitted to the corporation, which must take it into consideration in assigning work. On this fitness report, doctors write "fit," "unfit," or "fit with certain restrictions." They advise, for example: "fit with ear guards," "no work involving the loading of large kegs," "no carrying of heavy loads or posts demanding continual flexion-extension," or "fit for the post of controller if prolonged suspended efforts are avoided." In case of fitness restrictions, employers can be led to change their decision on the recruitment of an employee, modify his/her work assignment, or transfer him/her to another post, or they might even dismiss the employee. Doctors base their reports on "medical appointments." An annual check-up is imposed by law, but employees can ask to be seen, and their employers can request that the doctor see them.

Legally, the doctor's decision is binding, although the employee may appeal against the conclusions drawn by the employer insofar as the employee's assignment or posting is concerned. In the event of a dispute, particularly if the person judged unfit for work is fired, s/he can claim compensation by appealing to an ad hoc judicial body—in France, the Conseil des Prudhommes. In reality, any debate about medical fitness tends, from the employee's point of view, to involve his or her trust in the occupational doctor in the corporation. From the point of view of the employer, these conflicts bring into play not just the issue of trust in the doctor but, because of this, also issues such as the opportunity for the doctor to investigate what goes on within the corporation and, finally, his or her career. This brings us back to the more general question of the status of occupational doctors. Here we can distinguish two different cases. Large French corporations (roughly speaking, establishments with over five hundred employees) are obliged by law to set up and finance their own occupational medicine services. In this case, the doctor is an employee of the corporation. Smaller corporations must join together and set up an "intercorporation service," which then employs the doctor or doctors. The latter service functions as a private association financed by subscriptions paid by the corporations in question. Each doctor then divides his or her time between several corporations while his or her salary is paid by the association.[1]

Another responsibility of occupational medicine is to identify the professional risks to which employees are exposed (toxic risks, physical risks like noise, infectious risks) and to propose preventive measures for each case. This task brings several factors into play. The employer's legal obligations come first. In fact, the time that the occupational doctor is obliged to devote to a corporation depends partly on the number of employees exposed to one of the risks indicated on a statutory list and hence requiring "special medical supervision" (appendix A). Hence, the higher the number of persons judged by the doctor to require "special medical supervision," the greater the amount of money that the company will have to devote to occupational medicine, a point that can make this assessment controversial. In addition, the occupational doctor is seen as an "adviser" to both employer and employees in combating occupational hazards. In this capacity, s/he may deliver an opinion at the request of either party or take the initiative of alerting them to certain risks. Here again, these opinions are integrated into risk management on the part of employers and into the complex network of relationships that springs up between the partners around questions to do with working conditions and safety.[2]

These expert appraisal functions are guided by codified rules, which are more or less numerous depending on the case treated. We will see, for example, that there are regulatory norms for decisions on medical fitness. Occupational risks are defined in numerical terms of maximum and minimum values or through lists of potential risks collected in technical or regulatory texts. Over and above the particularities of this type of medical practice—notably, that it consists of medical appraisal, since occupational doctors are not empowered to prescribe drugs or treatment—occupational medicine is a good example of medicine defined by standards, which are sometimes very precise. A close study of the practice of occupational doctors can provide interesting data to demonstrate the pragmatic effects of the arrangements for framing medical practice by means of precisely codified rules, whether these rules are drafted for reasons to do with cost management or administrative or legal concerns, or to provide a scientific foundation for the activity. The existence of these rules does not tell us how they are actually used in concrete situations. This is the question that frame analysis allows us to develop.[3]

THE ADMINISTRATIVE FRAME

In the frame that I call *administrative,* the individual is depersonalized, in that s/he is treated according to a formal category or according to rules applying to a population to which this person is said to belong. Many occupational medicine mechanisms guide doctors' actions according to an administrative model. They generally use technologies of treating risks, described well elsewhere:[4] the monitoring, supervision, and advising of individuals; ascription and reparation of damages; and references to rules of behavior. These mechanisms entail a bureaucratic use of the notion of "risk factor." "Belonging to a category," in this case, signifies "belonging to a population defined by a risk factor." As soon as an individual is linked to a risk factor, measures are applied to her/him that are appropriate for any member of that risk population.

Let us begin by considering the events that precede an individual's annual occupational medical visit. The appointment fixes a date and an hour for an examination of a certain population: for example, this morning, the doctor will see "corporation X," "service Y," or "workshop Z." Risk factors determine the frequency of systematic visits: the job description (the risks that justify, according to the terms of governmental decree, special medical supervision),[5] the sector (for example, in the nuclear industry, employees are seen every six months), and so forth. Before the actual medical visit, a secretary asks the patient a series of questions and records administrative information in a file according to a standard schema (age, date of birth, profession, etc.). When there is a nurse working in the service, the patient undergoes systematic tests during a "previsit," including tests for vision and weight and analysis of the urine. The person then goes into a changing room according to a standard organizational protocol. He or she exits the changing room stripped of all personalizing items of clothing.

Evidence of the administrative frame is the use of *lists* for judging individuals during the visit. Many of the items are defined a priori. They are compiled through the use of questions on the medical file: family medical history, personal background (congenital diseases, illnesses, operations, accidents, history of intoxication, incapacities, occupational illnesses); education and professional experience; vaccination history; condition of hearing, sight, skin, mobility, weight, and the respiratory system; X-ray analysis; condition of the cardiovascular system (including pulse, blood pressure, varicose veins), digestion, genital organs, urinary system; levels of albumin and blood sugar; hematopoiesis; functioning of the reticular system (ganglion, spleen), endocrine glands, the nervous system (trembling, balance, reflexes), and the psyche; and information derived from complementary exams (tuberculosis test, hematological and serological exams, etc.). The doctor uses a systematic list of questions to gather much of this information from the patient during the medical visit: "Do you have digestive problems?," "Are your periods regular?," "No back pain?," "At the end of the day, does your lower back hurt?," "Do you get headaches?," "Do you sleep well?," and so on. The questions are not written up on a form; there are different ways to ask them, but they structure the visit. There are important differences among doctors: some measure blood pressure on both arms, others do not; some routinely ask questions about alcohol consumption, others do not.[6] These variations do not challenge the fact that the doctor, in each case, conducts an *inventory* of personal characteristics according to a list of items formulated a priori.

The patient's status during this portion of the visit is defined through his or her answers to the standardized list: the employee is considered as part of a given population. Being an employee is enough to justify a series of tests, which are part of the general physical exam. In certain occupational medicine services, for example, just the fact that one is a "male employee of 40 years of age" is enough to justify an electrocardiogram, and being a "crane driver" is enough to require psychotechnical exams. The fact that the employee belongs to certain targeted populations, defined a priori by specified criteria and "risk factors" (linked to age or sex, public health criteria, or occupational criteria) determines what lists of complementary items will be used. After these procedures have been completed, the doctor records the health of the patient in the form of a list of references: s/he fills in the boxes of a coded standardized form for the individual.

A device to oversee the indices can be added to these first elements. Belonging to a certain population necessitates a list of complementary exams (such as audiometries, biological exams, ophthalmologic exams). In the administrative frame, the value of each element is fixed from the outset, according to routine procedures that already exist at the moment of the encounter with the individual. An element prompts intervention if it is outside the established norms, which apply to every individual. A given occupational doctor, for example, conducts audiograms on all employees who work in the press workshops and proposes a transfer if their hearing is deficient in certain frequencies. Regulatory texts set, term by term, the incompatibilities between the individual profile and the employment category, according to "medical norms" or "fitness criteria" norms. This is notably the case in the transport sector, where a concern for public security has produced an abundance of rules and regulations. In a decree of October 4, 1988, from the French ministry of transport we find four types of disqualification for drivers of heavy-load vehicles. For example:

Type I: Eyes and vision. Candidates with a sum acuity in both eyes, possibly with correction, of less than 15/10 are disqualified. The acuity of the weakest eye cannot be less than 5/10; for the reactivation of a license, the required scores are 13/10 and 4/10 respectively. Type II: Ear, nose, and throat and pneumology. Auditory deficit. The referential limit for 2000 hertz is 35 decibels. (Astin and Wehbi 1991)

We can observe an identical form of transfer in the systematized production of preventive advice, as soon as the employee belongs to a population "at risk." In medical visits, for example, we find the following associations: "Decrease in hearing"/"Do you wear a helmet?"; "backache"/"Show me how you pick up an object"; "skin problem"/"Do you wear gloves?"; and so on. The individual is wholly assimilated into a given population when the examination ends with advice. This is also the case when a symptom is explained by the existence of a risk factor. Mentioning a risk factor, in this schema, completes the interpretation process. This type of explanation intervenes notably for symptoms that are particularly loaded with epidemiological correlations, such as lung problems with tobacco consumption. A blood pressure problem can also be attributed to cigarette smoking, as in the following example, which shows the capacity of administrative framing to eliminate lengthy questioning by identifying a person as belonging to a population "at risk."

The scene occurs in a burner factory that employs approximately one hundred people. The employees are primarily skilled steel industry workers. The medical office is located in the company itself but is too small to satisfy the statutory standards. The doctor, who is employed by an intercorporation service, comes approximately once a week to run a half-day clinic. Help in organizing the medical visits is provided by a secretary from the personnel department.[7] The case concerns the annual visit of an electrician, about forty years old, assigned to maintenance work. The following exchange represents my verbatim notes taken during this visit:

[The man, who is bearded, comes in. He speaks with a hoarse voice.]
Doctor (D): So what do you have to tell me?
Employee (E): I collapsed through overwork. I fainted, about forty days ago. I lost consciousness, my blood pressure was a little over 180. I was hospitalized at the Tripode [a city hospital], then I was allowed home.
[The employee gets out the results of analyses done three weeks ago.]
D. The analyses are fine!
E. Well, I've been resting. . . .
D. Was there something worrying you?

E. It's not so pleasant at the factory, but not to that extent! I was working hard helping my kids with their homework [he mentions that his children are working with computers]. I took a break and I took urbanyl [an anxiolytic]. I've stopped the drug now.

[The physician tells me that this employee had an obstruction of the bowels three years ago.]

D. This man is a fairly energetic type, perhaps overenergetic! And then, for no reason, he has this problem. . . .

[The employee came back to work one week ago to his usual electrical mechanic's job.]

E. I'm in the testing section [testing burners].

D. You're no longer working in the electrical department?

E. No, testing, it's interesting. . . .

[The physician asks him to weigh himself: (? inaudible)]

D. Same as last year.

[He examines the patient without comment and takes his blood pressure.]

D. 170/80. Keep still a moment [to take the blood pressure again. The employee rests.]

D. Do you smoke?

[The employee admits to smoking 15 cigarettes a day. The physician takes his blood pressure again, still 170/80.]

E. I feel better at 4.30 [that is, when he stops work].

D. Perhaps . . .

[The physician suggests that a solution would be to forbid cigarette smoking in the factory. According to the employee, they've already tried that but "the lads" were even more on edge.]

E. I still have rather high blood pressure. They expect you to turn out boilers at top speed, with breakdowns on top of it!

[The physician terminates the visit by declaring the employee "fit."]

Note the speed with which, at the end of the visit, the information concerning consumption of cigarettes sums up — via reference to a rule of prevention, that is, "No smoking" — a whole series of possible questions about the links established by the employee between his current condition and his family and occupational environment. This physician, on other occasions, would have brought up these questions. He has been trained in both occupational medicine and rheumatology. The reason he went back to occupational medicine five years ago was because his attempt to practice as a rheumatologist was a failure financially, and, as he puts it, he was not comfortable with the financial relationship between himself and his patients. He displayed a keen interest in medical psychology, and I noticed that on many occasions he stressed psychosomatic concerns and had a very flexible approach in listening to patients as a way of exploring the relationship between the working life and health of employees.[8] However, on this occasion, keeping things on an administrative level, he does not follow up these concerns and contents himself with referring back to a main point of relevance in such a framework: the consumption of cigarettes.

In all such judgments, the doctor identifies an individual by a list of items and applies systematic rules of judgment for each of these items. Either the individual belongs to a population that corresponds with a positive value of the item, in which case the doctor applies the value that applies to any member of that population, or the item has a negative value, in which case the doctor does not apply this value. The group to which the risk factors belong leads to a corresponding list of values that are applied to the individual. The risk factors create a bureaucratic transfer: the individual is characterized by a list of variables, each of them leading to the application of a given rule. The individual is defined by the sum of these rules, in the form of orientation, guidance, advice, and financial compensation. The consequence of this administrative status is depersonalization: the individual is considered the point of intersection of different rules. There is no obligation to integrate the different judgments. Individuals are the target of as many interventions as categories to which they belong. They accumulate series of judgments deduced from each of the administrative rules.[9]

These administrative mechanisms lead to strict judgments on individuals. In effect, they represent a way to treat the uncertainty involved in individual particularities. The reasoning involved is as follows. As soon as an individual belongs to a given population, the doctor assumes that s/he knows enough about the patient's situation. The patient is categorized as facing a given statistical risk. Regardless of other particularities, s/he will be treated just like all the other members of that population. Association with a population is considered sufficient to justify action. It allows the doctor to come to a firm decision. Therefore, strictly speaking, one cannot say that the mechanisms "do not take into account the particularities of the individual." They in fact do, by relying on properties that allow one to group the individual in certain categories. It is even completely possible that the doctor, in behaving in this way, manages to locate very precisely the appropriate population for evaluating the risks involved. A judgment will be even more precise if it assigns the individual to restricted categories.

The characteristic application of rules for this type of framing is a syllogism: a given rule applies to a given class of individuals, a given individual belongs to this class, therefore this rule applies to this individual. The particularity of the individual is limited to her/his actual existence. You have seen all there is to see of the individual once you have applied, like a label, her/his class membership. This is what makes this type of judgment at once rigid, rapid, economic, and systematic. It explains why the judgment is henceforth closed to all complementary information. As soon as you define your action as an application, through a succession of cases, of rules defined for a population, you do not have to concern yourself with the details of the particular circumstances. All individuals are equivalent, in terms of your action, as soon as they belong to this population: all workshop employees must wear a helmet, all roofers on scaffolding must wear a shoulder harness, all operators must wear such and such a uniform when going into a given nuclear center. Assimilating individuals into populations consists of making all roofers, for example, follow the same rules (e.g., make them wear a shoulder harness) regardless of individual characteristics to which they try to refer in order to emphasize particular aptitudes that could distinguish them from others in a reference population (such as seniority, qualification, residence, lack of previous accidents).

This type of action has repercussions on the relationships that develop among people in administrative institutions. In this schema, the individual actor, confronted with individuals, applies general rules to particular cases: s/he is subordinated to other actors in the center. This is characteristic of the classical schema of a bureaucratic organization, in which actors at inferior levels of the hierarchy are responsible for the application of general rules. For example, we find risk analysts, who study populations and delineate regulatory norms, on one hand, and local actors, who apply the regulation, on the other. This structure corresponds, in the important services of occupational medicine, with the establishment of a hierarchical relationship between the chief doctor, who commands the occupational medicine service on a central level, and doctors divided in different group units. The central service produces the regulations of the enterprise, which the local doctors are expected to apply in the units. The development of an administrative frame is part of an effort to standardize medical practice emanating from scientific or administrative centers.[10]

CLINICAL FRAMING OF THE INDIVIDUAL

Let us now put the individual into a *clinical frame*. This is not entirely possible in an annual occupational medical visit that addresses the individual, from the beginning, according to an administrative procedure. The first sign of straying from the administrative model occurs when the doctor, during the visit, comments on simple items of the physical examination. The personalization of the individual arises when the doctor refers to an individual's idiosyncratic characteristics in pinpointing areas that need attention. This signals that the doctor is assuming the existence of personal norms. In order to discern this attitude on the part of the doctor, you must pay attention to her/his brief comments during the visit: "79 kilos. You, your optimum, I think is 75 kilos"; "130/80, those are your usual figures"; "115/70. Those are totally your figures"; "For you that's good." The usage of the possessive (as in "your weight," "your blood pressure," "your optimum," "your equilibrium" . . .) or the personal pronoun ("for you that's good, that's perfect, that's disturbing, that's alarming . . .") disrupts the assimilation of an individual into a population. An alternative way of judging is employed. The individual's points of reference are no longer connected to general categories, but to personal norms. In this approach the doctor has to wait for the first signs. In order to be capable of judgment, the doctor must leave room for particularities. This is why an isolated factor has no value in a clinical frame: it is not enough to apply a rule to be able to deduce something. One must have additional indices for the individual.

In order to completely characterize the clinical frame of the individual, let us now explore the principles of the diagnostic process in the medical clinic. It is instructive here to read manuals to understand what doctors do during consultations. Explanations of the diagnostic approach, on which these texts focus, illustrate particularly well the relationship between general and particular involved in clinical framing.[11] A clinical table is presented as a group of signs that, when simultaneously present, indicate the existence of a pathological state. "Simultaneously" should be interpreted loosely. Not all of the signs have to be present at the same time to establish the diagnosis. In the case of an illness, certain symptoms are always present, while others are more rare: this allows us to assign symptoms degrees of "sensitivity." Furthermore, the same symptom can appear in several clinical tables. The "degree of specificity" refers to the probability that, for a given symptom, a given illness will be diagnosed. The more specific a symptom is, the more it will direct the exploration toward an explicit diagnosis. A clinical table is a collection of symptoms with variable sensitivities and specificities.

To employ a clinical model, you first consider one or several of an individual's symptoms that, according to the clinical model, "evoke" a diagnosis (an illness, a syndrome). You then search for the presence of other symptoms, in this individual, that are characteristic of the evoked diagnosis. If you find specific symptoms of the diagnosis, you are likely to be following the right diagnostic path. If, on the contrary, you do not find sensitive symptoms that are consistent with the proposed diagnosis, you must ask yourself if you should change your diagnostic path. The path is thereby strewn with symptoms, or groups of symptoms, that more or less strongly evoke diagnoses, and illnesses that more or less strongly assume the presence of certain symptoms. The principle of moving between clinical models is therefore the combination of many procedures: connecting different symptoms in order to make a group, pursuing a diagnostic path in the clinical table selected, exploring the symptoms that correspond to the clinical table, and backtracking and taking another tack when the presence of certain symptoms that you were not looking for, or the absence of symptoms that you were looking for, weakens the initial diagnosis. This approach thus involves relating different symptoms with others so that eventually the combination of symptoms can be identified as an illness.

Let us consider, for example, the section "Recognize a Hyperthyroid" in D. Sicard's manual, *The Clinical Approach* (1987, 48–49). The list of symptoms that, associated together, evoke a hyperthyroid are presented in the form of a succession of sentences: "Someone ill with a hyperthyroid should have hot, moist, and trembling hands. The pulse is rapid. This tachycardia does not cease with rest, unlike neurotonic tachycardia. No more is necessary for the hypothesis of a hyperthyroid to come to mind." Sicard's use here of the statement "No more is necessary for the hypothesis of . . . to come to mind" shows that one can pursue this diagnostic path. But many other expressions provide evidence of the same formal relationship that exists between the list of symptoms and the diagnostic path. In the manual, for example, we find that a symptom "evokes," "marks," "suggests," "is a good indication of," "translates into," "raises the possibility of," "is very suggestive of," "is more or less evidence of," "can be observed during," "can integrate itself into," "is caused by," "is evidence of," "of course makes one look for," "can precede," "refers essentially to," "is very evocative of" an illness. Let us continue with the example of the hyperthyroid: "Rather drastic weight loss usually occurs without sign of a decrease in appetite and can even be accompanied by polyphagia." The list of associated symptoms continues: a new collection of symptoms—weight loss, sustained appetite, polyphagia—have been added to the preceding list. The verb phrase "is accompanied by" is characteristic of the search for a series of symptoms simultaneously present in the diagnostic investigation. It makes explicit the simple juxtaposition of the symptom sentences used above.

A clinical table generally contains sketches of other possible diagnostic paths, "differential" diagnoses, mentioning supplementary symptoms that are likely to privilege one path over another. The brief passage on the hyperthyroid provides us with an example: "This tachycardia does not cease with rest, unlike neurotonic tachycardia." Or: "Certainly, when these signs of thyrotoxicosis are accompanied with an exophthalmic goiter, the diagnosis of Basedow's disease is clear and is never mistaken. But in the absence of this ocular and cardiac semiology, it is important to take into consideration the hot, trembling, and moist hands in attributing a hyperthyroid, and in a middle-aged or old person, an interruption in rhythm such as a heart attack or a stupefying or hallucinating seizure." Sicard states that a tachycardia that ceases at rest is not a sign of Basedow's disease, while an association with a specific other symptom ("exophthalmic goiter") makes the diagnosis stronger. He also adds to his table an entire series of additional symptoms and syndromes: "interruption in rhythm," "heart attack," and so forth, with other supplementary indications ("middle-aged or old person").[12]

Of course, different tendencies exist in the manipulation of clinical tables. Certain doctors prefer to accumulate many symptoms, without any a priori connection, before embarking on a diagnostic path. An example of this consists of constructing a series of complementary tests. Other doctors, on the other hand, quickly take off in a particular diagnostic direction, only to subsequently retrace their steps. The symptoms privileged in the individual approach vary: certain doctors rely essentially on objective clinical symptoms, others take subjective symptoms (what the patient says) more into consideration; the weight accorded to complementary exams also varies. We find differences in the group of symptomatological tables explored first. Occupational doctors in particular explore more or less willingly the psychiatric nosology. Finally, the degree of exhaustiveness sought varies. One can be very selective in deciding which points of reference to consider as real symptoms worthy of interpretation, or one can consider every point of reference a symptom and try to enter the entirety on a large table. When one uses clinical tables, certain signs are more or less significant depending on the diagnostic path chosen. The choice of diagnostic direction influences the passage from a simple "reference point" to a "symptom."[13] Let us consider the following example.

A thirty-one-year-old employee, a heavy-load vehicle driver, comes for his annual visit. This visit takes place in the intercorporation service van, which makes the rounds of companies that do not have a medical office for the doctor to use. The driver accompanying the doctor also acts as medical secretary during the visits. On this particular day, the doctor will examine fourteen people between 11 A.M. and 3 P.M., hours chosen because they overlap with the morning and afternoon shifts. This corporation is

active in industrial meat processing and employs around eighty people. It is a subsidiary of a large pharmaceutical group. During the medical questioning, in response to the systematic question about current medical treatments, the employee mentions the medicine that he takes for his chronic acne. The auscultation begins: the doctor comments on what he hears through the stethoscope in the lungs: "Ah! You can hear the cigarettes! Your left lung is not respiring well? I don't have an X ray to help me out. It's a bit of flu, but its also the cigarettes that are making all this uproar. We'll examine this lung, we'll do an X ray."
The examination continues: no digestive problems.
When the doctor palpates, he says that "it pulls a bit" at the left knee.
E: My meniscus was operated on.
D: Do you feel that pulling your muscle?
E: Yes, it hurts there.
D: You're overcompensating. You try to avoid what bothers you, but you carry it over to the other side.
[He proceeds to the blood pressure: 130/60.] Good.
[He examines the vertebral column.]
D: I have to admit that I don't really understand what's going on. There is a little scoliosis [sideward curvature], but that does not explain the difference! No, there isn't any shift. Oh, yes, there is, a little shift to the right, that could be a sufficient explanation. The scoliosis is a little bonus.

Some of the doctor's inferences in this visit are dictated by the general examination's systematic list of items (the doctor reviews the patient's medical treatments, lungs, digestion, legs, blood pressure). But other relationships are established: the flu and the cigarette smoking. He expounds his diagnostic exploration with a complementary exam, to finally gather other signs (the X ray). Another warning sign: the muscle "pulling" in the left leg. The doctor finds a concordance with a "subjective" symptom (the sensation of "muscle pulling") and, aware of a previous pathology, he sketches a diagnostic path (the work of compensation on one side after an operation on the meniscus). In order to consolidate this interpretation, the doctor looks for symptoms in the vertebral column. In principle, he should find a "shift." This is not pronounced, however: "No, there isn't any shift. Oh, yes, there is, a little shift to the right, that could be a sufficient explanation." As for the scoliosis, it is not strictly part of the table, but it is not incompatible either.
Let us return to an individual's physiological parameters (blood pressure, level of glucose in the urine, gamma-Gt number, etc.) and compare their usage

in a clinical and administrative frame. The medical texts delineate ranges and limits of normalcy. For example: "The urine glucose, on average 1.8 g/l, varies from 1.4 and 2 g/l depending on the individual"; "gamma-Gt: normal value varying according to the dosage technique (the laboratory supplies the norms), is generally less than 25 mU/ml" (Durand and Biclet 1991, 190). When the measurement result is outside of the range, it can suggest a problem: "Demonstration of glycosuria normally signals the existence of diabetes mellitus; nevertheless, the presence of sugar in the blood is indispensable in order to eliminate a tubulopathy" (ibid., 190); "In the diagnosis of chronic alcoholism, a normal gamma-Gt does not allow for the elimination of intoxication: combined gamma-Gt and vGM[14] only identify about 70% of alcoholics. On the other hand, elevated figures in the presence of hepatopathy do not allow for the confirmation of alcoholism because there are many other known or unspecified causes of augmentation (diabetes, hyperthyroid, nephropathy)" (ibid., 185). In both the administrative and clinical frame, the point of departure is identical: one uses statistical data that can delimit a range of "risk" values. In the administrative frame, the doctor uses the value as a parameter to decide if the individual is "at risk," and to act immediately. In the clinical activity, the doctor proceeds differently: before coming to closure, s/he will wait to have several values of one parameter for the same individual. In this way, the doctor aims to delineate the individual's personal point of equilibrium, while remaining open to conceding discrepancies with the ranges outlined in the texts. If the parameter normally has a given value for this individual, the doctor considers it an individual reference point. The administrative and clinical frame are two ways of dealing with uncertainty with regards to individuals. The first examines the individual's place with regard to reference points in the wider population; the second waits to be able to compare several individual reference points. And when clinical doctors have historical elements (an "individual file") at their disposition, they compare the present parameters to their values in the past. By reconsidering the file and judging the evolution of values, the doctor thereby appraises the significance of the present parameters.

One important characteristic of a clinical frame is the latitude that it allows the doctor for appraising the significance of a point of reference. A doctor can begin a diagnostic exploration by considering that a reference point is pathological, but change her/his opinion when s/he realizes that for such an individual, such a reference point does not signify an illness. On the other hand, s/he will be led to add another reference point to the clinical table, which did not seem very significant in the beginning. The same diagnosis can be attached to different tables, or the same symptom can orient the doctor toward different tables, depending on the individual. In a clinical frame, doctors may wait before giving their verdict on a given reference. Through their diagnostic exploration, after a bit of groping in the dark, and having integrated this individual's particularity, the doctor can retrospectively say whether one should worry about a given reference point in this particular case.[15] Through treating problems of a given individual, the doctor learns to identify the patient's particularities and is able to recognize, as I pointed out above, personal norms: the doctor becomes capable of recognizing *individual characteristics,* that is, stable corporal dispositions that are revealed after a series of successive accounts. His or her knowledge of these traits can be used to increase the speed and certainty of the diagnosis: the doctor would claim to "know" the individual in such a case.

Clinical judgments do not ignore "risk factors," notably by considering epidemiological results, but doctors do not use them in the same way as in the administrative frame. They become one of the reference points that the doctor can try to integrate in a clinical table, all the while associating it to others. The risk factor is no longer the source of the rule, relevant for an entire population, that will be applied to the individual. It is a salient point among others, which is more or less significant according to the case. In the clinical frame, there is no direct link between membership of a population vulnerable to a risk and the judgment delivered on a person in that population. The clinical judgment intercalates an exploratory stage between the identification of populations and the diagnosis, in which the group of salient points of reference are integrated for the individual. The individual is not assimilated into a population. Nor is the individual, as in the administrative frame, a compilation of a list of rules relative to different populations. The patient is, rather, the unity of integrated memberships of various populations. The doctor has the responsibility of determining and formulating the outcome of this integration, according to her/his judgment.

In an exploratory diagnosis, each symptom, taken separately, can contribute to the placement of an individual in a class, but the doctor waits to have other points of reference before acting.[16] The rules formulated for classes of individuals are not discarded but change status. Judgment does not consist of applying rules, but of putting them in relation with one another within clinical tables. "Following a rule" here consists of placing it within the significant reference points of the diagnostic transfer. Here, unlike in the preceding schema, the individual is not "reduced" by being treated exactly like any other member of the same class. The doctor acknowledges the individual organism's capacity to create idiosyncratic norms and takes these into account in his or her judgment. Furthermore, clinical doctors also formulate their own individualized rules.

This framing of the individual transforms considerably the relationships between the producers and users of rules. Here, the actors who must judge the cases are the "clinicians." Unlike the "agents" of the administrative schema, they do not apply rules. They are not subordinated to the agents working on a more general level. Clinicians integrate the general rules in their judgment, but in principle they have the initiative in the treatment of cases. They prove their objectivity by associating the symptoms within a clinical table. Nevertheless, the formal rules are not challenged. The clinician accepts that other actors produce rules, norms, and epidemiological indications and uses them. They serve as points of reference. However, the clinician does not feel obligated to "apply" them in her/his work. This clinical stance with regard to rules leads to a relativization of the import of administrative rules (medical fitness norms, thresholds of risk evaluation). These rules are suggestions—not prescriptions. Notably, security and public health rules, based on the identification of risk factors, constitute useful references but are not binding. The doctor weighs the import of these rules according to the autonomous normative capacity of the clinical individual. They are then submitted to the verdict of the case's particularities, as they emerge in the clinical encounter.

FROM FRAMES TO ETHOS

Each frame is based on concrete action through external components (objects, rules, words) situated outside of the person, as well as through internal components, people's capacities (Dodier 1993a). The relationship between frames can be looked at from two viewpoints: the distribution of each frame in space and the articulation between them. The first viewpoint is based on a structural approach. It addresses the question, What is the best way of identifying frames? This analytical framework allows us to categorize and distinguish between different "types" of occupational doctor. Some of them have genuinely chosen to privilege one frame over another in such a way as to build up a genuine *ethos,* that is, if we apply Weberian terminology, a set of durable predispositions. Consider the example of Doctor T.

In 1977, Doctor T began working as an occupational doctor in a pharmaceutical company in the Greater Paris region. He had already worked in another corporation in the same group, which manufactured basic chemical products. In this corporation, he had completely computerized the calculation of special medical supervision. Subsequent to discovery of cases of angiosarcoma due to the effects of vinyl chloride in 1970 in the United States, he systematically reconstituted the occupational trajectory of all personnel in the company. Since each entry represented a single, invariant production line, it was comparatively easy to have the machine memorize a list of toxic products for each work station and to have it calculate the degree of exposure of employees. Since 1980, Doctor T has been a member of a working group run by the Union of Chemical Industries looking into "computerization of medical files." He has implemented a complex procedure to identify all possibilities of exposure in the new plant, a task rendered difficult by this company's flexibility of production lines (the company wants to adapt its production of a wide variety of products to variations in short-term customer demand). Most of this doctor's energy is devoted to the financing, implementation, and statistical exploitation of the findings of this system, both on the local level and in terms of its national extensions (in the private sector and the Ministry of Labor).[17]

Here we can talk about an *administrative or bureaucratic ethos,* characterized by the determination to define — and rigorously adhere to — a set of precise rules. Note that such an ethos can only develop if it finds some outside support. In the French system of occupational medicine, this is traditionally found in the fact that it has been seen as a branch of public health medicine since its inception, and has been highly regulated by the administrative obligations defined by the state. However, several factors currently work in favor of the development of such an ethos: the development of epidemiology in the work environment, and, more generally, the desire of certain occupational doctors to acquire legitimacy by investing in scientific research (apart from epidemiology, a favorite concern is toxicology), and the setting up of vast preventive campaigns for "populations at risk." This type of occupational medicine is particularly suitable for the type of corporation described as "industrial," according to the terminology of Boltanski and Thévenot (1991): a corporation organized according to codified standards, and based on measurement, figures, objectification of findings, and reference to science.[18] Note that a minimal administrative ethos, based on systematic follow-up of several simple procedures (filling out boxes in the medical file, a limited list of questions on working conditions) may constitute the physician's response to significant constraints on his/her time.[19] Such doctors may have to see large numbers of employees within a short period of time, without getting involved in the unpredictable divagations of the clinical approach — open, even in terms of the questioning itself, to the diversity of individual experience, and hence unpredictable in duration.

As an example of *clinical ethos,* we may look at the activity of Doctor Y, at least, as it can be apprehended after two weeks of observation in his service.

Born in 1949, this doctor works in an intercorporation service in a large provincial town, which represents most of the companies in the department — it employs sixty doctors and represents 14,500 member firms and 180,000 employees.[20] He also represents the personnel at the joint works committee. He is often referred to as "Citizen Y," the nickname referring to his sense of civic responsibility. Although not harnessed to any political activity, this characteristic of his is nonetheless very obvious in his relationship to his own employer and company management. His activity in the surgery is characterized by a pronounced preference for the clinical approach, with in-depth medical examinations, displayed quite openly by expressing out loud the questions that occur to him, in his search for symptoms, his obvious pleasure in solving enigmas, and his use of a varied, colorful, and definitely personal way of speaking of the body ("that slides," "noble, fragile mucus membranes," "the guts," etc.). He is also completely uninterested in filling out computer listings, preferring to take a very vague approach to coding — indeed, his references to statutory requirements are extremely vague and inaccurate. On the other hand, he is absolutely firm about questions of confidentiality and refuses, for example, to routinely fill out the "additional examinations" column for each employee as requested by the management of his service. He tends merely to indicate this globally on a day-to-day basis. We could say that his clinical approach is combined with a definite stance in favor of the employees: he will quite easily enter into conflict with the employer or call for factory inspection in the event of a problem. Also, he is automatically suspicious of any attempt to augment the company's right of inspection vis-à-vis the health of employees and vis-à-vis his own practice. What is more, he cultivates a high degree of openness with respect to employees, commenting on his own notes, explaining his actions or gestures in the surgery itself. This commitment to the employees' cause corresponds to his political convictions (Doctor Y spontaneously mentioned "doing 1968" [a year of student and worker revolts] although he had not been a militant in any particular movement). Unlike other doctors like him, keen to defend the rights of employees, his stance did not involve taking an interest in working conditions. In this sense, he is first and foremost a clinician. Most of the time he stays in his office, the rightful domain of clinical practice. He makes very few factory visits, shows little interest in ergonomics and any of the devices to measure risk in the workshops and does not take part in epidemiological surveys — all these areas leave him indifferent.

The ethos of this physician is characterized both by a taste for clinical practice and a critical or indifferent attitude to anything that gets in the way of it — that is, both anything not related to the doctor's office and anything that tends to associate medical activity with routine, nonindividualized rules. On top of this, in Doctor Y's case, we can also note a relationship to employees (defending their rights, concern with being open) that is not characteristic of the clinical approach. Indeed, his approach could be more correctly characterized as a "civic" clinical ethos, which calls to mind certain aspects of the "democratic format" described by Silverman (1987), and which might be contrasted with the "conventional" clinical approach, itself characterized by a definite silence of the doctor vis-à-vis employees or patients. This more conventional approach is difficult for a sociologist even to demonstrate, partly because such a doctor is, as a matter of principle, suspicious of any outside observer and partly because the silence characterizing his or her practice makes it esoteric for the observer.

The foundations of such a clinical ethos can be found in an old and significant clinical tradition that doctors can refer to, which underpins most of their medical studies and is reflected in the usual nosological tables. It still provides a comparatively solid base — although one that may well be in the process of eroding — that can be contrasted with arrangements aimed at standardizing medical practice. Outside clinical medicine as such, other disciplines in France have developed approaches to the working population that are keen to respect the specificity of different situations. This is the case, for example, of the French school of ergonomics[21] and psychodynamics of work.[22] It is therefore not surprising that a fairly significant minority of physicians leans toward these complementary acquisitions of investigative tools in preference to the more standard epidemiological or toxicological approaches.

The clinical ethos can also be based on — and conversely be used to justify — the freedom of the occupational doctor within the company. We should point out that occupational doctors, even where they describe themselves as "executives" within the company, are the only employees that are legally free to refuse to justify their decisions, or at least their medical decisions. In the most extreme case, the radically autonomous clinician is the doctor who judges each case in the secrecy of his or her surgery in the company and who delivers his or her conclusions without reference to any other argument. This approach is characteristic of the ethos of the silent clinician. We might point out that it is not an easily tenable approach when applied to the field of working conditions, since neither reference to clinical medical practice nor medical secrecy can be brought into play (Dodier 1993b).

The clinical and administrative ethos should be seen as distinct and opposite codes of practice. In a complex universe, where schemes of reference are not unified, the two frames may, however, coexist in the same person or the same place. The dichotomy just mentioned should then be seen as an analytical tool useful for highlighting the equilibrium that can be established between frames, either in terms of the arrangements for integrating occupational medicine in the corporation or in terms of the persons themselves, of whom more complicated portraits can be drawn. At this point arises the question of articulation between these frames according to the dynamics of concrete activity. I will distinguish here three modalities of articulation between the two frames: temporal succession, controversies, and combination.

Temporal succession is the first schema of coexistence. Following an occupational doctor's work are moments when the doctor is clearly engaged in an administrative frame: s/he lists risks of exposition, fills in work condition forms, fills in items on a medical file, or applies an epidemiological or toxicological protocol. In the medical office, the structure of the activity sometimes changes and the doctor slides into a clinical exploration: we see her/him compare different symptoms of the same person, try to integrate complaints with objective symptoms in a coherent table, and deliver a diagnosis. Here, the two types of framing peacefully follow each other in the doctor's activity.

A second schema is the appearance of *controversies* between types of framing. This is notably the case when a debate develops concerning the import of codified rules in medical work. An example of this confrontation emerges in debates over regulatory medical norms of fitness. Some of the debates are over the solidity of rules proposed in texts, based on an evaluation of risk factors and a determination of acceptable thresholds (cf. Douglas 1985). In these instances, we are in an administrative framing of individuals, discussing criteria of medical fitness. We are trying to define rules. But in other debates the larger question is disputed. Doctors who do not want to have to "apply" rules, regardless of their content, here challenge the place of rules in the medical judgment. The question is no longer, for example, whether the threshold of auditive deficit should be set between 35 and 40 decibels in the decree on heavy-load driving. Here, the question is whether a threshold should be applied at all, rather than considering it as a reference among others, in a clinical approach. Partisans of an administrative frame will defend the first solution, willing only to discuss the level of the limits or the list of illnesses to integrate in the regulatory text;

partisans of a clinical framing will resist being required to systematically apply the rule, regardless of the limits or illnesses presented a priori.

Certain regulations, for example, consider all epileptic employees unfit to drive cranes or heavy loads for safety reasons. Some doctors refuse to follow this systematic rule, as in the following example, related by an occupational doctor during an interview. Here again, we are with Doctor Y, whose attachment to the clinical frame has already been noted. The following excerpt from one of our interviews gives an example of a decision concerning medical fitness:

> Doctor: I have an epileptic who drives cranes, and I'm just waiting for trouble. Normally legislation forbids those people to drive, but I have one of them who drives heavy loads. That's not allowed by the legislation. There are certainly medical restrictions that I am very firm about, but there are other restrictions that are legal and that are barely imposed upon us. My heavy-load driver and my crane driver, legally speaking, are unfit. I'm waiting to get caught, because I have good insurance!
> ND: You think it is best that this person continues to work?
> Doctor: Why should he have to stop working?
> ND: I don't know, one might consider that . . .
> Doctor: A legislator made the decision, not a doctor. Not all the doctors. I say that in such a case, those people have X amount of chance to have an epileptic attack. Epilepsy that is treated well and not aggravated, *in my soul and conscience,* does not pose a problem for such work assignments. Those people, if they have epileptic attacks, *of course in a certain number of cases epilepsy is not treatable, but in the case that I'm thinking of,* if the guys don't drink, if they follow their treatment correctly, if they don't party every day, I mean all that contributes to lowering their resistance, if they respect these factors that lower their resistance, they won't have an epileptic attack. So I generally put on their fitness report "It is clear that your fitness is contingent on following the treatment." [emphasis added]

In this example, the doctor refuses to conform to a general rule. He considers the details of the clinical case and decides that he has to judge case by case, "in his soul and conscience," whether the epilepsy justifies unfitness. So while someone using an administrative frame would refuse to take into account conditions that allow for the stabilization of the pathology (e.g., following a treatment, not drinking, not "partying"), this doctor takes into consideration the circumstances under which, according to him, the pathology is neutralized at work. The same debates emerge over drug addiction, cancer, AIDS, alcoholism, and so forth, for each case of which we find strict specifications of incompatibility between pathologies and positions in internal company rules and regulations.

Let me develop in greater detail another example of friction between the clinical and administrative frames, this time in relation to the import of codified maximum values in the medical supervision of employees. It involves the SUMER survey, a statistical survey of professional risks in France, instigated by the minister of labor.[23] In 1982, a work group composed of one of the minister's statisticians and six doctors came together to establish the survey questionnaire. The idea was to have occupational doctors fill out this questionnaire after each annual visit: each doctor was to code the risks to which the employee just seen was exposed at work. A debate broke out within the group about the utility of filling out numerical maximum values on the questionnaire. "Maximum values" exist in law or in technical recommendations produced by specialized agencies.[24] These maximum values seemed to be good candidates for obliging doctors to code risks carefully, notably in the case of measuring concentrations of chemicals in the atmosphere. Doctor Sabel,[25] a former occupational doctor and consultant for a large chemical company, protested against this use of maximum values in the questionnaire. The thrust of his argument was that in each case, the doctor decides, in terms of the particularities of the individual, which factors are dangerous and which are not. In the doctor's world, the meaning of the word "risk" takes on a specific meaning. Risk is not a characteristic of a job in isolation, but of a job with the particular individual at it. To standardize the list by dictating a numerical measurement of the work environment, as a criterion for decision, is to force the doctor to efface the specific person standing before her/him, in order to judge only in terms of the job. Let us examine more closely how Sabel defends the principle of *clinical judgment,* adapted to the particularities of each individual.

Sabel's comments reflect a larger debate over the relevance of maximum limits of exposure to risks in medical practice, of which the SUMER survey is part. Maximum limits are principally defended by "industrial hygienists," engineers or technicians, who praise recourse to quantified measurements as a means to objectify risks. Many occupational doctors, on the other hand, consider the importance of maximum values to be relative, to be taken into consideration with other elements in order to estimate the risk involved.

Sabel: To give you a concrete example, it is clearly stated that when a product contains less than 5 percent of aromatic carbide, people are not considered exposed. That is the statistical value of what is acceptable. For lead, less than forty micrograms of lead in the atmosphere and people are not exposed. So that was not taken into consideration [in the SUMER survey] — and so that's the regulation.

ND: When the regulation was being decided on, who made the final choice to say it's going to be 5 percent?

Sabel: That's Europe. It was the European experts that established those values. These were European values that were derived from American values and some values that already were in circulation. It had already been a while since the American industrial hygienists had set maximum values for everything. For them "maximum values" means maximum values of acceptable exposure, but also values under which people are not considered to be exposed.

ND: Right, absolutely.

Sabel: So, we didn't have all of that in France. Because in France we had difficulty accepting that people were not exposed when we knew that there was a toxin in the atmosphere. That's kind of how I see it; we are the only ones to take the health of individual people into consideration.

ND: Right, and you seem to be saying that this estimate is therefore . . .

Sabel: It is statistical.

ND: It is statistical . . . right, and that means . . . ?

Sabel: That means that, in my opinion, it covers most cases, but there are exceptions. When you have someone who works eight hours a day, if that person is part of the exception, I mean if he is really exposed to a risk, that's a problem.

This passage allows us to clarify the meaning that Sabel accords a "statistical" interpretation of maximum value criteria and how he judges the validity of this interpretation. The interpretation is "statistical" because it is not interested in people taken one by one but in populations. The maximum value is useful in action directed toward aggregated entities. In statistical logic, it is convenient to "cover most cases" without worrying about the exceptions. The relevant objects of action are in effect the populations for whom percentages of exposure are controlled. In the type of action that Sabel defends, on the other hand, each person is important. The doctor considers a succession of individuals, each time passing judgment on one person and considering each person an end in her/himself. By saying that an individual can be "truly exposed to a risk" without belonging to a population of individuals selected by a maximum value, Sabel shows that he regards this individual from a clinical angle: he considers the salience of the maximum value in the context of other reference points that can arise in a clinical exploration. To give a maximum value a decisive function in coding procedures is to concede that *clinical individuals* are not going to be considered but only *administrative individuals* assimilated to populations of association by the intermediary of risk references. Sabel defends here a clinical frame rather than an administrative one. The maximum value should not be a decisive rule in judgment but rather be a reference point to be associated with others. In the SUMER case, the tension between strict procedure rules and freedom of clinical assessment ended in a compromise: the questionnaire would include a standardized part (the list of risks in the decree of July 1977; see appendix A), concerning the medical supervision of employees, but it would not include a numerical limit of exposure. Also, the assessment would be done by the doctor "in her/his soul and conscience."

This resolution of tensions signals a third modality of articulation between clinical and administrative frames: a combination of forms of action, inscribed in the tools themselves. This is very common in cases where medical practice coincides with administrative mechanisms. It consists of reserving, within circuits of management by people oriented by rules applied in an administrative way, areas of judgment, where the doctor is allowed a clinical approach in a particular case.

The SUMER survey is a good example: the ministry of labor, in the end, collected sixty thousand files filled out by doctors "in their soul and conscience" on the basis of a list of risks that did not carry quantified maximum values. Friction between the two frames continues to arise over the status of SUMER's figures. Certain actors agree to grant significance to results collected in this way; they accept the SUMER figures as valid indicators of professional risk. Other actors refuse to accord significance to figures whose coders have flouted the administrative requirements for codified rules. For them (state engineers, industrial hygienists) an assessment based on the vagaries of the clinical process simply does not hold.

One of the coordinators of SUMER reports the reaction of a state engineer thus: "It is annoying. If we cannot take an accurate measurement, it does not exist. OK, either there is a risk or there isn't. I come with my instrument. I take a sample. I measure the dosages. There are norms that are unquestionable because they are European, so many micrograms per liter of air and it's dangerous, less and it isn't."

The merging of clinical and administrative frames creates complex ensembles, where a concern for strict rules coexists with the flexibility of the clinical frame. Consider the tables of occupational illness in French law, for example, the table "Illnesses Caused by Lead and Its Components" (see appendix B). In the column "Definition of Illnesses," there is a list of possible reference points. Each of them is either a symptom ("paralysis of the muscles in the fingers or in the hand"), the result of a complementary exam ("anemia confirmed by repeated hematological exams and accompanied by erythrocytes with basophilic stippling"), or a syndrome (a combination of symptoms, for example, "Biological syndrome characterized by a lowering in the level of hemoglobin to less than 13 g for 100 ml of blood, by a level of stippled erythrocytes greater than 1 per 1,000 erythrocytes and an elevation of delta-amino-levulinic uric acid greater than 20 mg per 1,000 ml"). In the column at the right is the "List Indicating Main Tasks Likely to Provoke These Illnesses." It consists of an inventory of types of work including, for example, "Casting type characters in lead alloys, working with typesetting machines, manual typesetting; fabrication and repair of lead storage batteries; lead tempering and wire drawing of steel tempered in lead," and so on. In the middle column is the "Time Limit for Medical Care" (thirty days, one year, five years . . .) for each "illness" on the list on the left. According to this table, in order for one's illness to be considered work-induced, the patient must, first of all, have at least one of the symptoms listed, secondly, have announced it in the designated time limit, and thirdly, have been exposed to at least one of the types of work mentioned in the column on the right, in other words, to at least one corresponding risk. If and only if the person satisfies those conditions is there an "assumption of imputation" and the illness is recognized as being of "occupational origin." The table therefore juridically codes a way of imputing a symptom, syndrome, or illness to a risk factor. It connects, term by term, two series of items: some relative to the individual, others to the job. This part of the regulatory tables of work-related illnesses establishes an administrative frame of individuals.

Now let us consider more closely the items found in the left-hand column of appendix B. Besides symptoms, we also find "Illnesses." The list of infections likely to figure on the table is heterogeneous: it contains the simple signs and syndromes but also names of illnesses ("ganglionic tuberculosis," "cutaneous or subcutaneous tuberculosis," "asthma"). In order to attribute pathologies to individuals, the doctor uses clinical tables. For a moment the doctor sets aside the administrative concern for codified rules and instead uses the diagnostic approach. Only once this work is finished does the doctor use the result to apply the rules to the signs that appear on the professional illness table. The regulatory medium orients the doctor toward an activity that tightly links the clinical and administrative frame.

MEDICINE BETWEEN CLINIC AND PROCEDURES

In this chapter, I have shown that occupational doctors' relationship to rules depends on the way in which they "frame" the people with whom they deal. In this respect, I have emphasized the coexistence of two frames: the clinical and the administrative. This analytical framework is more generally useful for analyzing arrangements, concrete activities, and for describing the dominant ethos of doctors, above and beyond the little-known but instructive example of occupational medicine developed in this text. I consider the coexistence of clinical and administrative frames an important source of heterogeneity in contemporary medicine, divided between the concerns to take into account individual particularities and to follow systematic protocols. The clinical frame is founded in devices largely present in medicine since the end of the eighteenth century (Foucault 1963; Armstrong 1984), and which endure in the core of medical instruction, as an analysis of current manuals would show. The administrative frame develops massively under the coupled effect of *law* and *scientific networks*. As Hart (1961) notes, a characteristic of legal rules is that they should be applicable in the same way to every person in a particular category. This lack of distinction between different people that is part of juridical categories is the prerequisite for a fair treatment of cases, even if actual judgments force a reassessment of the general principles. The framing of medical decisions by legal rules forces doctors to introduce an administrative frame that breaks with certain principles of the clinical frame. This ascendancy of law corresponds, on the one hand, with the increasingly strong bonds between medical practice and the mechanisms of social justice, controlling the distribution of care and goods in societies, and on the other, with the implementation of public health policy expressed as rules aimed at populations, as in the case of the prevention of professional risk examined in this chapter. The development of an administrative frame that adapts itself more or less well to the demands of the clinical frame also corresponds with the diffusion of scientific protocols in contemporary medicine. We have encountered these here in the form of epidemiological protocols, but they also take the form of therapeutic protocols designed for populations and required to be systematic.[26] The way clinical and administrative medicine encounter each other in daily action, influenced by both law and science, creates numerous examples of frictions among frames. This opens up a field of enquiry that we have only touched on in this text with the example of occupational medicine, but which is characteristic of the questions evoked by contemporary medicine.

APPENDIX A. THE SPECIAL MEDICAL SUPERVISION OF EMPLOYEES
EXPOSED TO OCCUPATIONAL RISK

Occupations Requiring Special Medical Supervision

Art. 1: For the jobs listed in this article: the doctor or doctors charged with the medical supervision of personnel routinely working in the jobs here listed will devote to their supervision a time period calculated on the basis of one hour per month for every ten employees:

1. Jobs involving the preparation of, use of, manipulation of, or exposition to the following products:

Fluoride and its components

Chlorine

Bromine

Iodine

Phosphorus and components, notably phosphoric ester, pyrophosphoric acid, thiophosphoric acid, as well as other organic components of phosphorus

Arsenic and its components

Carbon sulfur

Carbon oxychloride

Chromic acid, chromate, bichromate, alkaline, not including their aqueous diluted solutions

Manganese dioxide

Lead and its components

Mercury and its components

Glucide and its salts

Benzene and homologues

Phenols and naphthols

Halogen derivatives, nitrates and hydrocarbon aminates, and their derivatives

Charcoal, tar, and mineral oils

X rays and radioactive substances

2. The following jobs:

Application of paint and varnish by spray

Work done in slaughterhouses, quartering

Handling, loading, unloading, transport either of raw skins, hair, horse hair, pig hair, wool, bone or other animal hide, or of bags, envelopes or containers containing or having contained such hide, with the exception of bones from which the gelatin or fat has been removed and tanned leather

Collection and treatment of garbage

Work exposed to high temperatures, to dust or toxic radiation and involving the treatment of minerals, the production of metal and glass

Work done in refrigerated compartments

Work exposed to releases of carbon monoxide in gas factories, transportation of bottled gas, the synthetic manufacture of gas or of methanol

Work exposed to silica dust, to asbestos and slate (not including mines, mining, and quarries)

Work involving polymerization of vinyl chloride

Work exposed to cadmium and its components

Work exposed to iron dust

Work exposed to hormonal substances

Work exposed to hard metal dust (tantalum, titanium, tungsten, and vanadium)

Work exposed to antimony dust

Work exposed to wood dust

Work in shifts that take place entirely or partly at night

Work as a telephone operator, work on graphic-mechanic machines, on perforators, on a screen terminal or electronic hook-up viewer

Work of preparation, processing, preservation, and distribution of food products

Work exposed to a sound level greater than 85 decibels

2. The provisions of this decree do not apply to work listed in article 1 when this work is performed within tightly sealed, properly functioning environments.

3. When particular safety measures ensure efficient protection of workers from risks incurred in the tasks listed in article 1, the director of work and labor from the department [administrative district] can, following approval of the medical inspector of work and labor and of the company's committee or of the control commission mentioned in article D.241-7[R.241-14] of the Work Code, or, in the absence of one of these institutions, delegates of the personnel, relieve the head of the company of the requirement to ensure special medical supervision of personnel assigned to certain tasks.

4. The Decrees of June 22, 1970, and November 29, 1974, are repealed.

Source: France, Ministry of Labor, Ministerial Order of July 11, 1977 (establishing the list of occupations that require special medical supervision).

APPENDIX B. ILLNESSES CAUSED BY LEAD AND ITS COMPONENTS

Definition of illnesses	Time limit for medical care
Painful paroxysmal abdominal syndrome, without fever, with subocclusive state (lead colics), normally accompanied by a paroxysmal hypertensive crisis and an increase of erythrocytes with basophilic stippling	30 days
Paralysis of the muscles in the fingers or in the hand	1 year

Severe encephalopathy:
(a) Presenting in an individual who has had one or more of the symptoms of the table	30 days
(b) Not accompanied by these symptoms in the case of poisoning by alkyl derivatives of lead such as lead tetramethyl or lead tetraethyl	30 days
Azotemic nephritis or hypertensive nephritis with their complications	5 years
Anemia confirmed by repeated hematological exams and accompanied by erythrocytes with basophilic stippling	6 months
Biological syndrome characterized by a lowering of hemoglobin to less than 13 g per 100 ml of blood, by a level of stippled erythrocytes greater than 1 per 1,000 erythrocytes and an elevation of delta-amino-levulinic acid greater than 20 mg per 1,000 ml.	30 days

The diagnosis has to be confirmed by a repetition of the same examinations between 15 and 30 days after the diagnosis.

Main tasks likely to provoke these illnesses

Extraction, treatment, preparation, employment, manipulation of lead, of its minerals, of its alloys, of its combinations and of all lead containing products, especially:

Extraction and treatment of lead minerals and lead-containing residues

Metallurgy, purification, melting, rolling of lead, of its alloys and lead-containing metals

Recuperation of old lead

Welding and tin-plating by means of lead alloys

Fabrication, welding, filing, polishing of all lead or lead alloy objects

Casting type characters in lead alloys, working with typesetting machines, manual typesetting; fabrication and repair of lead storage batteries; lead tempering and wire drawing of steel tempered in lead

Metallization with lead through pulverization

Fabrication and manipulation of lead oxides and lead salts

Preparation and application of paint, varnish, lacquer, ink, putty, grease containing lead compounds

Scraping, burning, cutting with a cutting torch of materials covered with lead-containing paint

Fabrication and application of lead-containing enamels

Composition of lead glass

Fabrication and manipulation of alkyl derivatives of lead such as lead tetramethyl or lead tetraethyl, especially preparation of fuels containing such derivatives and cleaning of containers holding such fuels

Glazing and decoration of ceramic products by means of lead compounds

Source: Code de la Sécurité Sociale, art. R 461-3, Tables of Occupational Illnesses, Annexes to Decree no. 46-2949 (December 31, 1946), amended. Table 1, Decree no. 77-624 (June 2, 1977).

NOTES

Translated by Abigail Cope Smith and Philippa Wallis.

1 In 1986, 2,650 doctors practiced full time and 3,080 part time.

2 On this point, see Nelkin 1985 and Dodier 1993b. A general view of the position of occupational doctors working in companies in the United States can be found in Chapman-Walsh 1987.

3 A large portion of the material compiled is composed of direct observations of medical consultations. I include doctors' commentaries collected in situ in discussions that I initiated about their decisions. I worked with thirty-eight doctors; the period of observation lasted seven weeks. The main advantage of this survey was that I was able to build up a corpus of 210 accounts of medical visits and 259 case histories where the occupational doctor was obliged to mobilize complex resources to evaluate the medical fitness of the employee. These cases were taken either from observation or from accounts transcribed during interviews or a mixture of the two. For more details about the method used and for other developments concerning these doctors' methods, analysed in terms of a sociology of action, see Dodier 1993b.

4 See Castel 1981; Douglas and Wildavski 1982; Douglas 1985; Ewald 1986.

5 See appendix A.

6 A survey of occupational doctors at EDF (the French national electrical company) conducted by Imbernon et al. (1992) permits one to rank the frequency of questions asked and exams conducted during a systematic visit. Certain items are covered by almost every doctor (smoking, exercise, sleep, medication, heartbeat, weight, abdominal palpitation, pulmonary auscultation), while only a few doctors cover other items (5.6 percent claim to regularly ask questions about use of illegal drugs, 3.2 percent ask questions about the patient's sex life, 15.1 percent affirm that they perform a testicle palpitation, 11.1 percent measure the bilateral arterial blood pressure).

7 When doctors work in an intercorporation service, visits may take place in three different types of place: the service's own premises, which means that employees have to travel there but have access to all the service's technical equipment; medical offices located in the company itself, if it is large enough; the service's vans, which are designed to transport a mobile office to small companies.

8 On recourse to a psychosomatic frame in occupational medicine, see Dodier 1994.

9 Absurd situations characteristic of bureaucratic regimes, which have inspired many

(black) humorous pieces, are the consequence of this concept of the individual. Since the individual, in passing through different administrations, is attributed as many characteristics as populations to which s/he can belong, and since s/he must obey the rules that apply to each population, the individual can be pushed around among contradictory decisions.

10 Berg (1995) locates the advent of the major tools for the standardization of medical work in the 1950s and 1960s.

11 The merits of turning back to doctrinal texts to examine how people make the link between particular and general was stressed by Boltanski and Thévenot (1991) in their work on the ordinary sense of justice. In this case, I used Sicard's manual (1987) and consulted Bariety et al. 1981, Fattorusso and Ritter 1984, Bates 1985, and Hurst 1987.

12 The formalization of medical reasoning consists of transcribing this type of process in a logical or quantified language. The representation of the medical diagnosis as Bayesian reasoning (Fagot 1982) consists of transcribing the degrees of sensitivity and specificity of symptoms in the form of probabilities, and assumes the doctor will use calculations of probability in order to orient her/himself in the clinical tables.

13 I consider here a "point of reference" to be a characteristic of the patient that was simply noted during a visit, and I reserve the word "symptom" for references that the doctor tries to integrate in a clinical table. The "sign" is therefore a "symptom" once it is integrated in a diagnosis.

14 VGM: average globular volume, falling between 85 and 100 μm^3.

15 This explains why rapid judgment is considered "intuition" or "clinical sense," because the doctor is deemed capable of integrating through anticipation, naturally and unconsciously, singularities of the individual that have not yet been revealed. From the beginning the doctor chooses the correct diagnostic path from all the multiple possibilities, as if s/he had already perceived, without even being able to name them, the individual's singularities.

16 This attitude on the part of the doctor, of waiting and being open to diverse dimensions of the individual that can prove pertinent in the judgment afterward, is demonstrated by Mol and Law (1994), who comment on the "fluidity" of the associations thus constituted for each case.

17 The Ministry of Labor became interested at the beginning of the 1980s in the epidemiological possibilities opened up by this method of gathering information.

18 Boltanski and Thévenot (1991) contrast this form of coordination with the "domestic" form, based on reference to tradition, and the "commercial" form, based on reference to the laws of a purely competitive market.

19 The resources available to the occupational doctor depend very closely on the investment devoted by companies to safety and working conditions. One way of reducing these costs in the short term is to increase the number of employees monitored by each doctor in proportions that may sometimes exceed the statutory

limits (one hour a month per doctor for twenty-five white-collar workers, or for fifteen manual workers, or for ten white-collar or manual workers under special medical supervision). Where intercorporation services compete to attract members, one way may be to diminish the rate of subscription, here again by increasing the number of employees examined. The average length of an occupational medical visit is twenty minutes for a "normal" employee and half an hour for an employee "under special medical supervision," but some doctors may see a different employee every ten minutes in a given session.

20   The size of intercorporation services varies considerably. In the same department (administrative district), for example, another service was based on a limited area, around a subprefecture, and employed only five doctors. The principles of association between companies bring into play different bases of categorization: sectoral, geographic, linked to employers' associations, etc. Services may compete with each other where they have a licence to operate in the same area, which can lead to genuine commercial practices in terms of the relationship between subscription and medical service. This competition has important repercussions on the resources available to occupational doctors.

21   See Montmolin 1986 for a presentation of the opposition between this ergonomics of "real activity" and the ergonomics inherited from the Taylorian concept of the scientific organization of work.

22   See Dejours's work (1993) which has been attracting increasing interest on the part of occupational doctors for some years now.

23   For a more complete account of this survey, see Dodier 1993b. In Desrosières 1993 we find an in-depth study of the status of the individual in statistical arrangements and a glimpse of the resistance that this status has aroused at different times throughout the history of statistics.

24   For example, three Ministry of Labor decrees of July 19, 1982, March 12, 1983, and December 1, 1983 (amending art. L231-2 of the Code du Travail) set the acceptable levels of concentration of eighty-two chemicals in the work atmosphere.

25   For reasons of confidentiality, I used a pseudonym.

26   For an analysis of the effort to align doctors' practice by means of experimental protocols and the subtle negotiations that result between scientists and clinical doctors, see Löwy 1995b and Berg (this volume).

STABILIZING INSTABILITIES:
THE ROLE OF THE LABORATORY IN
THE UNITED KINGDOM CERVICAL
SCREENING PROGRAMME
Vicky Singleton

▼

The empirical focus of this chapter is the practice of an established medical program in the United Kingdom—the Cervical Screening Programme (CSP). The CSP has existed for almost thirty years and is referred to as a durable, effective, clearly defined medical process; from the woman who presents herself for a cervical smear test, to the general practitioner who obtains cervical cell samples, the cervical cells that change in predictable ways in relation to cancer, and the laboratory that detects and categorizes cytological abnormalities.

Drawing upon data obtained through participant observation, this chapter focuses on the role of the laboratory. It shows how the laboratory plays a readily identifiable, stable role in the program but is also a site of considerable instability. Like the other components of the program that the laboratory has contact with, the laboratory adopts a multiplicity of identities. The central argument that is developed below is that an established, stabilized practice does not require stable and unequivocal entities as its constituents. Contrary to what most recent science and technology studies would expect, the practice of the CSP is characterized by instability and multiplicitous identities. Moreover, this instability and multiplicity actually contributes to the continuity of the program.

INTRODUCING THE CERVICAL SCREENING PROGRAMME (CSP)

In the United Kingdom the CSP is referred to as "the largest, most ambitious public screening system to date carried out by the NHS [National Health Service]".[1] It is a preventive medical intervention that involves "testing" women for the presence of cytological (cell) abnormalities in the cervix (neck of the womb) that have the potential to develop into cancer. The cervical smear test is performed on women regularly and routinely. Cervical cancer is referred to as being "completely preventable" and mortality from cervical cancer as "unnecessary" and "avoidable" due to the ability of the CSP to detect treatable precancerous cytological changes.[2]

The U.K. CSP is a long-standing medical intervention. It was introduced as a national service by the British government in 1966.[3] Nevertheless, as was the case in 1966, on average two thousand women per year continue to die of cervical cancer (Roberts 1982; Johnston 1989). Some commentators praise the achievements of the program, stating that it has kept in check an otherwise devastating epidemic.[4] Indeed, in many of the health promotion leaflets and the books written for public sale about the CSP, the program is referred to as straightforward and unproblematic.[5] Consider the following excerpt from a standard letter sent to the homes of women inviting them to participate in the program:

> Dear Ms Singleton,
> I am sure you will know that it is strongly recommended that all women aged over 20 years have regular cervical smear tests. This is a simple check on the neck of the womb (the cervix). The test is straightforward and painless and enables doctors to diagnose a condition which may later develop into cancer of the neck of the womb, whilst it is still at a stage when treatment can prevent this happening.[6]

The CSP emerges from some of the texts written for women as a demonstration of the certitude and accomplishments of modern medical science. It is presented to the public as demonstrating the ability of medical science to triumph over one of its most persistent, reluctant and terrifying adversaries — cancer.

> The word cancer is an emotive one. For many years cancer was synonymous with death; the detection of the disease was usually at a late stage and the treatments were few and, for the most part, able only to relieve the suffering a little.
> During the last two decades, however, there have been enormous advances in the detection as well as the treatment of cancer. With the most modern screening techniques it is now possible to detect and to treat potential cancer of the cervix in its pre-cancerous state. Cervical cancer is therefore perfectly curable in its early stages. (Chomet and Chomet 1989, 11)

However, other writers are concerned about the "apparent ineffectiveness" and "failure" of the U.K. CSP, especially when programs in other countries appear to be achieving lower mortality (Roberts 1982; NCN 1991). Furthermore, some commentators suggest that the CSP might be doing "more harm than good," as it subjects women to an invasive procedure that is of questionable reliability, prone to false positive results, and can cause unnecessary anxiety (McCormick 1989; McTaggart 1990).

Hence, I begin this chapter about the practice and continuity of the U.K. csp, highlighting the contradictory discourses that coexist in regard to its validity and efficacy. On the one hand, there is a triumphant discourse about the successful introduction and expansion of a medical technology that effectively intervenes in the "natural" progression of cancer of the cervix to prevent mortality. On the other hand, there is reference to continued mortality and persistent failure that is accompanied by a discourse, which constructs the csp as problematic and ineffective.

Considering the above, it is difficult to provide one definitive history of the csp in the United Kingdom. Or rather, to do so would, given that any history is partial, be overly exclusive. Moreover, while the efficacy of the csp has been questioned by some, the program has continued. It is the nature of the durability of the csp that I am concerned with in this chapter, rather than the efficacy of the program per se.

DEFINING THE COMPONENTS OF THE CSP

In 1966 the U.K. Ministry of Health prepared a circular entitled *Population Screening for Cancer of the Cervix,* which describes the planning of screening services country-wide and defines the "parts to be played" by a diversity of entities, including hospital pathology laboratories, local health authorities, general practitioners, lay women, health visitors and midwives, and local and voluntary clinics (HC[66]76). That is, each of these components is given a specific role to play and a particular position in the program, the aim of which is to "reduce mortality from cancer of the cervix by ensuring that women at risk from this disease are screened at regular intervals in order to identify the early signs of the disease while it is still at the pre-invasive stage" (HC[84]17, para. 1). For example, and by way of outlining the procedures of the program, lay women are defined as at risk of death from cervical cancer. They are to attend their general practitioner or local clinic to take up the service on offer of a cervical smear test. General practitioners (GPs) are defined as the "ambassadors" of medical science. They have "an important part to play in taking smears from their patients", and "[f]rom their knowledge of their patients . . . are particularly well placed to encourage women in high risk groups to be examined" (HC[66]76, para. 9). They are also defined as responsible for following up a patient with a positive or abnormal smear test result by referring her to a gynecological department. On taking a cervical smear, GPs complete a record card that identifies the specimen and gives details of the patient. This record card accompanies the specimen to the laboratory. A copy of the record card is returned from the laboratory incorporating results of analysis and recommendations for follow-up care.

So, the part to be played by the hospital pathology laboratory, the most important component in the context of this chapter, is that of diagnostician. The laboratory is defined as "examining and reporting on cervical smears . . . efficiently and economically" (HC[66]76, para. 4). The laboratory examines the cervical smear specimens taken by general practitioners and in local clinics. It detects cytological abnormalities that are precancerous or have the potential to develop into cancer. Laboratories are defined as capable of "seeing" cell changes and of evaluating their meaning and, as stated above, they complete the record cards on which the GP or local clinic act. The laboratory is defined as a central node in the population screening program, as "[t]he basis for any screening service" (ibid.).

The laboratory is staffed by "a pathologist experienced in cytology . . . and fully qualified laboratory technicians trained in cytology" (HC[66]76, para. 5). A technician working full time is defined as capable of examining cervical smear samples from about seven thousand women per year.

The part played by laboratories in the CSP has come under scrutiny at various points in the history of the program. In the mid-1980s, several cases of "error" were publicly reported, such as that in Liverpool where it was claimed that nine hundred smears over a four-year period were incorrectly reported as negative (Chomet and Chomet 1989; Hopkins 1991). There was also considerable concern at this time that laboratories were being overstrained and smear samples were not being processed quickly enough. Consequently, in 1988 the U.K. government stated that "DHAS [district health authorities] must aim to ensure that laboratories can meet demand and avoid backlogs of cervical smears awaiting examination. Any delay in reporting results is unsatisfactory. Laboratories must aim to send results to the doctor who submitted a smear within a maximum of one month of receiving it" (HC[88]1, para. 14). Further, the government stated that all laboratories must have arrangements for quality control through external quality assessment schemes (HC[88]1). Regional health authorities were assigned the role of ensuring that facilities were available for adequately training NHS laboratory staff.

THE COEXISTENCE OF STABILITY AND INSTABILITY?

This chapter speaks to current debates within science and technology studies about how scientific and technological artifacts achieve longevity. For example, the actor-network approach suggests that those programs that achieve durability are the result of scientists and technologists successfully defining and positioning a diversity of nonhuman and human entities to form a specific network of associations — an actor-network.[7] It is possible to conceptualize the CSP as an actor-network and to consider how it is the result of the British government's defining and associating a diversity of heterogeneous entities to construct a particular process — a network of relations.

Importantly, the entities that are defined and juxtaposed are not just human or social actors. The government also defines and positions nonhuman entities in particular ways. For example, within the CSP cervical cancer is defined as a disease that leads to mortality. It is defined as progressive and predictable, visually detectable through microscopic analysis in its early stages, treatable, and preventable. Cervical cells are represented as easily and painlessly obtainable via a cervical smear test. They can be fixed and will maintain their form and nature. They can be observed and analyzed microscopically, and they have a specifiable structure that changes in predictable ways in relation to cancer.

According to the actor-network approach, in order for the CSP to survive as it has been constructed, and in order for it to achieve its defined aims, all the entities must adhere to the roles in the network that have been assigned to them. Various professionals, lay people and natural and technological entities each play a specific role. According to this approach, in order for the CSP to achieve durability, the network must be maintained through the stability of its components. And indeed, in the case of the CSP I have suggested how the program seems to have achieved at least a certain degree of durability. It has existed for almost thirty years and is referred to, at least by some, as a success and an optimistic area of modern preventive medicine. There is considerable commitment to the CSP as indispensable to women's health from a variety of groups, including health professionals and women's health activists, and the CSP is publicly presented in this light.[8]

Nevertheless, the CSP has also been the site of considerable controversy and, as I have noted, some commentators question its efficacy. By considering the work of practice of the laboratory within the CSP I hope to shed some light on how stability and continuity may and do interact with controversy and instability.

I could choose to focus upon any actor in the CSP, and elsewhere I have looked at each of the different actors (Singleton 1992; Singleton and Michael 1993). However, in this essay I want to look at the laboratory because it is positioned at a strategic point in the CSP. Ultimately, the validity and efficacy of the CSP depends upon the ability of the laboratory to detect precancerous changes in cervical cells. Only if this occurs is the concept of prevention of cervical cancer viable.

The role of the laboratory in the CSP involves the processing of cervical smear samples for analysis. When a cervical sample enters the laboratory it first passes through the "booking in" stage. The sample and report card are registered and the details recorded. The sample then passes through the staining process to allow subsequent microscopic analysis. Finally, the results of the analysis are recorded on the report card and a copy returned to the sample taker. By way of an overview, the following aspects of this process were described as a source of instability by laboratory workers.[9]

Report cards may not be fully completed by sample takers, or may not match the sample received. Samples arrive at the laboratory that are inadequate in terms of the amount and/or type of cells present. That is, some samples contain insufficient cells—"scanty specimens"—or contain excess cells—"if the doctor has taken the specimen with a trowel" (interview with EL). Furthermore, samples may not contain the "variety" of cells necessary for the laboratory to comment on the health of the cervix. Some areas of the cervix may not be represented in the sample and the laboratory frequently cannot determine the presence or absence of certain cell types. The analysis of samples is also hindered by the presence of blood and/or mucus in the sample. This may or may not be significant, and it obscures the screener's view of the cervical cells. Moreover, the significance of some cell changes is uncertain, and the recommendations to be made are ambiguous. For example, enlarged cell nuclei may be benign or may indicate malignancy. Further, differences between and within women affect analysis and diagnosis of degree of abnormality, and what is defined as abnormal or significant is continually renegotiated. In addition, the previous experiences of the screener may affect his or her evaluation of the sample.

Concerning reporting on the analysis, this is a further source of instability. How to word recommendations is problematic because a concern to detect and to treat abnormalities is continually balanced against a concern not to promote unnecessary treatment and anxiety through highlighting cell changes that are insignificant or may revert to normal without treatment. Awareness of the possibility of, and detrimental consequences of, "missing something" interacts with an awareness of the occurrence of false positive results and the unnecessary treatment, pain, and anxiety that could be caused.

Laboratory workers seem to engage in complexifying and destabilizing their role within the CSP and this, in turn, involves exposing the complexity and instability inherent to the roles played by other components of the program. For example, cervical cells are represented as adopting a variety of identities and structures, rather than as changing in predictable, easily identifiable ways in relation to cancer. So too, samples, report cards, sample takers, and women assume a multiplicity of identities through laboratory discourse and practice, some of which do not readily fit into the CSP as defined by the government and as publicly presented. The same is true of machines and artifacts that the laboratory depends upon to carry out the analysis of samples such as staining machines, mounts, and fixatives. The result is the impression of ongoing instability as inherent to the role played by the laboratory in the practice of the CSP. Such fluidity and movement could be seen as destabilizing the CSP and hence as a threat to the continuation of the program. However, below we will see how the laboratory actively constructs but simultaneously accommodates instabilities and multiplicitous identities — in the form of the diverse ways in which the various nonhumans and humans that are involved in its role in the CSP behave and interact — into its role in the CSP.

Management of the Samples

The work practices and discourse of the laboratory exposes various administrative uncertainties as inherent to the practice of their role in the CSP. For example, "the main problem that we experience in the lab is GPs not filling in forms or the specimen slides properly" (interview with EL). However, the majority of samples that enter the laboratory are processed — discrepancies are highlighted but accommodated. In cases of information missing on the sample slide or the report card, the laboratory notes the discrepancies and the slide continues in its process of staining and analysis. The laboratory staff have developed jokes that refer to the difference between what a report card "should" look like and what they receive in the laboratory. In response to a question about what the most important things on the report card are, from the perspective of the laboratory, one technician sarcastically stated, "Well, we like the name!" (interview with JuL).

Cross-contamination of samples during the staining process is also highlighted as a problem and explained as a consequence of doctors smearing the sample too thickly onto the slide, and of the inadequacy of the machinery available for staining. However, this "problem" was simultaneously deproblematized and incorporated into the role of the laboratory. For example:

If the doctor has taken the sample with a trowel, it is very thick and you have to look out for this, then carefully wipe off some of the excess with a tissue. Otherwise you may get cross-contamination. On the [staining] machine the slides are pulled along and excess cells on one slide may be dragged off and onto other slides. . . . You can usually see cross-contamination has occurred at the time of analysis because the alien cells will be at a right angle to the original: the machine smears the cells on across the width of the slide. It is not usually necessary to repeat the sample in such a situation because you can see and distinguish the original from the alien cells. You do nothing really because you can normally tell. (interview with EL)

The laboratory highlights the discrepancy between its defined role in the CSP and the work that it does. That is, the laboratory engages in problematizing its defined role by exposing the diverse identities that various other components of the program adopt. However, the lab technicians at once deproblematize their role through redefining their own identity within the CSP. They can analyze samples that are not "ideal" as well as those that are. They can construct ideal samples from nonideal samples. They adapt their own identity, and the identities of samples and report cards, as they ambivalently incorporate instabilities and other components mutable identities into the program.

Analysis of Samples and Detection of Abnormality

This aspect of the role of the laboratory was highlighted as the site of considerable uncertainty. For example, laboratory staff spoke of problematic "gray areas":

It's not easy to do screening. It is easy to pick up malignancy and normality but the gray areas are not so good. They are very difficult and it takes a trained eye to do it at any speed. (EL)

The problem in the lab now is that people want black and white — it's cancer or it's not — however this is rarely the case. In the lab most things are somewhere in the middle, they are hard to define. I hate them. It is easy to see cancer or normality but the gray areas are a problem. (Dr. M)

The aim of the CSP is to detect the "areas in between" — the precancerous cytological changes. The most important aspect of the role of the laboratory is to categorize cell changes into varying degrees of precancerous abnormality and on the basis of this categorization to make recommendations for the follow-up care of women. The laboratory follows guidelines for recommendations, and it must and does fit its diagnoses into the categories on the report cards. Cells are defined as "normal"; "mild, moderate or severe inflammation"; "cervical intra-epithelial neoplasia (CIN) I, II, or III" (degrees of precancerous change); or as "invasive carcinoma."

Nevertheless, the laboratory discourse quoted above suggests that detecting the degree of abnormality present is not as straightforward as presented by the government and public CSP. Even those cytological changes that are easily identified do not always imply clear diagnoses. One technician introduced "the problem of the BENS" (benign enlarged nuclei) (JaL). Enlarged cell nuclei are defined as indicative of cancerous changes. However, some cells exhibit enlarged nuclei that it is felt are nonmalignant. They were described as "the problem cases of abnormal enlarged nuclei with no apparent cause" (JaL). They appear problematic because, as one technician stated, "How do you report on these?" (EL). Not only can cell nuclei be enlarged to varying degrees, but this enlargement can have a variety of meanings.

Considering the reporting of CIN I, II, or III in relation to the stage of pre-cancerous abnormality, one senior technician highlighted one source of varied diagnoses: "How it is reported will depend on what you were doing previously. If you had previously screened all normal smears then any abnormality will seem very abnormal and vice versa. So some abnormal you might say are moderate one day but could be diagnosed as mild on another day" (EL). This technician went on to say, "It's impossible to standardize this. The only thing you can do is be aware of this and acknowledge its influence. It is difficult to deal with but in reality it does not make a lot of difference, in that the query is only on half a stage—mild or moderate—and this does not make too much difference, so you don't worry too much" (EL). While a source of uncertainty is identified, again the laboratory incorporates this and accept it as a part of its role, ambivalently saying that it is influential but that "this does not make too much difference."

Focusing on inflammatory smears, here again laboratory workers highlighted many possibilities for various interpretations. Inflammation present on samples can obscure the screener's view of the cells. Furthermore, it is difficult to detect the degree and significance of inflammation. According to one screener, "The degree of abnormality should be noted for the report. However, it is difficult to determine just what signifies mild, moderate or severe inflammation, and each has different treatment prescriptions" (JL). In addition, another technician added, "the majority of slides demonstrate some degree of inflammation. It is not possible to always highlight this, or rather, if you did you would be pulling out 90 percent of the slides" (EL).

There was considerable concern in the laboratory that many women were undergoing unnecessary treatment and that there was a tendency to over-reporting and false positive results. This was not only the case with smear samples demonstrating inflammation. As one technician stated, "Even when you feel satisfied with a diagnosis of CIN I, the problems do not end. In some cases this may clear without treatment. The problem is that some cases would probably be best left as normal for subsequent reevaluation, but this would mean that I would not identify the slight abnormality and hence the doctor would see no reason for follow up" (EL). Even when precancerous changes are confidently identified by the laboratory, they feel that this may best be left unidentified to prevent the woman undergoing potentially unnecessary treatment.

The role of the laboratory in the practice of the CSP emerges as far from straightforward. In addition to the above there is controversy over the presence or absence of certain types of cells on the smear samples. For adequate analysis the laboratory requires that "endocervical cells" are present on the cervical smear sample, as well as superficial "ectocervical cells." These cells can be difficult to obtain and frequently the laboratory cannot determine their presence. The concern is that the diagnoses they then make are based upon a sample that is not representative of the health of the whole cervix. Laboratories adopt different policies on this issue. "In this laboratory the policy is to write on the report card if the endocervical cells can definitely, or definitely not, be seen. Most frequently we are unsure about their presence and do not write anything. Generally we aren't too worried because the woman will have another sample taken at a later date. We adopted our policy in part to let doctors know that their sample taking needs to improve" (EL). The British Society for Clinical Cytology statement on this issue places the responsibility for submission of an adequate sample upon the doctor or nurse who obtains it, but adds that the laboratory should reject samples that are qualitatively or quantitatively inadequate.[10]

The laboratory has identified another area of ongoing instability that can affect the efficacy of analysis of cervical cell samples — the adequacy of the samples received. By doing so the laboratory indicates that the role of the general practitioner in the CSP — to obtain cervical cell samples — may not be as straightforward as is publicly presented. However, again the laboratory demonstrates how this instability does not question the validity of the CSP. Indeed, in this instance, the exposure of the adequacy of cervical cell samples as indeterminate can be seen to validate the procedures of the CSP — that women have regular cervical smear tests.

Diagnosing and Making Recommendations

Other areas of uncertainty and instability identified by the laboratory as inherent to the practice of their role in the CSP are uncertainty related to diagnosing cervical cell samples, to making recommendations, and to ensuring that the doctor follows the intended interpretation of the slide. One screener described the latter issue thus: "The report has to be strong enough that the doctor follows it, but not so strong that the woman is unnecessarily panicked" (JaL). A pathologist subsequently expanded upon this by describing the uncertainty inherent to making a diagnosis: "The main problem is that screening identifies many more potential cancers than one would expect. The problem is one of over-identification rather than under-identification. Basically, if you look hard enough you will find something, but you need to weigh up the costs and benefits to the woman" (Dr. M).

While this pathologist carried out sample analyses, he referred back to this issue and demonstrated how the laboratory bases its recommendations on more than just cytological analysis of samples. Incorporated into making a diagnosis on a sample was information on the age, marital status, and number of children of the woman. For example: "This is a mature woman, she has had her kids. It's probably best to do a follow up," and conversely: "This is a young woman, she hasn't had her kids yet. We must consider whether she can be treated early without risk of infertility" (Dr. M).

It seems that cervical samples are analyzed in different ways in response to the various identities of the woman from whom the sample was obtained. That is, instabilities that are deemed significant by the laboratory occur not only in terms of the constitution of the cervical cell samples that they receive but also at the site of obtaining the sample.

One further point that arises from the above laboratory discourse is the repeated references to "remembering the woman at the other end" of the process. In one laboratory I was introduced to technicians by the pathologist as "looking at what our results do to women, the number of suicides we cause" (Dr. M).

LIVING WITH INSTABILITY AND MULTIPLICITOUS IDENTITIES: THE AMBIVALENCE OF THE LABORATORY

While the above presents the practice of the CSP as rather unstable from the perspective of the role of the laboratory, the laboratory does play its assigned role in the program. That is, the laboratory does continue to analyze samples and to make definitive diagnoses and recommendations. Moreover, despite the above references to areas of uncertainty and instability, laboratory discourse included references to its role in the CSP as straightforward and simple. For example, in response to my request to spend time in one laboratory observing the process of booking in, analysis, and diagnosis of samples, a pathologist agreed access but stated: "I don't know what use it will be to you because analysis only takes ten minutes really" (Dr. M). Similarly a laboratory technician, during my time spent in a laboratory stated that "the process is quite straightforward. It will only take ten minutes to show you" (JuL). The official guidelines are that sample analysis should take ten minutes and hence that screeners should be able to screen thirty to thirty-two slides per day.

Many other comments directly contradicted the above. For example, "There's more to the process than you first think" (JuL), and "Screening is very difficult. It takes a trained eye to do it at any speed. At present we do not have enough staff in the laboratory to carry out the screening and to train new staff. You need to screen all the time to learn to screen quickly, y'know ten minutes per slide" (EL).

Furthermore, despite the numerous comments about "remembering the woman at the other end of the process," and considering her needs and anxieties, one technician stated: "In order to cope with the work you have to forget that it is a person at the other end of the sample. If you didn't, it would be too upsetting and you would never get anything done. You can guarantee that every year, just before Christmas, a sample for someone young is diagnosed as malignant. It always upsets me" (JaL). The technician stresses the psychological and practical value of divorcing herself from the human element of her work. However, she also vocalizes her emotional involvement, and she goes on to say: "Y'know we are not paid enough or valued enough because we're defined as not having any responsibility for patients, face to face. But how much more intimate can you get than playing about with someone's insides? Decisions we make here have a direct effect on people's lives" (JaL).

The laboratory is both capable and incapable of divorcing itself from the human at the "other end" of the process that it carries out. Indeed, while it is engaged in "objective," "scientific" work, it also wants to take responsibility for its direct effect on the women whose cells it observes and categorizes because this increases its status and value within the CSP.

EXPOSING INSTABILITY AS A RESOURCE FOR THE NEGOTIATION OF IDENTITY

The following conversation between two laboratory technicians demonstrates their commitment to the CSP but also their wish to redefine their role within it and how this results in their exposure of instabilities in relation to the role of the laboratory in the csp:

> JaL: I believe that it is every woman's right to receive a good service. They shouldn't have to wait for results, it's horrible waiting. I have friends who won't go along, and I say "You must go." But nobody thinks about the other end, of us, can we cope with the increase in screening.
>
> JuL: All this and the breast screening too. It's just implemented with no thought for, can we cope. We need time to train people up. We need an extra member of staff for the cervical cytology screenings [pause]. Y'know people think that lab workers are well paid, but we are not. The public perception is of well-paid scientists, but it's not like that. I think that they think we dunk something in a solution and look what color it turns. If it's blue, it's positive, and pink, it's negative. They are unaware of the process, it's difficult and lengthy.
>
> JaL: Yes, and in the past, just because we've kept it to a one-day turnaround, they think you haven't got enough work, so they give you more.
>
> JuL: Well, it's just going to build up, you can't rush it, it wouldn't be fair. There's nothing else we can do.
>
> JaL: Yes, but it reflects badly on the lab, personally. They don't understand the work to do and it just reflects badly on the lab.
>
> (JaL and JuL)

The above type of comment was common in laboratory discourse. The laboratory expresses its commitment to the csp as a valid intervention that is indispensable to women's health — "You must go." It stresses its concern for women — not to keep them waiting for results and the potential detrimental consequences of rushing sample analysis. However, the laboratory is also concerned about personal working conditions, staffing ratios, and the status of laboratory workers and the laboratory itself. The exposure of the analysis of samples as difficult and lengthy rather than as straightforward and quick is part of the process by which the laboratory attempts to negotiate and redefine its identity within the csp. The laboratory demonstrates how the practice of its role is oversimplified and hence how the laboratory is undervalued within the government and public csp. By redefining its role as complex, the laboratory emerges as worthy of increased status and resources.

However, this approach to negotiating identity can be dangerous for the laboratory and consequently for the csp. The laboratory exposure of uncertainty could indicate that the program is potentially ineffective in that it becomes doubtful as to whether the laboratory can reliably detect cytological changes that are precancerous. A conference for a newly emerged organization, the National Association for Cytologists (NAC), demonstrated that laboratories are aware that their exposure of uncertainty could pose a threat to their continued existence.[11] The association has been set up to give a voice to the role and responsibilities of cyto-screeners, to "allow cyto-screeners and cytologists a voice for uncertainties" (fieldnotes, NAC conference). The papers presented to the conference, and much of the informal discourse that followed, focused on the ambiguity and areas of uncertainty inherent to the role of the cyto-screener. However, there was ambivalent hostility toward voicing the indeterminacy and instabilities. Following a presentation to the conference about the reporting, but uncertain significance, of the presence of human papilloma virus on cervical smear samples, and the subsequent potential for overtreatment, numerous comments emerged similar to the following: "I'm not sure about all this. This feeling that screening isn't worth it, it's dangerous. We'd be out of a job." And "It's not right, it makes it sound like we do more harm than good and that's not true" (fieldnotes, NAC conference). Indeed, one public health physician, in response to a suggestion that there should be an attempt to increase public awareness of the complexities inherent to the CSP stated, "If women get a detailed letter explaining about the uncertainties in the test they will all be coming saying, Doctor, do I really need this?" (interview with Dr. CU)

While the laboratory engages in problematizing the CSP in order to redefine their identity within it, the exposure of instability could threaten the existence of the CSP and the laboratory. The process of negotiating identity through exposing instabilities and indeterminacy is a delicate and complex one that requires careful monitoring and management.

MAINTAINING THE CSP BY ADOPTING MULTIPLICITOUS IDENTITIES

I want to include one final example of ongoing instability as it occurs in relation to the role of the laboratory in the CSP. In the following discourse there is evidence of laboratory workers adopting the identities of other components in the CSP, and of how these multiform identities support the CSP. For example, one technician stated, "In laboratories specimens are often thought to be inadequate, but it's not understood that if it's a very obese woman, for example, it is difficult to see the cervix. Because we have a pathologist in our lab who is a GP, she highlights the problems that a GP might have. It makes things easier" (NAC conference). A consultant cytopathologist, who manages the largest cytology laboratory in Europe, commented, "I have a very good relationship with general practitioners. They ring me up and ask questions. This is not normal. I think it's because I was trained as an obstetrician and gynecologist—I'm not a pathologist" (interview with Dr. YC). He also stated that "screening is a woman's job. Men get more fed up easily. It's routine work. Women are more motivated because it's for women. It's for them" (Dr. YC).

Laboratory workers move about within the CSP adopting the identity of other components of the program, demonstrating how they inhabit various domains at the same time. Moreover, it seems that this multiformity lubricates the functioning of the program even though it can result in laboratory workers adopting a diversity of interests and identities that appear to be beyond the limit of their defined role within the CSP.

CONCLUSION: CONTINUITY THROUGH INSTABILITY

I have attempted to demonstrate how laboratory workers, from within the CSP, are engaged in constructing and exposing instabilities and to describe the character of those instabilities. The laboratory exposes the multiple forms that it and other components of the program that it has contact with (such as cervical cells and women) adopt. From the perspective of the role of the laboratory, the CSP emerges as composed of a series of interacting, complex, decentered identities and as characterized by ongoing instability. However, laboratory discourse is also fraught with ambivalence, for coexisting with the laboratory's exposure of indeterminacy, instability, and the mutability of components' identities, is reference to their role and the CSP as straightforward, stable, and efficacious. I will expand below on the suggestion that it is this marriage of two apparently opposite conceptualizations of the CSP that affords the program durability. Moreover, I suggest that the ambivalence of the laboratory is to be seen as a necessity and an inevitability, rather than as a source of threat and breakdown of the CSP.

The construction and exposure of instability, that is, its amount and character and how it is represented, is a feature of the laboratory negotiating its status within the CSP. Indeed, my analysis of the role of the laboratory in the practice of the CSP suggests that there is not a fixed amount of instability inherent to the CSP, nor are the instabilities of a static character. Rather, the amount and nature of instability is negotiable and emergent from the processes of negotiation that characterize the practice of the CSP. Elsewhere, along with Mike Michael (1993), I have written about how GPs in the U.K. CSP, in response to recent government redefinition of their role and changes in how they receive remuneration for cervical smear tests that they carry out, have redefined and complexified their own role in the CSP by exposing instabilities in the role played by lay women. GPs have constructed hitherto apparently coherent and unquestioned aspects of their role as problematic.

The suggestion that the source, character, and amount of instability is negotiated and flexible is not dissimilar to Wynne's (1987) conceptualization of uncertainty in relation to technological artifacts: "[T]here is not a fixed level of uncertainty 'out there', but different interacting perceptions of how much, and of what shape and meaning it has" (p. 95). Moreover, my suggestion is that instabilities are not necessarily "uncertainties," if uncertainties are construed as a threat to practice. Rather, the laboratory constructs instabilities in the name of continued practice of the CSP. The instability that the laboratory exposes affords negotiation of its identity within the CSP. The laboratory is represented as able to deal with uncertainty and ambiguity. It becomes an important complex component carrying out difficult and lengthy procedures and hence worthy of increased status and resources.

Put another way, there is an apparent paradox; the laboratory is engaged in exposing indeterminate identities and sources of uncertainty, and hence could be seen to be problematizing the CSP *but* it is doing so from its position as a component of the CSP. This, however, leads to "necessary ambivalence" rather than to conflict. The laboratory workers construct and expose instability and complexity in the CSP as they redefine themselves, but they simultaneously demonstrate their commitment to the validity and indispensability of the program. Indeed, the laboratory workers expose instabilities as inherent to the practice of their role in the CSP and as a part of negotiating their identity *within* the CSP.

We can consider here the words of Star that "People inhabit many different domains at once . . . and the negotiation of identities, within and across groups, is an extraordinarily complex and delicate task. It's important not to presume either unity or single membership, either in the mingling of humans and non-humans or amongst humans" (Star 1991b, 52). In our attempts to capture the intricate work by which scientific knowledge-claims and programs such as the CSP achieve durability and longevity, it is important not to assume that the components of these programs adopt stable identities or inhabit only one domain. To put it simply, a laboratory worker can also be a general practitioner and a woman recipient of the program. This habitation of a variety of domains at once has an effect upon the role played by the laboratory in the CSP. Indeed, we have seen how it can support that role and contribute to its workability. The CSP can be seen to be continually changing shape in its practice as it adjusts to the movement, insights, and changing needs of its constituent decentered components—both human and nonhuman. That is, further to Star, laboratory discourse has highlighted that it is not only people that "inhabit many different domains" because cervical cells, staining machines, and cervical samples can also be seen to be adopting a multiplicity of forms.

Programs such as the CSP that are long-standing can appear to be composed of a series of stable elements—as, for example, actor-network theory tends to suggest. However, as various writers are now suggesting, it is important to consider the functioning and stabilization over time of such apparently stable constructions.[12] My analysis of the practice of the CSP, focusing on the work of the laboratory, suggests that ongoing instability characterizes and lubricates the continuation of the CSP and that this instability can be seen as a consequence of the multiplicitous mutable identity of the components of the program. I suggest that components of the program must adopt a diversity of identities in order to maintain the CSP, because other components are demonstrating their multiformity and are exposing instabilities. For example, from the laboratory perspective, GPs must be good sample takers, capable of obtaining qualitatively and quantitatively adequate cervical cell specimens in order for the laboratory to overcome its inability to determine the presence of certain cell types. However, GPs must also be bad sample takers, whose specimens are inadequate, in order for the laboratory workers to prioritize their own skills and to redefine their role as a complex and difficult one that is, on the whole, undervalued and oversimplified within the CSP. Components of the CSP, at the level of practice, are perpetually moving around, exposing their instability and redefining their own identity and hence the identities of other components with which they interact. The CSP must, therefore, be flexible and unstable at the level of the interaction of its components to accommodate the complexity, indeterminacy, and negotiation that ensues.

I suggest that we can think in terms of the coexistence of two formulations of the CSP. One formulation of the CSP, for example that which is publicly presented, is composed of a series of textually and historically stable and identifiable identities. That is, the CSP appears to take on a distinct identity and to exist at an abstracted level, and the process of the CSP consists of a series of stable and distinguishable components each playing a specific role. Furthermore, as the discourse of the laboratory suggests, components emerge as trapped within these defined identities and this stable structure, inasmuch as their continued existence and future development is dependent on the continued existence of this clearly defined CSP. However, there coexists another CSP at the level of practice, which has different characteristics. In this formulation components are complex, decentered identities, and instabilities inherent to their interactions come into focus. My suggestion is that it is the coexistence of these two formulations that is necessary for the continued existence and evolution of the CSP. For example, if the laboratory was tied to its stable, historically identifiable, clearly defined role and could not negotiate and redefine that role, it could not incorporate ambiguous cell structures and contaminated specimens into the CSP. The existence of the CSP could be threatened as the role of the laboratory emerged as unworkable: its efficacy depends upon the ability of the laboratory to reliably and effectively detect precancerous cytological changes. In turn, laboratory discourse suggests that the ability of the laboratory to detect precancerous cytological changes depends upon its ability to accommodate instability and ambiguity. It seems that only by allowing and accommodating instability at the level of the practice of its role does the laboratory manage to maintain stability at the level of the CSP.

The above suggests possible ways of beginning to understand, and to analytically capture, the dynamism and development of stable and durable medical interventions. Pivotal in capturing this in our analyses is to recognize the potential multiplicitousness of components' identities while looking at the work of practice. We may then begin to see what was previously invisible— the negotiation inherent to work practices and the instability, indeterminate identities, and ambivalence that fuel this negotiation and emerge as inevitable and necessary rather than a source of conflict and threat.

NOTES

I want to thank the staff in the two laboratories that put up with me in 1990–1992. Annemarie Mol, Marc Berg, Dick Willems, and Mike Michael have commented on earlier drafts of this essay, for which I am very grateful.

1   Association of Community Health Councils for England and Wales 1989: 1.
2   Singer and Szarewski 1988: 121; Posner and Vessey 1988: 9; Johnston 1989: 1.
3   Great Britain, Ministry of Health Health Circular, HC[66]76. I draw upon various government documents referring to the introduction and development of the program.
4   National Co-ordinating Network for the National Health Service Cervical Screening Programme (NCN) 1991.
5   For example see Chomet and Chomet 1989; Quilliam 1989; and Singer and Szarewski 1988.
6   This is taken from a standard letter received in 1993.
7   Main texts outlining this approach include Callon 1986a; 1986b; Latour 1986; 1987; Law 1987; and Callon, Law, and Rip 1986.
8   See previous references to the health professionals and the public presentation, note 5. Examples of women's health activists demonstrating this commitment include Barnett and Fox 1986; Posner 1987; and Saffron 1987.

9 The information presented here is taken from data obtained through participant observation in two laboratories (1990–1992) and from interview transcripts with laboratory pathologists and technicians. The in-text references refer to interview transcripts.

10 National Association of Cytologists (NAC), The Inaugural Meeting, April 6–7, 1990.

11 Ibid.

12 Akrich 1992b; Callon 1991; Law 1991; Fujimura 1992; Star 1991b.

INHALING DRUGS AND MAKING WORLDS: A PROLIFERATION OF LUNGS AND ASTHMAS

Dick Willems

▼

Mais si elle n'admet pas des rétablissements, la vie admet des réparations
qui sont vraiment des innovations physiologiques
—G. Canguilhem

BREATHING

Steven had not come to see his doctor for breathlessness, which was the usual reason for his rare visits to the surgery. This time his complaint was a persistent cough. "I think I've just got a cold, but it doesn't seem to get any better." His asthma, he told the doctor, had been all right. He needed only about two or three Ventolin inhalations a day, sometimes even fewer.[1] And they helped him well.

After examining Steven's chest, the doctor said that the long duration of this cough was most probably an indication that his airways were "irritated," and that he needed more of his inhalations than he thought. "Although you do not feel breathless anymore, your Ventolin may still help to cure this cough. Therefore you should increase inhalations to four times a day."

Steven was surprised. "You told me that Ventolin opens up my airways. Why should that help me if I don't feel breathless?"

"I'll tell you why. You see, Ventolin distends the smallest muscles of your airways. The small airways, the ones at the outskirts of your lungs. If these muscles constrict too much, you may become breathless. But their constriction may also cause irritation. And if that is the case, you start to cough. Coughing is related to breathlessness, it is yet another symptom of asthma."

Though still somewhat puzzled, Steven left the office saying he would at least try some more Ventolin, since he saw no harm in taking a few more inhalations for a few days.

Carl came to see his physician not for any specific complaints, but for the half-yearly check of his airway problems. Keeping these appointments demanded quite some discipline since he felt in rather good health. But the severe asthma attack he had had a few years ago had, as Carl put it, "cured him of the idea that he could do without control." The drug Carl used on a daily basis was called Becotide.[2] It was packed in a brown, box-like inhaler device, and he used it twice every day.

Carl carried his drugs wherever he went. This didn't mean that he had no doubts about continuous treatment. He had been taking drugs for five years now, and began to feel uneasy at the prospect of having to continue doing so for the rest of his life. Carl said as much to his physician. The doctor said he could certainly understand Carl's worries, and then embarked upon an explanation of the working mechanisms of Becotide. "The reason you tend to get breathless is that your airways are in a continuous state of inflammation. This goes especially for the smallest ones, the airways in the extreme periphery of your lungs. They tend to overreact to comparatively harmless substances that reach them when you breathe: dust, smoke particles, cold air. Because your airways are continuously inflamed, not just from time to time, you need your anti-inflammatory drugs continuously, too. They suppress the inflammation and the swelling that comes with it. In that way, they increase the volume of air that can get into your lungs. And they also prevent your airways from constricting."

Carl insisted: "But is it quite sure it is safe to use these things for years and years?" The doctor responded understandingly: "I am as sure as one can be—years of research have never shown any adverse effects. You see, when you inhale drugs, they don't reach the bloodstream. They just reach the lung tissues. They don't get anywhere else in the body where they could cause side effects or other problems." Carl was only partly reassured. He couldn't entirely stop thinking that it must be bad for airways to keep on having steroids applied to them—he happened to know that it is bad for skin to constantly put steroid creams on it. The doctor conceded that this sounded logical. "But," he added, "it has never been proven to be true."

These two consultations are mostly different and partly similar. The main similarity is in the type of health problems, which have to do with airway obstruction, and in the diagnosis that is established to explain these problems. Both patients have breathing problems and have been diagnosed as suffering from asthma. But there seem to be more differences between them than similarities. They use different drugs in different ways, and what their physician tells them about their treatment is different as well. It is doubtful whether an outside observer would consider it probable that the diseases these men suffer from go under a single name — and yet they do.

This chapter discusses the meaning of the differences and similarities between Steven's and Carl's consultations. It starts by presenting the way in which these differences are accounted for in medicine itself. Here, differences such as these are taken to *reflect* the characteristics of either the disease, the patient, or the physician. The third section is devoted to a critique of this account. I will show that types of treatment (drugs and inhalers, in this case) are part of a *practice* around disease, and this implies that they have a role in the *making* of differences and similarities rather than simply *mirroring* these. The varieties of drug treatment against breathlessness, I claim, are not a passive *reflection* of given differences, but contribute to the *creation* of such differences. Thus, different treatment practices involve the making of different *diseases* — different asthmas — and different *lungs* as the locus of disease. Carl and Steven, I will argue, not only think and talk differently about their asthma, they *have* different asthmas — asthmas made different in the practices they are involved in.

The fourth section further develops one of the ways in which treatment practices create new differences in the body. Using Foucault's concept of a *geography* of the body, it shows how different drug forms create different maps of the body.

The last section discusses a problem that is crucial for the approach developed in this chapter: the fact that one and the same patient may be involved in different practices at the same time and, as a consequence of the analysis, would have several different diseases and different airways. Here, as in the preceding sections, the concept of "practice" proves to be crucial to remove the sting from this problem by showing that a practice creates not only differences between diseases but similarities as well.

The chapter ends with some remarks concerning the value of this type of analysis for the theory of medicine.

DRUGS REFLECTING DIFFERENCES

Let us consider in some detail the way in which medicine itself accounts for the differences between such patients as Steven and Carl who, although they receive the same diagnostic label, are treated quite differently.

A first explanation consists of asserting that the drugs act on different *aspects* of the same disease (British Thoracic Society 1991). Salbutamol, the active component of the medicine Steven inhales, is a bronchodilator and acts on airway obstruction. Carl's steroids act on inflammation. Both obstruction and inflammation are regarded as aspects of asthma that are more or less pronounced in different patients.

A second explanation makes a distinction between *mild* and *severe* asthma. This explanation supposes a hierarchical relation between the various drugs. It would state that the salbutamol Steven inhales when he feels he needs it, is used for relatively mild forms of the disease, while more severe forms need continuous inhalations — either with chromones (see below) or with the steroids Carl uses.[3]

A third account attributes the difference between two therapies to *individual reactions,* or *idiosyncrasies* patients may display. For instance, someone may show adverse reactions or counterindications to one of the drugs and therefore be treated with the other.

Finally, a difference in therapy may be attributed to the characteristics of the prescribing doctors. Some physicians always prescribe drug A, others have a habit of prescribing B and stick to that. Often, interphysician variation is taken to be a scandal. From outside medicine, the fact that treatment may seem a matter of habit or taste rather than the rigorous application of well-established knowledge, is denounced as a sign of irrationality (Payer 1989). From inside medicine, it is considered to be one of the main reasons for loss of confidence in the medical profession. The desire to counter interphysician variation is one of the driving forces behind the recent proliferation of consensus statements and treatment guidelines (Thomas and Rutten 1993).

These, then, are some of the explanations that medicine offers for differences in drug therapy for similar diseases. They relate that difference to the aspect of the disease that is most prominent in the patient treated; to the severity of the disease the patient suffers from; to idiosyncrasies of the patient's reaction to drugs; or else to particularities of the prescribing doctor.

These various accounts can be traced in the explanations physicians give to patients like Carl and Steven. But they are also inscribed in rules, articulated in books, and discussed in conferences. Let me give a few examples.

In both the treatment guidelines for the treatment of obstructive lung disease issued by the Dutch College of General Practitioners and in those published by the U.S. National Institutes of Health, the use of different drugs is presented as an incremental process. Mild forms of disease, the guidelines say, should be treated with bronchodilators only (these widen the airways, as Steven's salbutamol does), moderate forms with continuous antiallergic inhalations, and more severe forms with continuous steroid inhalations (like Carl's Becotide). But the very same guidelines also contain examples of linking up the different drugs with different patient characteristics. Regardless of the specificities of their disease, some patients may react better to one type of treatment than to another. Patients, moreover, may develop allergic reactions to specific drugs. Or they may have concomitant diseases that turn the use of some drugs into unattractive options (Van der Waart et al. 1992; U.S. Department of Health and Human Services 1991).

DRUGS CREATING DIFFERENCES

If one takes the prescription of different drugs as the reflection of other differences, either in the variety of the disease — as the above-mentioned guidelines — in the specific reactions of the patient, or in the habits of the prescribing physician, then, even if it is said to have different aspects, "asthma" stays the same — and so do the lungs. In what follows, I challenge the presupposition that these are given entities, and will point to differentiations that different drugs *produce*. Using the vocabulary that has been developed in the actor-network approach to technology (Callon 1986a; Latour 1984), drugs are among the elements in a consultation that *define* (at least partly) *what the other elements are*. A somewhat trivial example would be that the existence of inhalable drugs changes the definition of the doctor in the sense that, apart from many other things, s/he has to be an expert in inhalation techniques, and has to be able to explain these techniques to patients. Inhalable drugs thus define the role of the physician, just as much as the latter defines the role of the former. For the medications, as well as for the physicians, patients, and lung function measurement devices, the actor-network approach would state that "for any given actor, there is nothing beyond the network which it has created, which constitutes it, and of which it forms a part" (Callon, Law, and Rip 1986).

Building, more specifically, upon "the semiotics of technology" of Latour and Akrich (Akrich 1993; Akrich and Latour 1992), I consider artifacts (in this case medications) as a specific type of negotiator in the debates about what is the matter with Carl and Steven. In what follows I argue, first, that the very existence of different treatment substances is what generates, on the level of the *classification* of asthma, a division of asthma into subclasses fitting these treatment possibilities. Subsequently, I will show that various drugs against obstructive lung disease constitute not only different asthmas but also different lungs as their target.

Different Asthmas

Taking cardiac drugs as an example, Vos (1991) has shown that therapeutic innovations bring along new categorizations of disease. Using the example of the effect of β-blockers in postinfarct arrhythmias and infarct size, he argues that a new subdivision of the concept of myocardial infarction was produced by the drug: that between fresh and old infarcts. Because they show different effects according to the time elapsed after infarction, β-blockers introduce duration as an element of nosology. With the coming of cardiac drugs, thus, new subsets of heart disease came into being.

With drugs against obstructive lung disease, similar developments have occurred. Bronchodilators are a case in point. When asthmatic patients have their lung function tested (either in the hospital with a spirometer or at home with a peak flow meter), two measurements are taken: one before and one ten minutes after inhaling a bronchodilator. If lung function improves significantly after inhalation, the asthma is called "reversible." Various guidelines for physicians say that the difference should be at least 10 or 15 percent to indicate real irreversibility. Thus if Carl blows 355 instead of 345 liters per minute after an inhalation of Becotide, he may regard this as an improvement, but his physician should not. He is supposed to call Carl's asthma "irreversible."

Bronchodilators are indispensable elements of the differentiation between reversible and irreversible airway obstruction. Thus, as therapeutic agents, they also diagnose. But does that mean that they actually *construct* the classification of these two forms of the disease? Do they create a nosological difference, that is, a difference in disease definitions? Yes: without the existence of bronchodilators it would be impossible to reverse the airway obstruction, and thus it would be impossible to sensibly differentiate between reversible and irreversible asthma. Drugs construct the division in a very down-to-earth sense: they enter the lungs and physically produce a reversal of the obstruction of the airways — in "reversible" cases, that is, not in "irreversible" ones.

But drugs *do not*, of course, make classifications and differentiations all by themselves. A bronchodilator like salbutamol is able to construct a difference between reversible and irreversible obstructions only in conjunction with measurement devices, epidemiological researchers, and the laboratory assistants whose encouragement is indispensable for the patient to blow properly. Bronchodilators are elements, among others, in the reshaping of disease classification (nosology) into one in which *two* types of airway obstruction exist — they are part of a network of elements. Or, with a more dynamic term: they are part of the *practice* of making differences between forms of airway obstruction.

In a similar way, chromones such as cromoglycate are active elements in the creation of a second distinction within the disease asthma: that between "mainly allergic asthma" and "mainly aspecific hyperreactivity." Allergic asthma, according to this distinction, is the consequence of contact with specific substances such as pollen or house dust mites, while nonallergic or aspecific hyperreactivity denotes a general tendency to overreact to any kind of stimulus. Chromones are especially used to make this difference in young children with airway obstruction. In order to illustrate this, let me briefly introduce you to a young patient.

Denise is four years old, and already has a long history of airway complaints: continuous coughing and periods of tightness. In alternation with her asthma attacks, she has had frequent episodes of ear infections. For a while she was helped out with salbutamol on an incidental basis, but her need for the drug gradually increased. This augmented her parents' worries, and when she was about three years old the physician proposed trying a long-term treatment with cromoglycate. He said that Denise was too young to have allergy proven by blood tests, but that she probably was allergic. If so, cromoglycate would reduce the allergic reactions inside her lungs.

After a few weeks Denise and her mother came back to the office. "I am not impressed by the results," Denise's mother said. "She still asks for 'the blue one' several times a day, and although I don't always give it, I think it signals that she still has problems." The physician sits back for a while, looking at the computer on his desk which displays Denise's record. He then concludes that Denise may not be allergic after all, or at least not only allergic. The fact that cromoglycate does not help her sufficiently suggests that her airways have an aspecific sensibility. Allergy is cured by cromoglycate, but aspecific sensibility is not. "So she may have the sort of sensibility to smoke, to mist, to sudden temperature changes that we call aspecific hyperreactivity. In order to take care of that, she will have to start using inhaled steroids."

It may be clear from this description that cromoglycate is just as indispensable as the stethoscope, the peak flow meter, and, for that matter, the physician to establish a *diagnosis* of asthma in Denise's case. All these become elements of a practice in which Denise's disease is defined, controlled, and treated. Being allergic or hyperreactive means nothing else than becoming a part of this practice.

That the role of cromoglycate in diagnosis is not exceptional is testified by the fact that the Dutch guideline for the treatment of asthma in children advises taking a stepwise approach once continuous treatment is considered (Dirksen et al. 1992). Chromones, it states, must be tried out as a first step, serving simultaneously as treatment and as diagnostic tool. If cromoglycate diminishes complaints and reduces the need for bronchodilators, then the child has an allergic form of asthma. If not, a treatment with inhaled steroids is started, and the child has a nonallergic form of hyperreactivity. Again, the drugs are not the sole makers of this difference: they do so with other actors, such as a properly inhaling child, a parent who has the discipline to administer the drug, and a doctor who is prepared to give these drugs even to very young children.

To take the argument a step further, cromoglycate not only makes a diagnostic distinction, but also a nosological one: that it *creates* a difference between allergic and nonallergic forms of airway obstruction. Just as the reaction of the airways to Ventolin is part of the definition of (ir)reversibility, the reaction to cromoglycate and similar antiallergic substances becomes a part of the definition of asthma as either allergic or nonallergic.

Different Lungs

If the supposition that drugs contribute to the differentiation of asthma into various subsets has any validity, the question may be asked whether it is right to consider the *airways* as the unchanging substance, the stable stage on which various asthmas are performed. Let us look somewhat closer to see if the various forms of medication in asthma define not only the disease, but also the airways — which would mean that different treatment practices involve different lungs as well as different diseases.

Cromoglycate *treats* the lungs as a defense line against inhaled intruders: when Denise's doctor prescribed cromoglycate in order to treat her asthma, he thereby treated (defined) her airways as allergic, for instance to the house dust gathered in her favorite teddy bear. The use of cromoglycate pulls Denise into a practice that involves avoiding close contact with house dust, and therefore avoiding contact with her teddy bear and a ban on overnight stays with a friend who has too many of them. In this practice, the airways are a — sometimes unreliable — defense line against inhaled substances.

Salbutamol and other bronchodilators, on the other hand, define the airways as a system of variably sized and constrictable tubes that allow air to get in; the practice that these drugs are part of is directed to opening up the constrictable tubes that have a tendency to develop spasms — an entirely different activity from protecting the body against allergens. Inhaled steroids act upon airways that are a large surface of inflammable mucous membranes: when he asks what steroids do for him, Carl hears that his lungs are mucous membranes covered with a thin layer that tends to inflame and develop swelling. These different airways are not different mental images or theoretical constructions, they are different entities because they are part and parcel of different practices.

As in the explanation of the disease definitions that are part of the drugs, a classical explanation interprets these different definitions of the airways in a terminology of *aspects*. Being a defense line, or consisting of constrictable tubes, or having membranes that are prone to inflammation, are all taken to be "aspects" of the lungs. This terminology, however, suggests an outsider who can switch at will from one aspect to the other by taking a different point of view. All such a switch seems to require is that the observer "turn around" the object and "look" from different angles. But this visual metaphor, suggesting "all the aspects" can be "seen" by taking the right perspective, is treacherous. For the different narratives about the airways only exist as part and parcel of different *practices*, such as the various treatment regimens. In order to switch from one narrative to the other, one has to stop *doing* some things and start to do others. One has to lay down some tools and start using others. The number of different narratives and definitions of the airways and their diseases is limited not by our imagination in developing points of view but by the extent to which practices may vary.

In all asthma practices airways are treated—but they are treated as *different* airways. Some drugs strengthen entrance barriers, others open up constricting tubes, and yet others treat inflammatory membranes. If these were all "aspects" there would have to be one underlying or overarching unity: "the lungs." But if different practices each treat different lungs, and each of them defines its own *ontology of the airways*, then the answer to the question what kind of an object "the lungs" *are* starts to look quite different. For now this object does not precede medical practices, but rather follows from them. Objectivity is not *opposed* to difference in narratives, but the difference in narratives is part of what the objects in medicine are. And if medical practices shift, the essence of the lungs will alter with them. Thus, since the beginning of the nineties, the role of steroid inhalations has become more and more predominant in asthma treatment, at the expense of that of bronchodilators (Reed 1991). I would argue, then, that as an element of this change in treatment policy, the lungs are changing their character, too. They become more and more a surface of membranes with a strong tendency to inflammatory reactions and less and less a tree of tubes with a tendency to constrict.

Different drugs, I have argued, are linked up with different "lungs," and, going a step further, with different bodies. In order to clarify this idea, it may be useful to look at the work of Michel Foucault, especially his concept of *the body's various geographies*. In *La Naissance de la Clinique*, Foucault urged for a study of the different spatializations of the body that occur in medicine: "This order (of the anatomical atlas) is just one of the ways in which medicine is able to situate diseases in a space. When will it be possible to define the pathways of allergic reactions through the secret spaces of the body?" (Foucault 1963).[4] Whereas Foucault asks for the maps drawn by allergic reactions, I will look at another example: the way the treatment of such reactions with drugs makes connections and disjunctions between regions of the body. The question is, which differing maps of the body are made by either swallowing drugs or taking them through inhalation?

Inhalation therapy is advocated as preferable to pills (or injections) for what may be called geographic reasons: it is a form of *local therapy*. Other instances of local drug therapy are creams, eye drops, and drug patches. "Local" with respect to the inhalation of drugs, however, is something other than "local" with respect to creams. Creams are applied on the skin and are absorbed only to a small, but not always negligible extent. Where do inhaled drugs go? They form a cloud of either powder or gas that is drawn inside the lungs and goes on into deeper parts of the airways. In studies designed to find out where they go to, drug particles are made *visible* on their travel into the airways. In Foucault's terms: they make visible the pathways followed by medication — pathways that are, however, not only followed but created as well.

One way to make these paths visible is by radioactivity. Once drug particles are accompanied by radioactive substances (tracers), they can be seen on a radiographic screen. In this way, tracers trace a map, not only of the places the drugs reach, but thereby also of the airways. In making this map they literally go further than previously existing mapping technologies, like, for instance, bronchoscopy. They bring new areas inside the lung into existence. Thus, various medical investigations produce a number of superposable, but not identical maps, which are specific to the practice that the investigation is part of.

Drug inhalation creates a map of the airways as a tree with ever finer branches. In other practices, lungs may be no more than large bellows that pump air in and out. The different maps of the lungs are constructed in these practices, and roads into the lungs are opened. That this is hard work is evident in the fact that inhalation *skills* are so important in the use of these drugs.

Making this geography happen involves developing a skillful inhalation. Each and every textbook, guideline, and patient information brochure acknowledges that inhalation involves a skill that has to be practiced over and over, in other words: that this road into the lungs has to be opened by the patient, and kept open with repeated effort.

Each and every inhalation should be performed in such a way that the larger part of the airways, from the trachea to the medium-sized bronchi, should be passed by the inhaled cloud on its way down. However, tracer studies indicate that whatever inhalation technique is used, a large part of the aerosol is usually deposed in the throat and in the larger airways, while the smallest airways, the new area within the lung that comes into existence as it is depicted, receive only a very small portion of the spray. From the mouth to more than halfway into the lungs medicine may be lost — this is the wasteland of inhalation, so to speak (Dompeling et al. 1992). And in fact, as much as 90 percent of the medicine gets lost under way, however perfectly all the actors (patient, inhaler, carrier) behave and coordinate (Newman et al. 1989). Whether or not the gas reaches its target depends on the design of the apparatus, the skill of the inhaling patient, and various other factors. Inhalation thus introduces another division in the geography of the lungs: accessible and less accessible areas, central versus peripheral, high versus low.

There are noticeable differences between this "inhaler geography" and the way oral drugs make maps of the inside of the body. The ingestion by mouth of a sufficiently large dosage of salbutamol will forge a connection between the heart and the lungs. Salbutamol will both open up the lungs and quicken the heartbeat. Heart and lungs are thus connected in that they both have receptors for salbutamol. They are not so connected when salbutamol is inhaled, because then it remains "local" and never reaches the heart.

Moreover, the ingested-salbutamol connection between heart and lungs is another type of link than the one established in other geographies of the body. For instance, on radiological images of blood vessels (in which dye opaque to X ray has been injected), these go from heart to lungs and from lungs to heart and thus connect the two organs. But ingested salbutamol produces a connection that is made of drug receptors and that is particular to those drugs that find receptors in both organs.

So far, I have discussed the way in which treatment practices constitute new maps of the airways. However, the continuous use of inhaled drugs changes the airways in yet another way: drugs are not only constitutive for the geography of the airways, they literally stick to them and thereby form new entities. Continuous treatment with inhaled steroids turns Carl's airways into *hybrids* of living material and chemical substances. The production of hybrids in chronic disease has recently been discussed with regard to the continuous linking of children to ventilator machines (Kohrman 1994). In similar ways, the continuous use of medications is interesting for medical anthropology and students of technology precisely because they effectively, and almost visibly, construct new and durable links between bodies and machines, between humans and non-humans.

CONNECTIONS AND SIMILARITIES

Steven and Carl both have asthma, which means that they have similar problems with their airways. In taking different drugs, however, they are engaged in different practices and thus have, in practice, different asthmas and different airways. It happens, however, and with this disease it happens quite often, that one person is involved in various treatment regimens at once. This poses a problem for the ideas developed in this paper, because it implies that people live with different diseases and different bodies from one moment to the next. Let me present one such patient.

> Paul, a twenty-five-year-old man, has had asthma since his early childhood. He used to be hospitalized frequently. For a decade he has inhaled various drugs every day. This is his daily regimen: in the morning, he starts by taking an inhalation of salbutamol to fight his morning breathlessness. "It opens up my airways, usually they get obstructed when I'm asleep, you know. But not always. So I only use the salbutamol when I am breathless," he explains. Ten minutes later Paul takes two puffs of beclomethasone. "I take this against the inflammation. My lungs tend to get inflamed, a bit like other people get eczema. If I keep a layer of this stuff in my airways, that suppresses the inflammation. And I take it after the salbutamol. It has become a routine. They tell me that if I didn't do that, the steroid will probably not reach the smallest tubes of my lungs." At lunch time, Paul takes two more puffs of beclomethasone. In the evening yet two more. Then he also takes a puff of Serevent. He only got this one recently, it prevents his waking up from breathlessness. "It's the same as salbutamol, but it sticks to the airways a lot longer. And keeps them from constricting—at least somewhat."

Indeed, one of the consequences of saying that different practices produce different asthmas and different airways seems to be that persons who are involved in different treatment regimens, either concomitantly or in a sequence, have different diseases and lungs. Paul's airways are sometimes closed and have to be opened up or prevented from closing—his is what they are when Paul inhales salbutamol or Serevent. Ten minutes later, beclomethasone treats Paul's airways as being inflamed and swollen and in need of a covering layer of steroids. Apparently, Paul has to live with different airways.

How is this to be imagined? Do people indeed switch from one disease to the other, from one body to the other? Do their airways consist of muscular tubes on one moment and of inflamed mucous membranes on the next? Do they live with a disrupted body? Does the use of different drugs only imply a loss of unity, or does it install new links as well, thus contributing to a novel unity?

The central concept necessary to tackle these problems is, again, that of a practice. Drugs and devices do not operate in an isolated fashion, but as parts of a network. Paul's different airways do have relations between them. They are not independent. When Paul inhales salbutamol in order to allow the beclomethasone to reach his small airways, he forges a connection between the constricted pipes and the membranes that tend to develop inflammation. In Steven's treatment no such connection is made. Neither is it practiced in Carl's life. But for Paul there is one, because the treatment practice he is involved in may be complicated, but it nevertheless is *one* practice.

In a more general way, one could say that drugs and other medical techniques do not just make new differences: they also make new connections. Above, we saw that ingested salbutamol makes a connection on a different level: it connects lungs and heart in a specific way, different from anatomy or X rays. As soon as an asthma patient gets more air after ingesting drugs, his or her heart starts beating at a higher rhythm and s/he starts to tremble lightly. There are other such connections. Steroids, for instance, exist not only for inhalations in airways, but also in creams for the skin, and in injections for joints and tendons. The practice of using these drugs in these varying ways connects the parts of the body they are applied to. One patient may use the same steroid both for his asthma and for the eczema on his arms and for an inflammation in his shoulder. Being treated with steroids makes these different parts of the body become similar. Likewise, the act of inhalation creates a similarity between the mouth, the throat, and the trachea: while a patient inhales, the difference between mouth, throat, and trachea are put aside and they all similarly become roads drugs should pass by to get further along.

Similarities not only emerge within one patient, but also between patients. For instance between Carl, who has periods of increased breathlessness, and Denise, the four-year-old with recurring cough. The fact that they use an identical little brown inhaler makes them similar. Thus, the long-standing theoretical debate about the question whether their diseases are different or the same, is resolved locally, through the likeness of practices (Willems 1995). In an analogous way, salbutamol forges a connection between the occasional hay-fever patient with lung symptoms and the adolescent sportsman with a slight asthma: they have the use of the blue inhaler in common. The use of similar drugs contributes to the forming of distinct groups of people—a group that may be wildly dissimilar on other criteria but that is similar in this one respect: they all use a specific type of drug inhalers.

Drugs, then, are therapeutic agents, but as a part of their therapeutic action, they produce differences and similarities, divergences and connections. They do not merely help the body, or body parts, to resume old functions that are hampered by disease. They also define diseases and reorganize the body by creating new identities for it.

NOTES

1 Ventolin®: salbutamol, a bronchodilator. Reduces airway spasms.
2 Becotide®: beclomethasone, a corticosteroid. Hormone that reduces inflammation.
3 Chromones: antiallergic substance. The most common one is cromoglycate. Pre-scribed in order to reduce the severity of allergic reactions in the airways.
4 "Cet ordre (celui de l'atlas anatomique) n'est cependant qu'une des manières pour la médecine de spatialiser la maladie. . . . Quand pourra-t-on définir les structures que suivent, dans le volume secret du corps, les réactions allergiques?" The English translation is mine.

PAIN PHYSICIANS:
ALL ALIKE, ALL DIFFERENT

Isabelle Baszanger

▼

Associated with the emergence of a specialty or a new professional group is the idea of convergences—of problems, objects, and practices—upheld by the people involved, due to a gradual recognition of their similarities. However, at the heart of this movement of convergence, there is also room for differences that go hand in hand with the constitution of this new professional entity. These differences structure this new entity, shape it, and separate its members as much as the perception of their similarities brings them together. I will attempt to explore this dichotomy between similarity and difference, using the particular case of pain physicians in France in the 1980s. This small group was from the outset built up around differences, whether in their mode of segmentation, in the logic behind associations of physicians, in forms of cooperation, organization of treatment, or deployment of techniques. However, whatever the differences among them, these physicians today constitute a group, form a new professional segment, share an identity, refer to themselves as pain physicians, and work together in developing pain medicine. As a group, they seek actively to establish their legitimacy in the medical world within recognized boundaries. They take similar public positions with respect to general medical structures and in opposition to certain theories of pain that predominate in these structures. They participate together in many debates, whether academic or professional in nature and whether organized by the government or open to the general public. They are jointly and increasingly present whenever the question of "combating pain" arises, for whatever reason. This group of physicians, then, is united around common physical and theoretical boundaries and separated by two different approaches to the same subject: pain. This current situation is in my opinion neither ephemeral nor accidental. Quite the reverse: it can be seen as the usual modus vivendi of this group, at least until new developments modify this situation.

This stabilization of a group around its differences may seem surprising at first sight. Research into professional segments and their social and micro-worlds[1] has taught us that a clear definition of the central object of the segment or world, the activities centered around it and of the right and "authentic" manner of performing these activities is essential to the development and continuing existence of new groups. This is even more essential in that these groups are initially very fragile. They contain within them a tendency toward later segmentation around an ever more precisely defined object and the techniques associated with it. As we will see, in the case of pain physicians we can distinguish between at least two definitions of the central object of the group, associated with two ways of proceeding—yet this does not necessarily imply a movement toward separation or chaos. There is one particular point that allows us to clarify this seeming contradiction: the dual manner in which all actors involved treat a vital resource—the scientific theory of pain—that serves as a framework of reference for this group of physicians. The development of the first pain clinics by actors who were isolated from each other, subjected this theory to local practices that were strongly structured around one or other of its axes. On the other hand, and at the same time, all these isolated local actors also cooperated to establish the legitimacy of pain medicine and pain specialists—a collective task that was carried out in the name of this same theory. I will show that even though this group is structured around internal differences gradually fashioned in practice, this theory, acting as a "boundary object" between different local groups, is the source of its stability. In doing this, I use the term "boundary object" in a way that is slightly different from its initial definition (Star and Griesemer 1989). I use it to understand the preservation of major internal differences *within* a group being formed rather than to examine the cooperation of heterogeneous groups with different viewpoints and goals.[2]

Ilana Löwy (1992), drawing partly on the concept of a "boundary object," focuses on interactions between professional groups—in this case, scientists and physicians in the field of immunology. She shows how a "boundary concept" facilitates the development of heterogeneous intergroup alliances. "[S]uch alliances enable the members of distinct professions to work together and to develop areas of efficient collaboration . . . without, however, obliging them to give up the advantages of their group identities. In immunology, a 'boundary concept'—the immunological self—allowed physicians and scientists to elaborate federative research strategies," leading to the rapid development of immunology. In the course of her analysis, Löwy clearly illustrates the way in which this boundary concept brought together disciplinary groups hitherto too different to work together: to some extent, this boundary object was used to reduce at least some of these differences in order to develop a new field. The perspective changes with the example of pain physicians. People associated under this label have developed distinct forms of activity, limiting their collaboration to activities that increase their social visibility and allow them to establish their legitimacy in the medical world. Unlike immunologists — and because they all come from the same professional group, medicine — they seek to create for themselves a common identity that unites them and distinguishes them from the rest of the profession. At the same time, they develop and preserve separate areas of work that refer to the same boundary object.[3]

Given this subject of enquiry, I will present an empirical comparison contrasting the historical development of two French pain centers. These two centers represent the two poles of a continuum along which we can classify all pain centers in France. In the physicians' own terms, these centers are today perceived by the group as a whole as the incarnation of two ways of "making pain." The continuum — stretching from a pole of "healing through techniques" to the pole of "healing through management" — is not specific to France. According to my hypothesis, its existence is largely due to work done by physicians who started working with pain as a way of translating a theory into practice — into their respective practices.[4] This theory — the gate control theory of pain — has played a crucial role in the development of pain medicine as proposed by John Bonica. The proposals from this American anesthetist date from as early as 1944, but only became widely accepted in 1974.[5] In other words, the French physicians that this chapter discusses did not develop their activities in a vacuum. Because of a lack of space, I will do no more than give a brief summary, dissociated from its historical context, of some elements of the world of pain medicine to which these physicians claim allegiance.

First, with the concept of pain clinics launched in 1953 by John Bonica, physicians had access to an organizational model. By the end of the 1970s, this model was largely accepted in the world of pain medicine. It stipulated that lasting pain — chronic pain, a concept I will come back to — should be treated in specific pain clinics or pain centers by multidisciplinary teams whose composition might vary locally. An interest in the problems associated with pain brings together different people. It is the degree of individual commitment rather than the original specialty that governs the strength or weakness of the individual's links to the group. The justification for such a grouping of people stems from Bonica's 1953 book *The Management of Pain*, where he analyzes the complexity of problems associated with intractable pain that has resisted any traditional treatment in a number of disciplines. Such problems, his book argues, call for the pooling of multidisciplinary skills in order to arrive at a correct diagnosis centered on the pain itself (and not restricted to its initial cause) and to define a multimodal therapeutic proposal. The preferred tool of such a center is the multidisciplinary conference, which allows a structural confrontation of different disciplinary viewpoints until a multidisciplinary evaluation of a particular patient's pain emerges. Moreover, any pain center must count among its members a representative of a discipline covering the psychological field: a psychiatrist or a clinical psychologist. This results from the new definition of pain as a multidimensional phenomenon with physical, psychological, and social consequences ensuring that any evaluation of a pain problem must be carried out on both the physical and the psychological level.[6] As we shall see, this is an essential point — although it is handled very differently.

In addition to this model, the second crucial element that physicians keen to work on pain had at their disposal was a conceptual framework that was broad enough to be used as a basis for most of the techniques employed. An important aspect of Bonica's work in promoting the idea of pain medicine was to use all the data at his disposal to confer a new status on pain. That is, moving away from the idea of pain as a symptom toward that of pain as an illness — as an entirely separate problem requiring a specific treatment. Hence, chronic pain gradually became a new medical entity covering all pain that lasts longer than six months and does not respond to conventional treatment. Gate control theory considerably influenced this work by proposing a new representation of pain that led to a different type of therapeutic approach. Presented in 1965 by Melzack and Wall, the theory basically proposes that a gate-like mechanism exists in the somatic transmission system, allowing pain signals to be modulated before they evoke perception and response. The gate can be opened or closed by variable amounts, depending on factors such as relative activity in large and small peripheral nerve fibers, and various psychological processes such as attention and prior experience. By proposing a variable gate, it became possible to attempt to close the gate by various manipulations.

This theory runs counter to the representation of pain linked to the theory of specificity, whereby a system specific to pain (made up of pain receptors and peripheral nerves) transmits pain messages in a specific way from skin receptors (on the periphery) to a pain center located in the brain.[7] The fixed link between lesion and pain that the theory of specificity postulates has clinical consequences: tackling pain, here, implies trying to interrupt the channels by which the pain message is transmitted. Conversely, gate control theory postulates a variable link between lesion and pain. The therapeutic logic is transformed: we are no longer talking about interruption but about modulation. A new era, that of sensory control, has dawned. It should be stressed — and I will demonstrate the vital importance of this — that gate control theory, by postulating the existence of a modulable barrier in somatic transmission of pain, points to two possible, nonexclusive paths for obtaining a modulation in the sense of a reduction of the pain message. These paths are not mutually exclusive — indeed, the main merit of this theory is that it presents these in a single model. The first path involves acting on organic structures or chemical mediators (nerves, glands, bone marrow, synapses, thalamus, enzymes . . .) whereas the other makes use of mental processes — cognitive processes for example — via descending controls.

In this way, a theoretical basis was created for numerous existing techniques, allowing some of them to initiate a change in status — acupuncture or certain types of massage for example — from folk medicine to medical procedure. For other techniques, this theoretical basis allowed a reevaluation of their merits in pain treatment and, above all, a wider field of application. Here we find a broad variety of anesthetic techniques, some of which are used widely, alongside others that are more complex and are reserved for professionals: from temporary local anesthesia in its routine form, including the anesthesia procured by throat pastilles and that practiced by dentists, to increasingly complex techniques such as peridural or rachidian[8] anesthesia and the vast panoply of physiotherapeutic techniques — massage, manipulation, traction, compression, heat including ultrasound, cold, electrotherapy (whether faradization or galvanization). The methods for directly activating systems of descending control by electrical stimulation stem from experiments carried out before the formulation of gate control theory. Concretely, this involves stimulation of large peripheral nerve fibers using three different types of procedures: stimulation of nerves via electrodes placed on the skin; stimulation via electrodes implanted around the nerves and activated by subcutaneous radioelectric stimulators (what the media refer to as "pain pacemakers"); and finally, stimulation of the sensory roots that penetrate the bone marrow. The first procedure, TENS, or transcutaneous electric nerve stimulation, has become a basic weapon in therapeutic strategies of pain control in pain centers.[9] It can very easily be manipulated by patients themselves. The second method uses the same type of equipment, miniaturized and implanted in the patient's body. In addition to these physical methods, psychological techniques have been developed for treating pain, which find their justification in gate control theory. Here we find techniques coming from different intellectual horizons. From psychodynamic psychiatry comes the framework for evaluating personality and some principles of analytic treatment. Psychobehavioral techniques, however, are the most highly developed. These borrow from the findings of experimental psychology and

theories of social learning (Pavlov, Skinner, Bandura) and use techniques of relaxation, biofeedback, desensitization to stress, or modification of behavioral
reinforcement contingencies.[10]

All these techniques, whose logic of use is derived from a single conceptual
framework, are integrated very differently in the two major models for treating chronic pain. The hypothesis that I will advance here is that the existence
of these two models should be seen as resulting from the special ways in which
the concept of the pain clinic, with its multidisciplinary framework, and the
technical possibilities offered by gate control theory have actually been put
into practice. In other words, the specific ways in which these techniques have
been developed and the specific features of organizational relations developed
around them have led to distinct operative interpretations of chronic pain and
pain medicine. These internal differences are linked less, a priori, to the intrinsic characteristics of gate control theory (such as the existence of two paths for
modulating sensory messages, for example) than to the specific ways in which
this theory has been applied in practice. This is what I will explore in detail in
the findings of my ethnographic study. Subsequently, I will briefly examine the
parallel development of the collective work undertaken to form a group within
recognized boundaries.

The ethnographic study on which this chapter is based is part of a larger
research project on the "invention" of a new medical field: "the medicine of
pain."[11] The focus of this research, the conceptual and organizational developments of pain centers, differs strongly from the anthropological literature
on chronic pain. The latter deals more with the inner experience of patients
and is less interested in the historical and sociological developments of chronic
pain as a new medical entity.[12] This entity, however, has intellectual and practical consequences for medical work, for patients' courses of action, and for
the interactions between patients and physicians, and is therefore important to
study. As we will see, this very entity shaped and was shaped by the practical
implementation of pain centers.

CENTER 1: HEALING THROUGH TECHNIQUE

The First Steps

Founded officially in 1984,[13] this center gradually developed from an encounter
a few years earlier between three people from two medical specialties often associated in practice—anesthesiology and neurosurgery. In this development,
these physicians gradually differentiated themselves from their original special-

ties. The two anesthetists, working in the field of urology, dealt with terminal (cancer) patients' pain, and were keen to try out some of the various technical possibilities of which they were aware. Hence, they became involved in pain medicine through techniques associated with their disciplines, which they sought to master and use in the more specific framework of pain treatment. They studied neurophysiology in the faculty of science and set up a "small pain practice" in the urology department. Gradually, they started to include patients not suffering from cancer and not treated in the hospital itself. During this first phase, they associated themselves with a neurosurgeon "who worked in the urology department treating problems of pain on the surgical level." He had been dealing with pain for a number of years, notably in the case of facial neuralgia, where a neurosurgical treatment is possible when drugs are ineffective. This technique, "thermocoagulation of the semilunar ganglion," uses certain anesthetic practices and offers a possible extension of the anesthetist's sphere of action. The three physicians began to collaborate around this technique: the two anesthetists increasingly collaborated with the neurosurgeon on cases of facial neuralgia, while the neurosurgeon started to include patients suffering from intractable pain of various origins.

Gradually, the idea emerged of working together more specifically. To improve their overall training, one of the two anesthetists spent time in two European pain centers run by neurosurgeons or anesthetists. Their approaches were based on technical interventions using traditional anesthetic and surgical procedures. In other words, they saw pain in terms of the techniques belonging to the first approach stemming from gate control theory, that is, techniques for modulating pain messages. They were using these techniques as pain specialists, since their application requires a specific diagnosis centering on pain and not on any causal pathology. These techniques were therefore the starting point for the multidisciplinary approach, based on the need for self-training. This stage of self-training recurs in the history of every center, where physicians learn together (and from each other) how to approach, diagnose, and treat patients with chronic pain.

Moving toward a Hierarchical Multidisciplinarity

This learning phase is internal to the group: it does not call on other specialties. Hence, the problem for these physicians is to learn how to match the techniques with which they were familiar with the types of pain that they could alleviate systematically. Naturally, not all pain could be dealt with by these techniques. If pain did not respond to these specific treatments—which they tended to describe as "mixed" pains—it was necessary to call on other specialists better equipped to deal with these cases: "Then you have all that mixed pain that you can do nothing for, pain in the tongue or gums after teeth have been pulled out or [resulting from] nerve damage, [what we call] glossodynia; coccycodynia [pain in the coccyx], allodynia [pain due to a stimulus that normally does not trigger pain]. It's amazing, all those cases of causalgia [pain syndrome after a traumatic nerve lesion]. . . . I prefer to leave all that to the neurologist."

In one sense, there are thus two types of pain: the kind for which you can do something, with the aim of curing it, and the other where the only remedy is new treatments specifically developed for pain. From this division arose a particular type of multidisciplinary approach, which we might call the hierarchical multidisciplinary (or two-tier) approach. The first tier (referred to by the physicians as "the hard core") was forged in the first three-physician consultations, which emphasized the first path for modulating pain messages, as suggested by gate control theory. In line with their desire to transform the initial practice of pain consultation into a pain center (and following Bonica's recommendations), they rapidly sought to develop regular collaboration with different specialists. This was achieved in November 1984, when the center was officially opened.[14]

In its first incarnation—this changed over the years—the team consisted of the original two anesthetists and the neurosurgeon, joined by two neurologists, a rheumatologist, and a psychiatrist. The "hard core" spent one and a half days a week carrying out the major technical operations, but focused primarily on consultations. The two anesthetists each devoted four half-days to consultation, the neurosurgeon two half-days; one of the two neurologists did two half-days, the other one half-day, while the psychiatrist and the rheumatologist each did one half-day. The anesthetists were therefore responsible for almost 50 percent of the consultations. They dealt with much "mixed pain," for which the first line of treatment is generally antidepressant therapy (as prescribed for "minor psychiatric treatment" by almost all physicians in their daily practice).

In the method of organization adopted, we can see a concept of a pain medicine whose central object is virtually defined by existing technical capacities. These range from the use of drugs or the simplest physical means to increasingly sophisticated anesthetic and neurosurgical techniques practiced by only a few physicians working in specialized centers. According to the pain clinic model, patients are received on receipt of a physician's letter. These letters serve as a basis to sort out which patients will be seen by which physicians, a task that can be done by any one of the three "core" physicians. This aspect highlights the existence of two different groups of physicians—a "core" composed of "real" pain physicians, and another group of specialist consultants, who receive patients for whom the hard-core physicians are unable to offer an original pain treatment.

> There is a huge pile [of letters] every day. We read all the letters and one of us sorts the patients out in terms of the main orientation but . . . with a little experience, it comes quite quickly, you see very well whether they should be seen by a rheumatologist or, rather, by a neurologist. Someone with multiple sclerosis with pain will be seen by the neurologist. A scar-induced fibrosis after an operation for sciatica, in theory, is external stimulation that might respond to peridural posterior cord stimulation, or an implantable stimulation with a pain pacemaker. . . . In that case, any one of us could take the patient.

A Short Follow-up, a Hierarchy of Treatment

This division of labor defines different statuses with respect to pain, with the hard core shifting, as it were, toward a new specialization around the pain object defined by a specific technical capacity. The other specialists retain their identity with respect to their specialty: the neurologist continues to work as a neurologist, the rheumatologist as a rheumatologist. These consultants do not redefine their specialty, neither individually nor collectively, even if they are very aware that the fact of working in a structure specifically set up to deal with pain has led to a change in their attitude to their work as specialist.[15] Logically enough, we encounter this double status again in the manner of conceiving the treatment and its place in the overall health system. The average follow-up envisaged is three consultations with a referral back as quickly as possible to the patient's personal physician—usually a general practitioner—who will continue the treatment. In this sense, the center is seen as one stage in the medical process and not as a place for long-term follow-up or a follow-up system as such (compare center 2, below).

However, the duration of the follow-up will depend on the nature of the problem to be dealt with and the degree of difficulty encountered. In all cases, there is a progression to be respected and established protocols to be followed. In many cases, an initial treatment will be proposed in the first consultation. This treatment will then be adjusted in a second consultation, whereupon the patient will be referred back to his or her personal physician. The main issue here is that in many cases patients have not even been prescribed the basic treatments, or they have had them, but at the wrong dosages. But there are cases when this general therapeutic progression does not yield the expected results, cases when the patient is suffering from truly intractable pain. Here, the follow-up is lengthier—and the method of seeking a solution the same as in all hyperspecialized hospital departments. These pain centers do not define a method of treating pain that is totally different from the approach of other specialties, including those from which they originate. They make well-reasoned attempts to reproduce findings obtained with data that are still not very well known, or that are still experimental. Or, when it is possible to exploit certain avenues opened up by gate control theory, technological innovations are attempted with which other teams have already experimented.

Some types of pain do not respond to these treatments, even though they focus directly on the pain. The core doctors, who have by now exhausted all the possibilities open to them, then envisage looking at the problem in other terms: "At a certain point, when we have exhausted all the possibilities in terms of drugs or physical treatments or infiltration (which are never iatrogenic at this level, because with a bit of experience you very quickly realize what's going on) . . . you say to yourself: maybe the psychiatrist should see the patient to make sure there isn't something else underneath and that we're not right off target."

The psychiatrist is the only physician in the center to intervene at a second stage, thereby overlaying the hierarchical multidisciplinary concept of pain with another concept of pain, again dual, stemming from the classical organic/mind dichotomy. To be clear, Bonica's work to establish chronic pain as a new medical entity inevitably leads to a recognition of the psychological dimensions of the pain phenomenon. This center, like all centers, sees this assumption as central. However, in the recourse to a psychiatrist as practiced here, there is no intention of activating the second path for gate control theory. Rather, the patient's pain situation is redefined within the framework of the organic/mind dichotomy. In gate control theory, psychological factors and cognitive processes intervene in the somatic transmission of messages. They are conceptually integrated as a component of the multidimensional pain phenomenon. In the context of this center's approach to the theory, however, they constitute an alternative dimension:

> Before you say glossodynia, coccycodynia, you do all the examinations. You can block ganglions, you can do rachianalgesia, they'll still complain of pain. It's terrible. You do phenolization, you burn the sacral nerves, but it doesn't work, they're still complaining of pain. [IB: So what do you do then?] We call it pain sine materia. When you can't find anything, when you've cut all the afferentia and everything that could trigger this pain . . . , then you have to envisage the possibility that the problem is elsewhere.

What is defined here is a two-tier approach: the first being purely medical and somatic and a possible second phase, which is psychiatric (upon which the patient will or will not agree to embark). For the core physician, the problem then no longer enters directly into his or her sphere of competence, which explains the way these physicians define themselves with respect to other centers: "We are somatic specialists."[16] Professionally speaking, this phase no longer concerns them. It is not part of what they consider to be their work. Conversely, a pain center should be competent to deal with it, and this is why a psychiatrist is essential. Up to a certain point, this is also part of the task of the neurologists who "have a closer relationship" with patients. The follow-up here is longer: "There's not just a need for brief therapeutic contact, you also need—there are people who need—a more lengthy kind of follow-up." However, this shouldn't become routine. "The system would seize up" since you would effectively be limiting the number of potential new patients.[17]

The presence of different specialists in the same place is justified by the need to deal with all pain-related problems and fulfill the role of pain center. Pain—rather than the need for medical work—plays the federative role. In fact, although consultant specialists and core physicians discuss problems from time to time and find these discussions mutually enriching, as in any hospital department, there are no routinely organized interdisciplinary work meetings. However, the core doctors are continually in contact with each other. The work done to translate the aspects of gate control theory into practice is structured around the first path for modulation of pain messages. Without being ignored, the second path is not developed as such. The psychological approach used is based more on a classic psychiatric analysis of psychogenic pain than on an attempt to integrate the data of gate control theory.

CENTER 2: HEALING THROUGH MANAGEMENT

The First Steps

Integrating the two avenues created by gate control theory, the second center gradually built up an approach to chronic pain based on achieving control or management of pain rather than on curing it. In this respect, it differs not only from the first center but also from the dominant schemas in medicine, which are concerned much more with acute than with chronic illness (see, e.g., Strauss 1975; Baszanger 1986). It started up in 1977 within the framework of a functional exploration laboratory in a teaching hospital. At that time, a neurophysiologist became interested simultaneously in "the practical application of gate control theory, [that is], methods for treating pain by peripheral stimulation . . . and techniques of acupuncture" (whose effects had found a new explanatory framework with gate control theory). He set up a small practice based on individual consultations, with the aim of repeating in clinical practice findings essentially discovered in the laboratory: "At the very beginning, when a patient was seen for a functional exploration . . . we prolonged electromyograph stimulation to see whether the pain was modified by stimulation at that particular instant. . . . To begin with, we were mostly concerned with the mechanism but [we wondered] how we could make it work effectively in clinical practice."

Patients were mostly referred by surgical and neurosurgical departments that hoped these patients would benefit from these specific techniques. At this point, the question became what to do with people who were not really helped by these techniques, or for whom such techniques were not advisable. From this preoccupation came the idea of a pain consultation and then a pain center. First came an attempt to set up informal multidisciplinary meetings between the heads of the neurophysiology, psychiatry, and anesthesia departments in the hospital. This was rather short-lived, since each specialist continued to practice his own specialty in his own physical space and the multidisciplinary "blend" failed to "take." [18] Then, the neurophysiologist organized multidisciplinary consultations. His main weapon was his experience, gained in 1977, when he participated in the early stages of a multidisciplinary consultation group for patient orientation in another teaching hospital.[19] There he took part in discussions organized between guest specialists after the patient had been seen by a neurologist and a psychiatrist. In October 1980, he set up a group comprised of himself, a neurologist, and a psychiatrist, seconded by their respective departments. At this point, the anesthesiological component had disappeared: "We took people in the afternoon, three patients, three for each physician. We all came at two o'clock, and each physician took a patient; we swapped around and then around five or six o'clock we had a meeting." After this consultation, the patient was referred for follow-up, either by the neurologist or the neurophysiologist (who had been joined by a young woman general practitioner studying neurophysiology). At this time, the psychiatrist was not involved in patient follow-up, although his diagnostic role was very important and his advice a valuable contribution to the therapy.

Opening Up toward Another Approach to Pain

This preliminary collaboration soon seemed inadequate. Here, however, the setup was extended not by taking in other specialties, as occurred in the other center, but by redefining the very concept of chronic pain and the manner of

treating it. The small initial group very quickly became aware of the reversi-
bility of the results obtained. "We saw people whom we apparently succeeded
in curing only for three months, since as soon as they were once more exposed
to unfavorable conditions, they were back again." This was how these physicians came to question the idea of an objective seen in terms of cure and to
move toward a new model of pain and a new work object: the management of
chronic pain.

> At the beginning when the neurologist and the psychiatrist joined the
> team, we said: It's going to be great, we'll really be able to solve problems.
> . . . Then we realized that things were not so clear-cut. We began to lose
> the habit of thinking only along these lines and realized that there were
> many patients whose initial pain was, say, somatic or neurological, but
> once there was no guarantee that the pain would definitely disappear . . . ,
> you also had to take into account the person, his or family environment,
> problems with work etc. . . . We had wanted to get rid of the pain, we saw
> the pain as something we had to fight, something we were going to cure.
> But over the last two or three years, we have developed another aim: we
> will first of all teach people how to deal with pain, teach them how to live
> with it, whatever its original cause.

This gradual shift from "cure" to "management" was achieved by incorporating new dimensions: the person and his or her personal and professional
environments. The concept of pain as a lesion was replaced by the concept of
pain in terms of the person in pain. Indeed, at the same time as he observed the
temporary nature of the results obtained, the initiating physician also became
aware of a rift between two types of approach (somatic and psychiatric) and
the fact that psychodynamic psychiatry was unable to breach this. Therefore,
there was a need to seek another theoretical framework:

> We felt that there was a huge rift between the somatic approach and the
> psychiatric approach. We just couldn't figure it out. There was a kind of
> vacuum and we didn't know how to fill it. First, there were ways of ex-
> plaining the illness to patients, helping them visualize the pain, which
> are strictly verbal techniques. The second point was to educate patients
> a little so that they could make a choice, adopt the most appropriate
> attitudes, whatever the origin of the pain. Here too, we weren't really
> talking about psychiatry in the conventional sense, it was a psychologi-
> cal approach. Later there were more physical techniques beginning with
> relaxation . . . whatever the origin of the pain, whether organic or psycho-

logical, or rather of organic or psychological origin. There are moments when people are defenseless. A sort of panic reaction sets in. The idea was to give them some sort of defense against this pain. This was more or less the origin [of our use] of relaxation techniques, which were not supposed to be a psychotherapeutic choice in the sense of doing analysis through relaxation. In this way we came to develop a way of stimulating patients so that they became responsible for themselves; something more complex than simply saying: "Don't think about it, take up your normal activities" — that kind of advice. So, starting from the point where we were keen to structure our actions a little by saying: "We have to target these particular objectives," we were no longer in the field of psychiatry. . . . It was at this point that we put our finger on what would eventually become techniques [cognitive-behavioral techniques] about which we could theorize in a conceptual framework.

The progress made toward defining a new conceptual framework, as described in this lengthy excerpt from an interview, implies an application of the second path of gate control theory. This approach was anticipated by the literature: the theoretical models proposed (especially in Bonica's *Pain*) implied a blending of very different approaches as a way of changing one's perception of disciplinary boundaries. As one of the leading physicians commented: "I believe that the borders defining specialties have disappeared. You read medical journals or conference reports and almost without realizing it, you find yourself reading the words of a psychiatrist and straight afterwards those of a behavioral psychologist or a neurophysiologist. There are some very significant overlaps. . . . I'm sure I've been 'contaminated' [by other kinds of knowledge] in this way."

Toward an Integrated Approach

Gradually, an approach to the patient and his or her pain emerged that integrated the two paths suggested by gate control theory: working on physical processes through drugs, stimulation, acupuncture, and so forth, and working on cognitive processes through a cognitive-behavioral approach. Sometimes, the two paths blend, as in certain relaxation type techniques that act both on the muscles and on the content of the person's thoughts:

At the beginning . . . we used mostly explanations . . . , drugs, and techniques like acupuncture, stimulation, and it's true that we came to a bit of a standstill when they didn't work. But there was a kind of psychotherapeutic approach, after all . . . and people began to discuss things. . . . [T]hen there was the introduction of behavioral therapies, relaxation, and so on, and then two years ago, the [patient] groups. This was the beginning, the start-up period. . . . Things have changed, now we tend to give people a whole package. . . . In a way, we gradually adopted an approach more specifically focusing on pain itself.

This "package" corresponds to an "integrated, extensive" treatment of chronic pain (in fact, less of chronic pain than of a person who is then referred to as "a person in chronic pain"). According to this concept, pain is defined as "poorly adapted behavior." Within this framework, a new diagnostic category, the "chronic pain syndrome," is defined as being a "set of attitudes and behavior that will increase and sustain pain." In other words, this new diagnostic category is no longer based only on understanding the cause of the painful stimulus, but also on analyzing the response to the painful stimulus (the reaction of the person to his or her pain), thus allowing plenty of room for the idea of the variable link between stimulus and response developed in gate control theory.

An Integrated Multidisciplinarity

In contrast to the hierarchical multidisciplinarity of the first center, this development redirected the way in which work was organized toward an integrated multidisciplinarity. The team was joined by new members and the work of each member was more precisely defined.[20] As in the first center, there are differences between the members, but the organization of the work as a function of the final objective does not involve a break between a hard core of practitioners and other specialists acting as pain consultants.[21] Each physician, as an individual, gradually came to modify his or her practice as his or her involvement with problems of chronic pain evolved. In addition, modifications also occurred as a function of changes in the group's theory and practice under the influence of the coordinating physician. The latter's role was to act as a kind of "scout," who "routinely initiated work in new fields." The two general practitioners, while being trained to handle a specific medical field, were also trained on the job to use the basic drugs used in a pain center. As the research of the coordinating physician evolved, they received additional training in the use of cognitive-behavioral techniques. At the same time, the neurologist became interested in stimulation, and the psychoanalyst, when treating a patient, noted that her "psychiatry-based approach now takes in some of the other elements I've learned here." At least once a week, some time is set aside for team members to work together "with the aim of bringing our concepts and our ways of doing things in line." In other words, there is a definite will to broaden the specialist's outlook and the ever-present idea is that to deal with pain you need to take an approach that differs slightly from your traditional approaches. In this sense, all the team members gradually learned to take "this wide-based behavioral approach."

Various areas of overlap and transfer of tasks emerged in the course of this development:

> The problem is one—how can I put it?—of degree of difficulty. So, if we're talking about a problem to do with drugs, say prescribing an anti-depressant . . .—everyone here knows how to prescribe it. But if the problem is to find the right drug for a person suffering from side-effects or anticholinergic effects, this means finding an antidepressant that has an analgic effect. . . . The same technical act becomes a little more complex and you might prefer to ask the advice of the psychiatrist . . . or alter-natively the internist. So, we're not talking about separate fields, there's an important overlap. Another example, if the neurologist notes that a patient has a stimulation problem, he will see the patient and prescribe this for him or her. But if the problem is more technical in nature, he'll discuss the matter with someone else. I believe that these exchanges occur more or less in the same way for all problems.

According to this way of looking at the problem, each person loses his or her identity as specialist X or Y to become a pain specialist.[22]

A Lengthy, Specific Follow-up of Chronic Pain

In this second center, there is no initial sorting of patients. Routine multidisci-plinary consultation—a neurologist, a psychiatrist, the coordinating physi-cian—has been abandoned in favor of a preliminary orientation consultation, usually done by the coordinating physician. The diagnostic phase focuses on evaluating the "chronic pain syndrome." The origin of the pain is verified from a physiological point of view, but the main point here is to examine the situa-tion of the person with respect to the overall pain phenomenon: "If on the one hand you have a well-investigated, precisely defined lesion, and if you have the elements of chronic pain syndrome, that is, if you can understand the persistence and amplification of the pain via a whole series of pathological variables . . . from that point on, the choice is made as far as we are concerned."

This evaluation decides on the orientation of the patient toward the different therapists according to a certain theoretical logic. A first referral may be decided on as a function of the skills of the person involved (internal medicine, psychiatry, technical specialization) and, as we have seen, the degree of difficulty of the problem in question. However, the gradual implementation of a treatment more specifically aimed at chronic pain as defined in this center may lead to treatment by two therapists working together, or two therapists working individually, or one therapist working with a group of patients. After the first consultation, the coordinating physician may organize a multidisciplinary consultation with the neurologist and the psychiatrist to define a therapeutic orientation. These multidisciplinary consultations are more likely to be set up if the physician responsible for the patient encounters some sort of blockade. It is impossible to describe a typical follow-up, although its purpose can be defined: to give patients a useful way of visualizing their pain, to help them try new ways of reacting to pain and learn how to use the available techniques. In other words: to help them manage their pain. They learn how to do this by using cognitive-behavioral techniques alongside the other available physical and chemical techniques — and the process requires time. An average follow-up lasts several months, with one consultation a week, while the follow-up for the most difficult cases lasts some eighteen months.

According to this center, their type of behavioral treatment, aimed at helping patients manage the pain, is the essential characteristic of a pain center. This definition helps us understand the position adopted by the center with respect to the question of diagnosis and especially with respect to its place in the overall health system. "We don't see ourselves as a diagnostic structure," or "The function of [pain centers] is not to establish a somatic diagnosis for a given pain," the coordinating physician states (Boureau, Luu, and Koskas 1985). This diagnostic dimension, in the classic sense, is done at an earlier stage. Close links with other hospital departments have developed, such as with the gynecology department. This department will refer patients experiencing pain for whom it no longer has anything to offer in terms of gynecological treatments. The pain center is seen as the end of the line (a last recourse): it will not waste its time establishing yet another gynecological report but will evaluate the pain itself and the person experiencing it.

CREATING A GROUP WITHIN RECOGNIZED BOUNDARIES

At the same time that these physicians were busy setting up their own pain centers, they were also working in a more collective way. Despite the internal differences between the two extremes of the continuum represented by the two centers examined, they cooperated in an attempt to establish a role for pain medicine within the medical world. Generally speaking, as soon as physicians attempt to begin practicing as pain physicians, they encounter a dual difficulty in defining their place. This difficulty is linked to the successive transformations of the status of pain. Briefly, we can identify a long period in the history of medicine during which the doctor dealing with pain generally established a diagnosis and a prognosis, and then treated the patient essentially by treating the symptoms.[23] With effective therapies such as sulfonamides or antibiotics came a second phase, in which physicians believed it was necessary "to respect the pain." As a symptom, it allowed them to discover the origin of the disease. The next step was to treat the disease — which would in theory lead to the disappearance of the pain. Any treatment that focused on treating the pain directly became reprehensible, to say the least, and symptomatic medicine was stigmatized as charlatanism. This was especially true since at the beginning of this period, medicine as an institution still had to fight to establish its exclusive right to deal with the problem of pain. Bonica and gate control theory ushered in a third period, in which pain is defined as the target of medical action. The context of this action has changed, however: here the task at hand is to tackle "pain as disease."

Examining this development, the risk that this approach to pain will be confused with "alternative therapies" defined as dangerous (since they are interested only in symptoms) by hospital and academic medicine becomes evident. In addition, by defining their central object as any pain that has lasted for three to six months and that has resisted the usual treatments, pain physicians introduce a second difficulty with respect to the logic of traditional medicine. They propose a transversal break in the order of specialties, which might cast doubt on the current categorization of pathologies and hence of patients. If, for example, back pain has lasted for over six months, by whom should the patient be seen: a rheumatologist or a pain physician? Pain physicians have to convince the medical world that they should be granted their own place within this world. As a group, they have to modify the boundaries of the general medical world, without however transforming it too far: they must also avoid the risk of rejection through assimilation with symptomatic medicine or various "prescientific healers." Pain physicians believe that pain medicine should evolve as a scientific medicine in the hospital framework — in medicine's "hardest" segment. The remarks of these physicians reflect their initial fear of being discounted, of "being taken for some kind of clown," to use their own words. When addressing conferences that are not specialized in pain, they hesitate about how to present pain as the target of medical intervention, no matter what their particular concept of pain is. Especially when they were not yet very

well known, certain strategies proved to be effective when faced with these difficulties. They often began their address by referring to the treatment of pain
associated with cancer, whereas in fact this was far from being the major aspect
of their activity. As I myself witnessed, they adopted this strategy even when
dealing with an audience that was very little concerned with cancer, such as a
psychiatric service attached to a major teaching hospital. Cancer pain is then
used as an instrument of legitimation,[24] serving as a basis for subsequent and
perhaps much less consensual messages. In this way, potentially controversial
techniques can be presented, the use of which they believe can be justified scientifically. Hence, when they present a technique such as hypnosis, they not
only redefine it as "deep relaxation," but also literally submerge the presentation of the technique in refinements of gate control theory, thereby giving it a
solid, scientific base.

But it is first of all in the world of actual practice, in the hospital, that each
physician must try to define his or her role, demonstrate his or her legitimacy. I
will briefly indicate the main strategies they use, which can be seen as processes
of legitimation based on claiming worth (e.g., Strauss 1982).[25] Pain physicians
develop a service-based strategy by presenting their work as an additional
space for patients to whom medicine has nothing more to offer. By highlighting the "scandal" involved in letting patients suffer, they can both reaffirm their
specific worth with respect to a shared ideal of relieving suffering and demonstrate their own expertise as physicians who have developed new techniques
around an original theoretical body of work. Gate control theory here serves
as a resource for delineating boundaries with the rest of the medical world and
defining a common identity.

In addition, information is a tool used to give greater visibility. It is directed
at other physicians in different ways: physicians working in the hospital where
the centers are located are offered familiarization meetings or receive person-
alized mail, while other physicians hear from this group's work through post-
graduate teaching, conferences, books, or magazine articles. The greatest boost
to the group's social visibility is undoubtedly due to the information directed
at the general public—as illustrated by the increasing number of articles, programs, and books that appear every year. Indeed, through communicating with
potential patients and their families and friends they also communicate with
their physicians, since a consultation in a center can only be obtained through
referral by a personal physician. Note that whatever the origin of this information, it benefits the group as a whole—internal differences are never highlighted in these attempts to communicate with the general public. Physicians
representing very different approaches often participate in the same events,

whether professional or directed solely to the general public. It is better to participate than to be absent—and, despite the real internal differences, what is good for one is also good for the other.

However, differences cannot always be submerged and can also have negative consequences. Based on the initial results obtained, the collective work initiated to gain legitimacy in the medical world was extended to take in more specific objectives. Attempts were made to create a body of teaching specifically concerned with pain or to collaborate with the authorities to define the quality criteria that would govern official recognition. Internal differences, however, have greatly hampered—and will continue to hamper—these efforts. Local teaching methods, for example, are sanctioned by a national diploma. In other words, the first stages of official recognition of pain medicine acknowledge these major internal differences instead of minimizing them. This insistence on differences takes its toll, however, as can be seen from the attempt to produce a report for the French Health Department. Here, the government asked the profession to define criteria that would allow control or development of these centers in the future. No internal agreement was reached, since the representatives of each approach promoted their respective models to the exclusion of the others. The final agreement, oriented toward the outside world, was based on major principles such as multidisciplinarity, presence of a psychiatrist or psychologist, and the referral of patients by a physician, leaving the way open for many forms of organization around different definitions of pain. But although the report constitutes a success for pain medicine, it cannot, because of its lack of precision, serve as a basis for encouraging the authorities to take steps to develop this area. Despite the official definition of a program to combat pain, the problem of pain plays a minor part in their preoccupations.

CONCLUSION

Comparing the development of two pain centers, we can understand how the emerging group of pain physicians takes form around pronounced internal differences. In the work of creating a medical practice to deal with pain, different physicians, confronted with the same need to enlarge the basis of their initial practices in order to tackle the problems related to pain, interpret the same conceptual resource in a different way. The fact that these divergent interpretations are all *based on practice rather than theory* tends to make them more stable. Similarly, the fact that the creation of techniques for treating patients and the methods of collaboration (type of follow-up, of multidisciplinarity, recourse to certain techniques of treatment) are closely associated with the elaboration of an operative definition of chronic pain and pain medicine also has a stabilizing effect. For example, we have seen that it is by focusing on the importance of certain dimensions (such as the individual, his/her environment and his/her behavior) that a group is encouraged to adopt techniques capable of addressing these dimensions. When these techniques are put into practice, they in turn tend to modify the objective of the treatment (from healing pain to managing it), thereby redefining chronic pain around the person and his or her pain (or the chronic pain syndrome). In this sense, the elaboration of techniques structures practice, which in itself cannot be dissociated from the definition of its objective.

Parallel to this work of development, the very mechanism of which tends to separate those involved in it, there is the attempt to position the profession with regard to the medical world as a whole. Using the same theoretical references and deploying common strategies, this attempt contributes to the constitution of a group identity. This double movement highlights the role of a boundary theory: to federate the whole while tolerating pronounced internal differences. Within this framework, differences occur at two levels: on the one hand, in the process of segmentation, allowing practitioners to move away from their original discipline and toward a new specialty. On the other hand (and this is less known) differences occur at the heart of the work of internal legitimation. This rather strained situation may, because of the mechanism involved, last for quite a long time, and indeed is its normal modus vivendi. We can thus understand how a community of practice may, from the outset, be made up of micro-groups with different definitions of the central object of their practice, without necessarily splitting into further segments. The legitimacy of the new segment can then be seen as having a dual aspect. It appears solid when used to establish boundaries with neighboring worlds and at the same time fragile within these boundaries whenever it must be decided whether pain medicine has a single legitimacy or whether there are multiple practices that represent it. That a stable, unconditional form of legitimacy established around dimensions that are the same for all can coexist with an open, virtually conditional form of the mutual recognition granted between peers is exactly what a boundary object can authorize.

NOTES

Translated by Philippa Crutchley-Wallis. I want to thank Adele Clarke, Charis Cussins, Annemarie Mol, and Marc Berg for their help and comments.

1   Cf. Strauss 1978a; 1982; 1984; Bucher 1988; Bucher and Strauss 1961; Clarke 1990a; 1991.
2   The concept of boundary object was proposed by Star and Griesemer (1989) as a

way of illustrating how to articulate activities at the intersection of different worlds and understanding how heterogeneous interactions can be effective. For them, a boundary object is an object that simultaneously inhabits different worlds and is capable of responding to their varied demands. These objects are both flexible enough to respond to the local needs and constraints of the different groups using them and also hardy enough to preserve unity around a project over and above the diversity of its areas of use. In other words, they are hardy enough to maintain unity and flexible enough to allow differences. They are loosely structured when used as common objects and highly structured when used as local objects.

3 As we will see, these physicians come from different branches of medicine — but the different approaches they develop are not necessarily related to their original specialty. For example, we find anesthetists working according to either of the two approaches.

4 The classification of American pain centers by Csordas and Clark (1992), although undertaken for quite different reasons, illustrates this cleavage between two approaches.

5 See, e.g., Bonica 1953. I will not go into detail here about his untiring efforts to promote this new field, but we should note that this theory, first presented in *Science* in 1965, allowed him, with the support of Melzack and Wall, to literally create a world of pain. They brought together scientists, physicians from a wide variety of specialties and clinical psychologists in an International Association for the Study of Pain (IASP) in 1974. The extension of pain medicine to different countries — at varying rates — only began in earnest thereafter. Various other elements made a vital contribution to this movement: transformations in medicine linked to the extreme development of specialization, the "psychologization" of society, developments in anesthesiology, the beginnings of a transformation in ways of dealing with death are some examples. It is not essential to look at these matters, since I am interested here in some practical realizations related to this movement, which in any case they help to reinforce by their very existence. On Bonica and the beginnings of pain medicine, see Baszanger 1995.

6 This pain center model is represented by the Washington University center directed by John Bonica, who referred to it constantly in the literature — in its different forms — since its creation in 1961. Along with other centers, it also served as a reference in the first conference in 1973, which was a basis for the creation of the International Association for the Study of Pain. Subsequently, different guidelines were published, although these focus on institutional matters and only mention the practical content of pain medicine in passing.

7 The theory of specificity (1894) has always been contested by another theory known as pattern theory, according to which the sensation of pain results from special patterns of intensity of stimuli and interpretation by the brain and no specific nerve ending is necessary to transmit the influx. The theory of specificity has dominated medical practice and teaching right up to our own day (cf. Rey and Wallace 1995).

8   This is the whole panoply of nerve or nerve block infiltrations (introducing a needle into an underlying structure and injecting certain substances or heat with the aim of blocking a nerve fiber temporarily or definitively, depending on the case). With the development of these techniques, the field of intervention of anesthetists was transformed; in certain cases, they became "remote" surgeons, that is, operating via needles and without direct contact with the organ in question.

9   This is a small box, around the same size as a Walkman, to which are connected two or four electrodes placed at certain points on the skin, according to certain principles and in relation to the pain. This box, which is in turn attached to a belt, is often referred to by journalists as the "antipain battery" or the "antipain black box."

10 For a description of the principles behind these cognitive-behavioral techniques and their medical use, see Baszanger 1993.

11 For a historical analysis of "pain medicine" and a detailed observation of medical practices, physician-patient relationships, and patients' logics of action in this new field see Baszanger 1995.

12 See for instance Kotarba 1977; Hilbert 1984; Corbett 1986; and Jackson 1992.

13 It started much later than others, notably much later than the second center. However, I am examining it first since it represents an option very frequently developed, the logic behind which can be smoothly integrated in that of usual medical practice in hospitals.

14 By demonstrating their usefulness for the hospital and for patients (through, e.g., activity reports), they succeeded in having all services relevant to their work participate in setting up the center. At the same time, this guaranteed them a certain autonomy, since no particular service (primarily anesthesiology or neurosurgery) can today claim it as its own. This method of constitution quite closely reflects the possibilities of and limitations to the independence of a pain center carrying out anesthetic and surgical activities. The center is structured around a hard core of three physicians who, in order to carry out their work, circulate between different places: the consulting rooms, three hospital departments (neurosurgery, digestive surgery, neurology), and various places where technical operations are carried out (i.e., a neurosurgical operating room, and the postoperative room in the anesthesiology–intensive care ward for blocks and infiltrations). These different places are available to them according to a fixed calendar and they are not obliged to negotiate on a case-by-case basis for hospital beds or operating theaters and so forth. Conversely, only a specialized pain department would allow them to bring all these places together in one location. This is not on their agenda, however.

15 For example, talking to one of the neurologists: (IB: Do you do other neurological consultations?) Yes, I have one other consultancy. (IB: Is your practice different here?) Yes, it's very different. Well . . . if I hadn't got involved in antipain consultation, I would have missed out on something in terms of contact with the patient and then in terms of the therapy. I think this type of patient really irritated me before. . . . When I saw the pile of prescriptions, I used to say to myself: Well, this

looks pretty hopeless. . . . But at some point, I said to myself: this is a pain consultation, I'm here to deal with this type of patient. . . . I'm sitting in this room and my job is to treat people in pain. You obviously can't have the same attitude as in a conventional consultation where you're in a hurry and your priorities are different."

16   This of course does not exclude using a certain degree of psychology to deal with somatic problems, which, because they have lasted for a long time, have psychologically affected the patient. These physicians also draw upon an everyday psychiatric framework in dealing with pain that they decipher as not completely organic. For the way in which physicians in the center distinguish between these pains and those requiring psychiatric treatment, cf. Baszanger 1992.

17   It is clear however that the "core" physicians, that is, primarily the two anesthetists, are constantly called on to practice this type of follow-up because of the type of patient they receive (see the preceding footnote).

18   There were structural reasons for this, since the anesthetics department was at this time obliged to handle increasingly diversified services within the hospital and tended to be more easily isolated. This was especially true since, at the same time, the change in the neurophysiological specialty of the functional exploration of pain allowed redeploying activities and resources to pain.

19   Quite deliberately, this consultation group was never developed into a center. See Baszanger 1987.

20   The team is made up of the coordinating physician, a neurologist who comes two days a week, a psychiatrist-psychoanalyst who comes one day a week (corresponding to one of the neurologist's days), two general practitioners who have gradually specialized in the techniques (one more particularly in nerve stimulation, another in relaxation), a consulting-room nurse who plays an important role in receiving the patients and who has them fill out a series of questionnaires, and a second psychiatrist specializing in behavioral psychology, who does not play a diagnostic role. Finally, there is an associate anesthetist who intervenes on a case-by-case basis.

21   Except in the case of the anesthetist, who is presented as an exception to the complete integration of the team, since she has chosen to work differently from the rest of the group: "She feels that she is there to carry out technical procedures, that is, if we need a morphine catheter, we can have it, if we need an anesthetic block we can have it, but she doesn't feel that by carrying out this technical operation, she must necessarily take responsibility for patients, or if you like, take complete responsibility for the patient for whom she is carrying out the operation in question."

22   This is why we find other centers that have developed the same approach as this one. In these centers, managed by anesthetists or neurosurgeons in which other anesthetists may work, each of these specialists will have moved away from his or her original discipline. Not gradually, as in the case of the first center (which has remained very close in spirit to the original discipline of anesthesiology or neurosurgery), but in a more abrupt way that is similar to a rupture. On these segmentation processes see Strauss 1982.

23   For the history of pain, see Rey and Wallace 1995.
24   That the pain linked to cancer serves as an instrument of legitimation is not with-
     out irony. This group of physicians and others still have to fight very hard to ensure
     that it is treated effectively by the different hospital departments and by liberal
     physicians who, very often, request advice and intervention from the pain center
     very late, in some cases much too late.
25   On this point and for a more detailed development of the whole of this part, see
     Baszanger 1990.

MISSING LINKS, MAKING LINKS:
THE PERFORMANCE
OF SOME ATHEROSCLEROSES

Annemarie Mol

▼

This text is about the multiple ontology of the body and its diseases. It is also about the way atherosclerosis is handled in present day—how to call it: Western? cosmopolitain? scientific? allopathic?—medicine.[1] It uses empirical stories to tell a philosophical tale.

Various medical disciplines tell different tales about atherosclerosis. They stress the thickening of the intima of the vessel wall, vessel diameter reduction, changes in blood flow, pain, necrosis. They talk about thrombus formation, high-density lipoproteins, age of onset, smoking, hormonal protection. It is possible to try to link these entities together, to call some of them causes, and others effects; to say that some are symptoms, while others are the underlying disease. It is possible to say that all these stories point to aspects of a single object: that of atherosclerosis.

But medicine doesn't handle "atherosclerosis" by means of storytelling alone. Hospitals brim with all kinds of other activities, too. Doctors interview patients, do physical examinations, judge the outcomes of diagnostic techniques, insert needles in vessel lumina, cut open living bodies in the operation theater and dead ones in the dissection room. Patients describe their histories, lie flat, walk, swallow pills, mobilize their strength. Technicians use ultrasound, X rays, electron microscopes, and ballpoint pens, to make pictures and to generate numbers. And researchers cut pieces out of vessel walls, write down numbers, dilute fluids, feed their computers, read, and present others with their findings.

In writing or talk one may try to answer the question "What is atherosclerosis?" But the activities that fill hospitals also have to do with "atherosclerosis." Not just by pointing at it, saying what it is, where it is, or whether it is, but also by handling it. Acting upon it, transforming it, they *do* atherosclerosis. They *perform* it.

Anthropologists interested in native knowledge, may ask the people they study what they think. And hope to hear interpretations of reality.[2] But anthropologists may also try to investigate what people do. Ask them about, and observe, their activities. The latter method makes it possible for researchers to reconstruct the world not through a grid of attributed meanings, but through a series of interventions carried out—which allows them to talk about realities that are performed.[3]

"Atherosclerosis" is a disease of blood vessels. There are blood vessels everywhere in the body. My study, however, starts off from atherosclerosis as it manifests itself in the lower limbs, the legs. I didn't want to be side-tracked too much by the complicated consequences bad vessels may have in brains, kidneys, or the heart. I preferred to start off from a relatively simple place, for I expected the complexities to abound. Moreover, where so many philosophers—especially ethicists—focus on dramatic questions of life and death, I preferred to study more banal deliberations about day-to-day life, which had the additional advantage that it made my role as an observer a little easier, and less disturbing to the people I observed.

"Western medicine" is a grandiose category. The site of my study is far smaller: it is a single Dutch university hospital. The textbooks and journals in its library are mostly in English. The medical doctors and researchers who work in the hospital attend Dutch, European, North American, and world conferences. Someone from Portugal may work for a while in a lab, collaborating with a Chinese refugee. A Swiss may come and see how a new endovascular procedure is done, and the speakers at a local conference about this procedure are from Brazil, Britain, Germany, California. Meanwhile routine handling of patients with atherosclerosis in the next Dutch hospital, thirteen kilometers away, is markedly different. I investigated my "site" as an ethnographer, attending meetings, investigations, operations, consultations, and other kinds of work. But I also read medical texts and talked with practitioners of various kinds. My aim was not to map as many details as possible, but to begin to unravel patterns in the coexistence of a variety of "atheroscleroses."

AN ABSENT LINK

In the textbook they may be printed on a single page: a list of patient *complaints* and a picture of a *thickened intima* of a vessel wall. A story articulates a link between the two by putting several intermediaries between them. It tells that the intima may grow so thick that the *vessel diameter* gets smaller and smaller. At some critical point, it becomes so small that too little blood reaches the downstream tissues, and *oxygen supplies* fall short. If the muscles move with too little oxygen, this leads to *pain*. There we are: the story starts out with an intima and needs only a few lines to end with the pain complained about by the patient.

Presenting the textbook as a place where links are easy gives me a point of contrast that allows me to show how difficult it is to make links in the hospital. But is it fair? Textbooks aren't smooth. They contain gaps and frictions. A small amount of serious text analysis is enough to find this out.[4] Medical textbooks, after all, talk not only of entities such as "vessel diameter" and "oxygen supply." They are also about practice. They say such things as: "Peripheral vascular disease is assessed by a careful history and clinical examination for signs of ischaemia, absent pulses, audible bruits over the proximal arteries, poor skin nutrition, low skin temperature, and loss of hair, and then by blood pressure measurement" (Souhami and Moxham 1990: 448). Textbooks are not only about the body, but also contain a wealth of information about how diseases are—or should be—"assessed."

How are *complaints* and *the intima of the vessel wall* linked in hospital practice? In order to answer that question, I'll take you to hospital Z and tell a few stories.

In the *consulting room* a vascular surgeon has nodded a welcome to a patient, and now asks some questions. I sit in a corner and listen. "Where does it hurt, can you say, Mr. Stenis?" The patient answers, "Yes, doctor, down here it starts, down here, in my calf, beneath my knee, in the left leg, in this leg only." Doctor: "And can you also tell when it hurts? Is there a pattern?" Mr. Stenis: "Oh, sure, sure there is, it's when I walk, doctor. When I stop, I'm fine. After just a few minutes I'm fine again. But then it starts, after a while, when I walk along, it starts all over. Again and again." Doctor: "How far can you walk before it hurts, I mean, what kind of distance?" Mr. Stenis: "Now I have to think, doctor. How far is it? I can get from our place to the park alright. That's where I walk the dog, you see. And when I rest, I can cross the big lawn. That's, I dare say, what is it, 100 meters, 150 meters, something like that." The doctor nods. "Now, Mr. Stenis, could you now take off your trousers, please, and lie on the bench? You can leave your underpants on, yes."

By asking questions, the vascular surgeon makes his patient tell about pain and impairments. These are the complaints that go by the name of *intermittent claudication*. There are varieties. This patient walks one hundred meters, the next three hundred. Yet another reports that her pain doesn't stop when she rests: that is a worse case. Talk about pain that only begins upon resting, however, or about pain that markedly differs from one day to another, makes a "wrong" story. With such talk a disease may be articulated, but it is not atherosclero-sis in the leg vessels. In the outpatient clinic the performance of atherosclerosis depends first and foremost on the doctor's eliciting and the patient's expressing the complaints called "intermittent claudication": pain after walking a specific distance, that makes one stop before walking on again.

Maybe I shouldn't put quotation marks around utterances, for I didn't record the conversations. I made short notes between the visits by patients and wrote down long notes a few hours later. I also noted down—some of—what I saw. Mr. Stenis sits slightly bent forward. Then undresses in a corner. He doesn't close the curtain. His saggy body doesn't look like any photo you'd see publicly printed. The surgeon's pockets bulge with useful objects. Like him, I wear a white coat and a name badge, but I have no stethoscope. But such details are endless. If I were to start to make them relevant, I would lose the line of my story.

In the pathology department there are no patients. But there is "patient ma-terial." It's been cut out of a body, sliced thin, put on a glass slide, fixed, colored, covered with a protective glass sheet.

A pathologist in training looks through the microscope. He sees disease and points it out to me. "There, that's the lumen. It's shifted a bit—that's an artefact of making the slide. Here, this line of cells, they're fairly dis-tinctive—that's the endothelium. Now here, where the pointer goes, you see, here's the line between the intima and the media. So there's the in-tima, all this bit. That's impressive. Okay, now you've seen what you came looking for: there's your atherosclerosis!" He sounds as if he were pleased for both of us. Takes out a bit of paper and a pen and produces a short de-scription of the vessel wall, noting down carefully from which vessel part the pieces of wall were taken.

Atherosclerosis is performed in two ways at least. One that is clinical, which involves talk and physical examination, and another, having to do with pathol-ogy, in which one looks at a slide through a microscope. In the clinic, one could say, atherosclerosis *is* claudication. While in the department of pathology, atherosclerosis *is* a microscopically enlarged thickening of the vessel wall. But how do these two objects relate?

Sometimes it is possible to move practically from one to the other. The slides that the pathology resident looks at are made from a thin slice of an artery cut out of an amputated lower leg. When this leg was brought into the pathology department, it was accompanied by a paper form. On this form someone had written a few lines about the "clinical condition" of the patient whose leg was amputated ("Clin.: severe rest pain, cold feet, very poor skin condition, several ulcers"). Thus there is a link. If need be, it can be enlarged, for the patient's name and hospital number are also on the form. This allows the pathologist to trace the patient's file. Or to ask the treating surgeon for a more detailed report on the clinical condition of the patient at the moment the leg was amputated and the vessels that are now under the microscope were separated from the rest of their body.

This account does not locate the atheroscleroses performed and the links between them inside the body. Instead, they are presented as a function of a wide range of habits and materials. Forms, knives, pain, hands, gloves, telephones, slides, what have you. Links of many natures. Heterogeneous links.[5]

However, it isn't always possible to make the link between clinic and pathology so easily. A patient has told a story indicating that his claudication is deteriorating rather fast and asks: "Is there anything you can do, doctor?" According to the surgeon the "clinical picture" is clear: this is a serious atherosclerosis. However, a decision about treatment will only be made with additional diagnostic information. The clinical existence of atherosclerosis is a necessary step on the way to invasive treatment, but not enough to reach there. Stories have to be backed up with pictures.

Is this the moment to ask for a pathological examination of the patient's vessel walls? Not at all! To do this someone would have to open the patient's leg up and cut a bit of vessel out. Since the whole point of additional information is to decide whether invasive *treatment* might be a good idea, such extensive invasions aren't used in *diagnosis*. Moreover, it is not clear from the story alone *where* the vessel walls with the atherosclerotic deterioration are located—the narrowing of the vessel that might "explain" the patient's problems. Even if the site of the pain—buttock, calf—may give some indication, the question about location, about "where," isn't sufficiently answered by the clinic. Thus no direct links from "claudication" to a "vessel wall with a thickened intima" are made. This link is missing.

A surgeon may *imagine* a bad vessel wall upon hearing a patient talk. He may even *draw* one when he explains it to the patient. But there and then the vessel wall of this particular patient is hidden. And the strength of the association between his complaints and his vessel wall thickening is *unknown*. Pathology cannot be practiced while a patient's skin is closed.[6] Skin can be cut through. Knives and anesthesia make this possible. Indeed, in some diseases this forms a part of diagnosis. In many patients who have complaints that sound like cancer, for instance, pieces of tissue are cut out of the body and these "biopsies" are carefully inspected by pathologists. Thus whether there are links between clinic and pathology is not a question of principle. It is a question of practice. And in the day-to-day practice of deciding how to treat people with lower-limb arterial disease, there are none.

A LOOSE LINK

A surgeon who needs to decide whether or not to propose invasive treatment to a patient with claudication, doesn't turn to pathology. There are other places to go to — to pressure measurement, for a start.

> The technologist adjusts a cuff around Mrs. Galis's arms. Inflates it. Then allows the air to escape slowly from the cuff. Meanwhile she listens through the stethoscope to sounds of blood flowing irregularly. When the blood pressure starts to be capable of resisting the cuff pressure, murmuring becomes audible — the systolic pressure — and when the cuff no longer hampers flow during the entire heart cycle this sound disappears again — the diastolic pressure. Both numbers are noted on a piece of paper. Then another, larger cuff is put around the ankle of Mrs. Galis' right leg. Inflated. Deflated. Instead of the stethoscope, the technologist now uses a Doppler apparatus. This also generates sound, but a different kind of sound. A Doppler apparatus makes blood velocity audible by emitting ultrasound, receiving its reflection and sending the difference between these signals to a speaker. As soon as blood pressure is able to resist cuff pressure, we hear "pshew, pshew." As long as this sound doesn't disappear, blood is still going to the foot. Thus it is possible to note systolic ankle pressure, even if a stethoscope cannot be used. Diastolic ankle pressure remains unknown if this method is used.

If ankle pressure is lower than arm pressure, the patient is said to have atherosclerosis in the aorta or the leg vessels. Measuring *pressure drop* is another way in which atherosclerosis is performed. The result is usually expressed as a number, the "ankle/arm index." The textbook story links pressure drop to bad vessel walls on the one hand and to complaints by patients on the other. One: poor walls are enlarged and encroach on the vessel lumen and, beyond a critical point, increase resistance to blood flowing through the vessel. And this resistance leads to a drop in pressure. Two: low blood pressure is bad for perfusion of the tissues, the oxygen supply starts to fail, this causes complaints. But how do these links work in hospital practice?

The link between the complaints of the clinic and a poor ankle/arm index is fairly easy to organize. While the patient is still in the consulting room the surgeon phones the vascular laboratory. If the technician and the Doppler are free, the patient is sent up from the outpatient clinic to the laboratory immediately, carrying a form along. Otherwise an appointment is made for a better moment. So the arrangement is easily made — but despite this, the atheroscleroses performed in the clinic and in the vascular laboratory are not always easy to map onto each other.

> "Did you see that man?" one resident says to the other while they're waiting for a meeting to begin. The resident picks up the form where the patient's ankle/arm index is written down. "He came to the hospital all alone. Unbelieveable! On his mobilette. And he said he had some problems walking. Some problems! Do you see this ankle/arm index? It's unbelievable the man can walk at all. I cannot believe it. He has no blood! If we're to believe these numbers, there's hardly any blood in his feet at all."

The object discovered by clinical means doesn't parallel the severity of that found by pressure measurement. The complaints are bad, but the ankle/arm index is a lot worse. The pattern repeats itself when more diagnostic techniques are added to the list. Yes, there are links. But time and again these reveal gaps, loose ends, complications.[7]

No, there aren't always gaps. Sometimes all findings "point in the same direction." In which direction? That of the patient's "atherosclerosis." If the various "atheroscleroses" performed, map onto each other, they may be taken to be aspects of a single entity. This single entity is then projected as a virtual object *behind the "aspects" that "surface."[8] This virtual object resides inside the body. The techniques "approach" it. There are epistemological discussions about how closely they approach it, which explore the link between virtual objects and what is known of them. Does what is known express the truth about the object, approach it asymptotically, or simply offer one out of a series of possible representations? Here, I am not exploring these questions, but looking instead at new ones. I try to shift theoretical attention from objects that are represented, to objects that are performed.*

When several "atheroscleroses" in a single patient do not coincide, it becomes difficult to believe that they can all be trusted and yet still be about a single object. At that point there are several ways to go. The first is to make a decision to trust one of them — in which case the practitioners can hold on to the idea that there is a single object-out-there. A nonvirtual one. The discrepancy between the various things said about it is glossed as a *controversy* about this object. For if two techniques say different things about "the" atherosclerosis of a single patient, only one of them can be right. Intermediate variables may disturb the validity of the other technique. For instance the sensitivity of patients with diabetes may be so poor that they hardly feel any pain even if their legs get very little oxygen. In such cases clinical complaints do not tie up with lack of oxygen. Pressure measurement may do so better. If, that is, the vessels haven't become so stiff that a cuff can no longer compress them, and if the patient is thin enough for the procedure to work. The list of possible obstacles encountered by techniques on their way to a virtual object is long.

A resident asks in a meeting: "If the *duplex* [an apparatus that combines Doppler and echo imaging] still shows flow, while on the *angiography* there is an occlusion, which one of them is right?" Upon which two surgeons reply, as if in a single voice: "The duplex." And one of them backs up the answer. "In hospital [N], when I worked there, I picked out a series of cases like that. And then, when we saw them in the operating theater, when we *opened up* the vessels, the duplex proved to be right over and over again. No exception, I think it was a series of thirteen, so that's not a lot, but there was no exception."

In this example two techniques, duplex and angiography, disagree, and a third technique, observing a vessel in the operation theater, is turned into the arbiter.[9] Looking with the naked eye at a temporarily emptied blood vessel that has been cut open with knives is said to "really" distinguish between little flow and occlusion, while duplex and angiography are more approximate in their measure of atherosclerosis. The arbiter decides duplex was right in the current controversy.

However, the diverging outcomes of various "approaches" do not necessarily lead to a debate about which "really" depicts atherosclerosis. Sometimes such diversity is treated as a simple consequence of the technicalities and interpretations involved, and it is assumed that different techniques delineate something different in the complexity of the human body. The question is no longer "Which of these outcomes is right?" but "Which of them should be taken as a lead for further action?" There is no controversy over truth, but a negotiation about *practicalities.* Take the following discussion about the question whether or not to operate on Mrs. Visser.

An X-ray picture hangs on the light box visible for everyone attending the weekly meeting of radiologists, vascular surgeons, and others involved in the diagnosis and treatment of vascular patients. The X ray shows the white shadows of dye injected in the vessels. Where the white strand gets smaller, there's *diameter loss.* That's Mrs. Visser's atherosclerosis such as depicted by angiography. The clinical story is present, too, represented by the surgeon who knows Mrs. Visser from her visits to the outpatient clinic. The negotiations start. "It doesn't look that impressive, does it?" one of the surgeons says, pointing at the light box where the X-ray pictures are suspended. "You could wait and see what happens, or that's what I'd say when I see those pictures." The treating surgeon both nods and shakes his head: "No, well, yeah. But she's really bothered by it, she is. You see, she may be seventy-nine, but this is a woman who is used to going to places. She's always traveled a lot, and now she can't, because it hurts too much. She can't walk along with others. So she's hampered, she can't do what she likes about life. So I want to try, I want to give her a chance."

The severity of the clinical complaints put in the context not of the patient's body but of her life, may outweigh the lack of severity of angiographic pictures. What is at issue in this discussion isn't whether complaints or diameter loss are closer to a hidden "real" atherosclerosis in the body. Instead, the issue is which object to intervene in: in impairments that affect the quality of life; or in a loss of vessel diameter? The question is not which is the more *real,* but which is the more *important.*

There is no once-and-for-all answer to this question. It's hard to find a general rule. Instead the issue of "what to do" is a matter for negotiation. And the result will differ from one disease to another, from one patient to another, and from one hospital to another. From one day to another, even — as the results of negotiations do.

So in hospital Z the results of techniques are not always projected back onto a single virtual object taken to be nonvirtual. Sometimes, no one tries to argue about what is "really" the case inside the patient's body. Instead, there is discussion about practicalities. In terms of technical specificities, therapeutic possibilities, priorities, amount of suffering, wishes. But the implication of this is that what I write is neither above, nor outside, my field of study. For the epistemology I am trying to undermine (which takes atherosclerosis to be an entity within the body) and my nonepistemological alternative (that a variety of different atheroscleroses are practically performed) are both defended, or better, taken as a lead for action, by some of the "natives" some of the time.[10]

In the above example, a patient had severe complaints while her doctors didn't take her angiographic picture to be very impressive. It may also happen the other way around.

An angiographic picture of Mr. Grol has been made in a small hospital, hospital W. It hangs on the light box in the decision-making meeting of hospital Z. It shows severe diameter loss. The patient's complaints, however, aren't very strong. The supervising surgeon explains: "I show it because it looks bad. But I've talked to this patient, he's hardly bothered. He walks more than one hundred meters without pain. He lives in a home. Can go and play cards in the common room. In short: I think there's no reason to intervene. I wouldn't like him to run the risks of an operation—he doesn't have enough to gain. He's pretty old. He's seventy-nine." Another surgeon nods. "If it looks like he's going to risk his leg, it's early enough to do something." The first one: "That's what I thought, but I wanted your support, for I'll have to tell something to our colleagues in hospital W. They thought we'd operate on such pictures. I'll have to explain why we won't."

A case where angiographic pictures are bad while the patient has only minor complaints is rare in hospital Z. This isn't because complaints tend to be more severe than diameter loss. But precisely because the surgeons of hospital Z consider invasive treatment only when there is severe "impairment" and do not take "diameter loss" by itself as a reason to intervene. This implies that angiographic pictures are only routinely made in hospital Z if a patient's complaints are so severe that invasive treatment is being seriously considered. Without severe complaints there are no pictures.

Outcomes can only clash if they are present. Performed. Made to be. It is only in testing that a link can be found to be loose. When a link isn't made, then it can't be loose either. It is simply missing.

A HIDDEN LINK

That the various performances of atherosclerosis do not always match, that there are gaps between them, implies that acting in terms of one may be different from acting in terms of the other. Either complaints are treated, or diameter loss is, not because either is more real than the other, but because it is more important.

Yet it is more complicated still. For even when clinical severity is most important in the *decision* about invasive treatment, surgical *treatment* deals directly not with complaints or walking capabilities, but with the vessel. The vessel lumen is stretched or stripped clean, or a bypass is made that allows the blood to avoid a long stretch of narrow lumen. All these strategies increase total vessel diameter. However, they do so in order to bring about clinical improvement. Invasive treatment isn't primarily evaluated by assessing diameter increase in angiographic pictures. Instead, the patient is asked how she's doing and how far she's able to walk without pain. So success is measured in clinical terms again. The aim of the treatment is to reduce complaints.

Interference in one object, the lumen, must do something to another, walking distance. This assumes the existence of an intimate link between the two—perhaps that they are aspects of a single object. It assumes the presence of an object to which many techniques relate, even if no single technique can tell everything about it. An object in which many techniques intervene, even if no single one has a firm hold on it. A common object. This means that when the surgeons of hospital Z attempt treatment, their epistemological position has shifted again. They project the object of their intervention and the object that requires improvement onto each other. They create a virtual object and call it real, while hoping that a patient's walking distance is improved by enlarging her vessel lumen.[11]

The strength of the link between an operation on a blood vessel and the patient's ability to walk is a matter for assessment. Indeed it is something that can be tested in practice. In the Dutch context it is fairly easy to organize a routine visit of the patient to the hospital a few weeks after invasive treatment to ask how well things are going.[12] And the results? These again range from disappointment to improvement, from complication to success. The relationship between enlarging the vessel lumen and the pain-free walking distance reported by the patient may be perfect. There may be no correlation at all. Or any shade of gray between these two extremes.

Often, however, it is more difficult to test the connection between the "atherosclerosis" that requires improvement and the "atherosclerosis" operated on. The link is hidden.

The general pracitioner lifts her eyes from what she's been writing in the patient's file on her desk and looks at Mr. Mançevic who is sitting opposite her. He has a mild claudication, his legs start to hurt after some five hundred or maybe seven hundred meters. The doctor has examined him and he's dressed again. "The problem, Mr. Mançevic, is that you have high blood pressure and you smoke. Both are what we call 'risk factors.' That is, they may cause your vessels to gradually silt up. And it seems that they've started to do so. So you've got to do something about them. You must stop smoking. That's the most important thing, that you stop smoking. And I'll give you something for your high blood pressure.

Let's start with a low dose, one pill a day, and let's see what happens."
Mr. Mançevic looks worried. Then the doctor even makes it worse. "Don't
expect that your pain will go away. It will not. If you want to be able to
walk better, you'll have to do exercises, you'll have to walk, I'll explain
about that later. But first this: if you don't take this medicine I'm prescribing, and if you don't stop smoking, you're very likely to get worse. You
may not be able to walk at all, not even a short distance, at some point
in the future. I don't want to make you afraid. But it may be the near
future."

In this conversation the talk is about pain upon walking. We've seen that before. But a new element is added. What is linked to the complaints is not the
poor wall of a vessel, or a loss of lumen hidden in the body the way it is now, but
a future. Atherosclerosis is performed as a disease that may be "mild" first and
later become "severe," as something that changes over time. The interventions
proposed by the general practitioner are interventions in this development.
The patient is urged to stop smoking in order to prevent the deterioration of
his disease. He is advised to take a medicine that will not alleviate his complaints but only prevent them from getting worse in the future.

Talk about smoking or high blood pressure doesn't have to do with complaints, or blood flow, or the width of the vessel lumen. Instead it hints at the
biochemical processes of deterioration of the intima and plaque formation.
These processes cannot be touched or smelt, nor made visible, audible, or pal-
pable in the general practitioner's office. The link between giving up smoking
or lowering blood pressure and the future development of atherosclerosis, is
hidden.

"Are you sure it's that urgent, doctor, that I stop smoking? I mean, if I
have to, I have to. That is, I would try. But my father used to smoke, he
smoked a lot more than I do, and he only died when he was eighty-seven.
I'm seventy-one now, and, well, I would like to live a few more years, but
eighty-seven is all right with me. Hah, I'd go for eighty-five, if I could go
on smoking cigars. I think I would."

In any particular case the doctor cannot be sure about the link between preventive intervention now and the future prognosis. If the patient's claudication
gets worse, there is no way of telling whether this is because of smoking, or
high blood pressure, or something else yet again. If there is no deterioration,
this may also have many causes, and none can be shown to be more true than
any other. In principle links through time are possible. But more often than
not, they simply cannot be made in routine medical practice.

*My original focus on the legs implied that I followed the clinical work of vascu-
lar surgeons treating claudication, rather than that of cardiologists attending to
angina pectoris, or neurologists taking care of patients with cerebrovascular accidents (CVA), or nephrologists dealing with kidneys lacking oxygen. But this focus
starts to lose its relevance in places where atherosclerosis is performed as a process over time. For this performance has to do with blood vessels all over the body.
The consequences of smoking or high blood pressure do not restrict themselves to
leg vessels. Thus, what at first seemed to be a simple methodological choice, risks
starting to side with some performances of atherosclerosis—those that are local-
ized—rather than others—those that are historical.*

General practitioners and internists often treat atherosclerosis as a process in
time. Surgeons may also urge patients to stop smoking. But their invasive treatment intervenes in vessels here and now.

> A young doctor in a hematology research job: "It's a miracle that these
> invasive treatments help at all. For what do you do? You mess up vessel
> walls, strip the intima away, bring in strange objects, do all kinds of things
> that provoke the atherosclerotic process. You do things that risk making it
> worse. But it helps. Somehow it often does. For a while. For of course no
> surgeon ever treats atherosclerosis. They only take away the symptoms."

First the relation between the surgical performance of atherosclerosis and its
developmental version is posed in terms of friction. The mechanical interventions of invasive treatment may lead to the formation of plaque. Subsequently,
however, the relation starts to shift. The loss of vessel diameter treated by the
surgeon is called a "symptom." And the gradual deterioration of the vessel wall
over time is called the "underlying disease."

*It isn't easy to sustain atherosclerosis as a virtual object. For such an object must
encompass and absorb all these relations. It must not look too confusing, even if
intervening in one of its alleged "aspects" clashes with intervention in another.
And even if a little later this clash has disappeared and the vessel lumen that has
been treated becomes the "symptom" of an underlying atherosclerotic "disease."*

Intervention that fits short-term concerns, may be a long-term risk. But the
converse is also possible. An attempt to improve the future, may lead to deterioration here and now.

> A neurologist in an interview: "And then these old people with athero-
> sclerosis, when they're found because of a claudication, and have a high

blood pressure, they get treatment for their hypertension, because high blood pressure is a risk factor. But people may have come to depend on it. And thus, when it's lowered, their claudication gets worse. Usually it's not only their leg vessels that are bad. Their carotids are stiff, too, and who knows how little lumen there's left. So in the morning, when they get up, paff, they fall. Or they fall getting out of a chair they have been sitting in. For with a low blood pressure, the blood supply to their brain falls short. If it's long enough: there's your CVA. So sometimes they only break a hip. Sometimes it just kills them."

Lowering blood pressure may be a wise preventive act. It may be a wise thing to do as part of the process of performing atherosclerosis as something which develops over time. But it may be foolish here and now because atherosclerosis is already hampering blood flow in all vessels, including those that lead to the brain. How to handle this? It does not necessarily lead to discussions about what atherosclerosis "really is." Atherosclerosis may well be deemed to be both this bad artery here and now *and* all arteries closed off in the future. And what matters is not which reality is more real, but which is more important. What is played out is a trade-off between several possible futures. One is deemed to be more undesirable than the others. And thus, so far as possible, it is prevented.

Is this, then, what attending to the local performance of objects is about: shifting the discussion from the facts of bodies to the values of lives? For when attention pivots around virtual objects inside bodies, practical intricacies of diagnosing and intervening are devaluated as "mere" practicalities, while talking in terms of performances, brings practicalities to the front, and turns living them into what matters most.

A TRANSPORTABLE LINK

Links that are hard to make in routine practice, may be practiced in a specific setting with careful monitoring. Thus, even if it isn't a routine practice to make angiographies of all patients a few weeks after their operations, this may be done for a few hundred patients. Even if it isn't possible to know if it will help Mr. Mançevic if he stops smoking, it is possible to evaluate the histories of large populations of people and see if there is a correlation between smoking habits and the onset, severity, and course of atherosclerosis. If such links are monitored and noted, they may be published. In this way, mobile connections are created that can later be quoted somewhere else.[13]

A researcher: "It isn't easy. Take smoking: you cannot create random research populations. Some people simply cannot stop. And if people can
manage to, well, then they ought to, if not for their blood vessels, then
because there's cancer to take into account. So the only thing you can
do is follow those who claim they quit and the others, who still smoke.
And if they are all willing to co-operate, and if their doctors are willing
to tell us what these patients died from if they die, then you can follow
them. For a year, three years, five years — or even more if you have the time
and stamina and money. And then if you see those numbers — in the case
of atherosclerosis, they're so impressive. So then you can say something,
even if you have no clear-cut controls. No random populations."

If when monitored, complaints, diameter loss, and death rates among those
who have stopped smoking are milder, less and lower than among those who
haven't, the link between smoking and atherosclerosis is established. A physician cannot test this link in every single patient. But there is no need to do so.
Quoting an article or two may do the job. Thus a link practically made in one
setting, can legitimate practice in another.

Correlative links are important legitimations for medical practice. For some
forms of treatments, for instance drugs, they are even legally required. While
for others, like surgical treatment, they are not encoded in the law, but have
recently become a part of professional standards. Moreover, links other than
those between a form of treatment and its results may also be measured. It is
possible to try and find "wild" links, and ponder about the implication they
may have for future action.

A research presentation. Talk, slides, drawings. A lot of graphs. A researcher from the department of clinical epidemiology presents her
findings. She has looked for links between estrogens and atherosclerotic
plaque. In order to do so, she didn't isolate estrogen in the lab, nor did she
observe plaque under the microscope. Instead, she measured the correlation between the age of onset of menopause and death from a vascular disease. "Onset of menopause" stands in for "loss of estrogens" and "death"
stands in for atherosclerosis. And she tells: "It's interesting. For there *is* a
link between an extremely early menopause and death from atherosclerosis. But then we talk about a menopause that starts well before forty.
Once a woman has passed that line, there's nothing. No correlation at all.
Forty-five, fifty-five, sixty: it makes no difference. Look at this slide, look:
all these lines run parallel. Now we don't know yet how to interpret that.
But we do know, or, eh, I should say, we have good reasons to suspect,

that the link between estrogens and atherosclerosis isn't as strong as it is sometimes suggested in the literature."

A good correlation between estrogens and atherosclerosis might legitimate a new treatment policy. If estrogens "protect" against atherosclerosis, prescribing estrogens to postmenopausal women might be indicated not only for those with menopausal complaints or osteoporosis, but also for all women who belong to a "risk group for atherosclerosis." The clinical epidemiologists of hospital Z think this shouldn't happen. Or, in other words, their study suggests that the link between estrogens and atherosclerosis is so thin that it should not be transported from research setting to treatment policy.

That "death" can stand for "atherosclerosis" implies that complaints, diameter loss, pressure drop, intima deterioration, and death are all treated as aspects of the same object. Death is simply the most severe manifestation of this object, or, in the language of epidemiology, its most accessible "indicator." In the meanwhile, however, correlation studies tend to be strikingly indifferent toward the nature of objects. They link one event to another. They correlate one practical occurrence with another. One could say they don't study objects, but events. Thus, if a strong link between "onset of menopause" and "death from atherosclerosis" were established, it could influence treatment policies even in the absence of any sensible story about the way in which, inside the body, estrogens act upon vessel walls. It could be turned into an action lacking its virtual object.

In research settings some things can be practiced that are hard or impossible elsewhere. Research practice is a matter of establishing difficult links: links that require time, large numbers of subjects, or only become discernible if "intervening variables" are ruled out.

In the hematology laboratory of hospital Z, the aggregation of platelets on vessel walls is investigated. Small steps in the development of the formation of plaque and thrombi are singled out. Each step can be isolated from the next one, and the influences on the outcomes of the presence, absence, or concentration of hosts of constituents are manipulated — and measured — one by one.

In the flow chamber platelets are allowed to aggregate on a thin layer of tissue. The platelets are elements of a fluid that looks like blood. But it isn't blood. Its constituents are slightly different. This fluid is composed of the plasma of one donor, and the red cells of another. The plasma has been altered. Some ions have been washed out, others added. This red fluid flows through the chamber with a pulse: the heart beat is imitated by a pump, the speed of which can be adjusted. The temperature is turned into a manipulable variable, too. It's usually set at 37°C.

Blood composition, flow, and temperature are difficult to manipulate in living bodies. Thus it is hard to link them to one another and to other events such as platelet aggregation. In the lab setting, this is possible. If washing the calcium out of the blood changes the behavior of the platelets in the flow chamber, a link between calcium and platelet aggregation is forged. If a specific reaction is more pronounced at high velocity than at low velocity, it is more strongly linked to the vessels feeding the heart, than to those of the legs. Other experiments make and unmake other such links. Variable after variable is related to endless others, the astounding possibilities fill volume after volume of research journals. Young researchers get Ph.D.s for making a link or five. Sustained relations may be turned into story bits that end up in textbooks, which then securely state that "a high calcium concentration facilitates platelet aggregation."

More often than not, the practice of manipulating variables in the lab cannot be repeated in living bodies. Changing the calcium concentration in a living body's blood, for instance, may be just a bit too risky. Even so, laboratory facts can be made mobile. They are transported in talk called *explanation*. They are mobilized in stories about what happens between here and there, between intervention and reaction. They are virtually projected into bodies. These transported projections, however, become a lot stronger if they are incorporated in a practical vehicle which sustains them.

The hematologist: "As hematologists we do a lot of atherosclerosis research, but we see no patients. The vascular surgeons see the patients. And the general practitioners and internists who do preventive work in risk groups. But we play no part. So far we have nothing to offer. I don't blame the surgeons that they don't know all the biochemical details of plaque formation or thrombus formation. It doesn't make any difference to what they're doing. They unplug the clogged pipes, like plumbers, and that's their task. But once we've found a drug, it will all change. A drug will get at some step in the process of plaque formation or thrombus formation. So with it, biochemistry will start to matter." The interviewer: "You think you'll find a drug?" The hematologist: "Of course I do. I have to, haven't I? I put it in all the grant proposals. It may take a while. But remember what happened with ulcers. Ulcers used to be treated surgically. First they got at the stomach itself, later at the innervation. But now it has become completely obsolete to operate on ulcers. There are several good drugs, now. Several."

As it is, the biochemistry of plaque and thrombus formation is a story in a text-book taught to students. Practicing doctors may know this story. They may teach it. They may explain it to their patients. Thus, as a legitimation, this link is transportable. But links such as these are only *practiced* insofar as they suggest something to do: something to do or to avoid doing, something practical.

Links are just like objects. They don't lie inside the body, but in practices. Or: in order to turn a link from a practical matter to a characteristic of the objects inside a body, a lot of work needs to be done. Blood tapping, centrifuging, cleaning glass-ware, noting down numbers, calculating. Or: writing prescriptions, going to the dispensary, taking pills. Or: talking on the television—with impressive pictures to show.

A general practitioner: "With cholesterol it went very fast. In the lab a relation between plaque formation and cholesterol was established. The shorthand for this became: cholesterol causes atherosclerosis. So every-body was warned against eating eggs and lard and what have you—for years, and very loudly so. The problem is that now there's doubt again about whether it's so very important, the intake of cholesterol. Even if the cholesterol level in the blood is still important, intake isn't necessarily so. There are so many other factors along the way. So you have to be careful. We cannot go on changing life rules from one year to another."

Making or dissolving links in research practice differs from doing it in the hospital or in public health campaigns that try to reach out to all potential patients. The weight of the factors involved is multiplied along the way. Manipulating the many variables of a fluid pumped through a fluid chamber built out of plastic and metal components isn't easy: technicians and researchers have fascinating stories to tell about the complexities that may arise. But manipulating even a single relevant variable in thousands of human lives tends to be even more complicated.

THE MULTIPLICITY OF OBJECTS

Atherosclerosis isn't one, but many. This diversity may be taken as a matter of different *aspects* revealed or different *meanings* attributed. Here, however, I have argued that atherosclerosis is *performed* in a variety of ways, or, better, that the name "atherosclerosis" is used for different objects—which also have names of their own: claudication, thickening of the intima, loss of lumen, pressure drop, plaque formation, and so on. They differ. The material manipulated, the concerns addressed, the reality performed, all vary from one place to another. The ontology incorporated and enacted in the diagnosis, treatment, and prevention of atherosclerosis is multiple.

Meanwhile a single "atherosclerosis" is often mobilized or cited. I've shown that this requires a lot of effort. The projection of a virtual object "atherosclerosis" behind the variety of "atheroscleroses" performed, depends on the ability to make links, links between one local atherosclerosis and another. I have shown that it is often difficult to make such links. They get established here, but they are missing a little further along. They are partial and erratic.[14] The obvious questions to ask next are: What difference does it make to show that making links is hard work, and that single objects are virtual entities? What difference does it make to say that medical practice performs bodies and diseases locally, and that its ontology is multiple?

Some responses: A first difference is that the disciplines of anthropology, sociology, history, and philosophy of medicine are freed from a dreadful dilemma. It is the dilemma of either believing that the body and its diseases coincide with what medical textbooks tell about them, or agnostically bracketing away the flesh to study only the meanings attributed to it.[15] Studying the practical performance of bodies and diseases may be a way of attending not only to the body as it is experienced or interpreted, but also to the body as it is manipulated, measured, observed, cut into pieces — or grows and decays. It is a way to attend to the body and its diseases "themselves." Realism no longer entails a submission to medical doctors if "the real" isn't mapped onto the singular virtual objects they talk about, but is, instead, taken to coincide with the multiplicity of objects they practically perform.[16]

A second difference has to do with the political style of the social sciences in relation to medicine. As things stand, it seems to be necessary to choose. One may side either with or against "medicine." One may take it either as a source of salvation or as a monstrous beast. Of course, it is possible to say that medicine has its "good and bad sides." But often this remains an empty statement, for it has been hard to find ways to name these sides. It has been hard to express normative views *inside medicine*. It is here that stories such as the ones told here may help. For they open up medicine's dealings with bodies and diseases: they open up an inside. And once inside, it may become possible to find ways to assess the local value of the various performances of bodies and diseases that coexist in medicine: something that can, I think, not be done in either awe or hatred of medical power, but only in serious dialogue with those who work inside the hospital.

Which brings us to the third difference. Discussion inside medicine is implicated too. This text strengthens a specific style of talk. It strengthens talk in which the central question is not which of various "atheroscleroses" is the more *real* but which is the more *important*. Discussion that mobilizes an array of concerns, from the patient's pain to her desire to walk, from her cardiac condition to the alternatives open to her in daily life, from the success rates of the local team of surgeons to the costs of operations, from the joys of smoking to the ethics of care. Discussion that attends to the possible gains and losses of any activity, measured on as many shifting scales as are made relevant by the participants. As it is, such discussions are often devalued as "merely pragmatic." Here I state that practices are all we have, that there is nothing above or underneath them. Which is a way to delete the "merely" and hold on to the "pragmatic."

So foundationalism is undermined. If it is true that it performs many bodies and many diseases, medical practice can no longer be defended through its foundation in the body and disease. But neither can it be attacked any longer as a practice that reduces human beings to fragments while forgetting about the patient as a whole. There is no whole that can be reduced: the variety of objects locally performed do not add up to form a single picture. They go this way, that way, the other. To act in one way does not simply differ from another possible act. Instead it may even be at odds with it. The question, therefore, is not "What is a human being?" or "What is life?" The question is "*What to do?*" How do medical practices perform and change our bodies, diseases, lives, and how to balance between the various alternatives?

But wait a minute. If it is complicated to transport the links made in — say — the hematology laboratory to — say — treatment practices, transporting the tales of empirical philosophy isn't likely to be a simple, straightforward matter either. It's not a question of what follows logically, but of what may practically ensue. And in order for the differences I mention to practically ensue, it is not enough to write down words. More solid vehicles are required. A larger variety of them. But who will build and maintain these? Will you, the reader, incorporate my words into your actions? Or is this text a complicated articulation of what — with little fuss — you were already doing?

NOTES

I would like to thank the Netherlands Organization for Scientific Research for its generous grant; the doctors, technologists, nurses, researchers, and patients of hospital Z for showing me their work, for their help, discussions, and in some cases their reactions on an earlier draft of this text; and Marc Berg, Nicolas Dodier, John

Law, Jan Mol, Jeannette Pols, Ab Struyvenberg, and Dick Willems for their contributions and comments. I am grateful to John Law also for correcting my English.

1   None of these names is satisfactory. It is awkward to still call "Western" a medicine that has spread all over the globe, even if it isn't hegemonic everywhere. Should this medicine then be called "cosmopolitan"? But that hides both that it is the product of a specific cultural tradition and that it is practiced in sites that one wouldn't want to call "cosmopolitan" in many other respects. "Scientific" indicates the intertwinement between this medicine and the modern sciences. But then again, it may all too easily be read as a sign of approval, or, at least, suggest that this medicine is "based on" science. Which it isn't. "Allopathic" contrasts with "homeopathic." It is a word used to mark out this genre of healing in discussions about the so called "alternative" medicines, discussions I do not engage in here at all. So maybe we need a better word. Which one?

2   While I do not take this road, I do want to stress that it may yield fascinating stories. For an example that is sensitive to the differences between the accounts of various people and in the accounts of the same people over time, and that stresses the fluidity of the answers given to an anthropologist's questions, see Pool 1994.

3   For a sustained defense of shifting our attention from thinking to practice in analyzing medical research, see Latour 1984.

4   For an example of a related analysis of differences in medicine in which only journal articles and textbooks are used as material, see Mol and Berg 1994.

5   "Heterogeneous engineering" has become a standard term in science and technology studies. It points at the way in which material and social activities intertwine in all technology. See Law 1986. Here, however, I talk not only about technologies and engineering but also about bodies and pain. And for the implicated notion of "heterogeneity," see Law and Mol 1994.

6   Let me stress again that this study is not about "styles of thought" that dominate medical specialties or individual doctors. A surgeon may well *think* about atherosclerosis in a pathological way. The question I ask is what he or she *does* and which atherosclerosis is incorporated in the activities he or she's engaged in. Which is not to say that my analysis doesn't build on earlier studies that do use "styles of thought" as an analytical category. See for the classic example Fleck 1980 [1935].

7   And the complication grows if a historical dimension is included in the analysis. For every technique is historically shaped and altered. Not just "hard" techniques, but those of the clinic, too. And the way patients feel their bodies from the inside cannot even be taken as a constant either. See for a historical account of their transformations Duden 1987.

8   For the usage of the notion of "virtual object" in this sense, see Law 1995.

9   For an analysis of the way techniques may *both* define each other *and* clash, with the example of Doppler and angiography in the diagnosis of atherosclerosis in the leg vessels, see Mol 1993.

10   The relation between epistemological or social scientific reflections by outsiders

and "native" self-reflections is shockingly understudied. For an example of a study (of health economics) in which this question is systematically dealt with, see Ashmore, Mulkay, and Pinch 1989.

11   There is yet another treatment strategy, walking therapy. When patients go for long walks three times a day for several months, their pain-free walking distance often increases impressively. Their vessel lumen on an angiographic picture, however, doesn't enlarge. And even if collateral vessels may grow, many studies fail to show serious increase in flow. The attempts made to explain the therapeutic effects even so, are interesting material for someone studying the gaps and links between various atheroscleroses! See for this Mol, forthcoming.

12   These "givens" are important. In a setting where distances are large, traveling is expensive or insurance limited, routine control becomes more difficult. "Come back if there are any problems," will be the more likely advice.

13   About making facts transportable from the place where they were originally practiced to many elsewheres, see Latour 1987.

14   Throughout this text, I have normally used the word "link" and not possible alternatives that come close to it, like "association" or "connection." For the former see Latour 1984; for the latter, and especially the notion "partial connections," see Strathern 1991.

15   This dilemma faces the social sciences in many guises, from that of the sex/gender distinction (Haraway 1991) to that of the distinction between blood tie and social kinship (Strathern 1991).

16   In his study of experimental sciences, Hacking attends to the way techniques locally perform objects and yet defends this as a realist epistemological position. Hacking also signals the implication of "disunity" — as he calls it — that this entails. See Hacking 1992.

ONTOLOGICAL CHOREOGRAPHY: AGENCY FOR WOMEN PATIENTS IN AN INFERTILITY CLINIC

Charis M. Cussins

▼

INFERTILITY CLINICS AS SITES FOR UNDERSTANDING WHY AGENCY REQUIRES OBJECTIFICATION

The Argument

Infertility medicine has been a massive growth industry since the birth in 1978 of the world's first "test-tube baby." These reproductive technologies, as they are often called, have captured the public imagination in an unprecedented way. On the one hand, the popular press regales us with photos and stories of happy heterosexual couples flanked by a white-coated physician proudly displaying the long awaited miracle baby. And more mundanely, almost everybody has now had, or knows someone who has had, a baby conceived with the help of these technologies.

On the other hand, we are bombarded with lousy statistics, the use of women's bodies as experimental sites, the ardours of being an infertility patient, the ill effects on surrogate or donor gamete children of confusing their genetic descent, the exclusivity and expense of treatments, and the scary eugenic vistas into which the technologies so easily play.[1] And there are more everyday concerns about the role of medical infertility clinics in determining attitudes to childlessness and womanhood. Patients and public express concern that pressure to pursue the technological approaches of the clinics increases the essentialist identification of women as childbearers in our culture. Likewise, a worry is often expressed about the role of the clinics in enforcing a genetic idiom for parenthood. Does the presence of the clinics as an apparent option thereby worsen the stigma placed on those women who choose not to, or cannot have children?

In amongst these tensions, in some ways so typical of new technologies, resides the woman infertility patient.[2] According to many public presentations of reproductive technologies, and in much critical work in medical sociology and interdisciplinary feminist studies, the woman infertility patient is paradigmatic of the objectified patient, supposed either to be helpless and saved by the technologies, or to be victimized by them. If she is supposed to be helpless, then the technologies and the predominantly male physicians come to the rescue of the woman otherwise unable to achieve the pregnancy she desperately wants.[3] Since the patient has no agency on this view, all the value and virtue accrues to the doctors and the technology. Whereas, if she is supposed to be a victim, she is driven to seek exclusive and expensive medical intervention, not because her life is threatened but to conform to a norm (becoming a mother). On this view, she is turned into an object of study, experimented on, and reduced to a mere physical presence in the name of procedures that rarely work. Since the patient has no agency, all the criticism and debunking accrues to the doctors and the technology.

In these ways, the woman patient is thought of as someone who has no voice in the shaping and application of the technologies. She is at best someone who happens to benefit from her objectification in the clinic by being one of the lucky ones to get pregnant. Contrary to this, I argue that being a multiply objectified user entails neither being helpless nor being a victim. I suggest that the woman's objectification, naturalization, and bureaucratization involve her active participation, and are managed by herself as crucially as by the practitioners, procedures, and instruments.[4] The trails of activity (see below) wrought in the treatment setting are not only not incompatible with objectification, but they sometimes *require* periods of objectification.

The position against which I am arguing, then, operates with the view that the use of medical technology entails the objectification of the patient, which entails her loss of agency. There are two motivations for taking up the question of personhood and objectification that have structured this essay. First, the argument takes on one element of a long tradition that sees objectification as alienating, with technology in imminent danger of usurping selfhood.[5] Where objectification is theorized as an important part of understanding modern personhood, it is still metaphysically opposed to subjectivity.[6] This tradition is also exemplified in a number of writings directed specifically at infertility medicine, most notably, the many powerful critiques of reproductive technologies for their objectification of women produced by feminist scholars.[7] The aim of the essay is not to deny the subjugating and disciplining effects of many technologies, including reproductive technologies, on those who work with or are monitored by technology. The aim is rather to question whether it is the various forms of objectification per se that are antithetical to personhood.

Taking on this tradition is a political as well as a philosophical move. Philosophically, it contributes to recent attempts to animate ontology and to explain rather than start with binary opposites such as subject and object.[8] Politically, this essay takes inspiration from the writings of a new generation of feminist scholars of technoscience who do not reject science and technology but try to negotiate a critical politics in use and development, paying attention to the possibilities of places of scientific, technological, or medical practice for different women.[9] As Franklin has argued, in reproductive technologies in particular patients and practitioners are bound up with the technologies in question, so a politics of "just say no" is unconvincing.[10] Some remarkable recent literature on gender and technology has combined the philosophical and political strands in historical and contemporary accounts of the co-construction of the subject and the technology.[11] My argument offers a further illustration that the components of one's subject position and the power of technologies are negotiated in a heavily constrained manner, together.

The second motivation for taking up the question about objectification and agency and personhood is that it promises to contribute to the discussion of the relations between humans and things that is an important topic in contemporary science studies. The dependence of science and technology on social, individual, and political factors has been quite extensively worked out, but the connections in the other direction (for my purposes here, the dependence of selves on technology) have not received so much attention. In the last few years there has been an interdisciplinary revival of the Maussian anthropological inquiry into culturally specific configurations of the self.[12] The exploration in this work of the multiplicity of selves—the different kinds of face or personae or social roles we routinely switch between as we go about our daily lives—has opened up the possibilities of meaningful conceptions of the self that are not tied to the essential unity of the self. This essay hopes to contribute to extant work in medical sociology/anthropology on the changing self in medical settings.[13] It draws on these literatures that take the construction of the person seriously and attempts to link the initiatives of science studies and the literatures on the self by adding an ontological connection between technology and selves.

Agency and Selves

This essay is not about agency or selves as preexisting philosophical categories. For many philosophers, agency just is the power to act, and action and agency are almost indistinguishable. By contrast, I am using "agency" to refer to actions that we attribute to people or claim for ourselves, actions whose definition and attribution make up the moral fabric of our lives, and in line with which we assign locally plausible and enforceable networks of accountability.[14]

In one philosophical literature, debates about self and personal identity revolve around the conditions for the unity of a life. On what does the continuity of a person from one time slice to the next depend? What are the necessary and sufficient physical and mental conditions for the persistence of self-hood?[15] In this essay I take the self to involve a much longer range project than that implied by the Lockean and Humean tradition. Personal identity is here taken to have at least these elements: a long-term orientation to the good, to be essentially in movement, and to have an irreducibly narrative character.[16]

For the women infertility patients, whether or not they remain the same instance of the same sort is not at stake, just as our own continued existence is only extremely rarely the subject of our own or anyone else's doubt. In an investigation of agency, as I understand it here, what it is to be a subject changes in ways that are the result of, and simultaneously proof of the person's agency. To understand this interdependency it is necessary to look at the local achievement of identity, without deciding beforehand what may or what may not be an element in that achievement.

The defining aporia of current discussions of agency is, perhaps, the following: the constructed nature of the unitary human subject is a datum for the social sciences, but it is difficult to account for agency without presupposing the unitary human subject.[17] This aporia is particularly salient in medical settings where we have become accustomed to thinking of patients as disciplined subjects *par excellence*—anything but active agents—and yet where it is clear that there are different descriptions of the patient at play, at least some of which require acknowledging agency.[18] My essay aims to shed some light on this apparent tension in infertility medicine by showing that the subject is dependent on the constant ontological dance between ourselves and our environments that changes how many descriptions we fall under, of how many parts we are built, and how integrated we are or need to be. In this site we cannot presuppose an ontology of the unified subject precisely because a coherent self narrative requires ontological heterogeneity.

Why This Site?

An infertility clinic is a rich site for an examination of agency and the ontological commitments that go with it. The clinic deals on a daily basis with human gametes and embryos, which function in this clinical setting as questionable persons, potential persons, or elements in the creation of persons. Embryos, for example, can go from being a potential person, as when they are part of the treatment process, to not being a potential person, as when it has been decided that they can be frozen or discarded, and even back again as when they are defrosted or a patient's religious convictions require treating an embryo that would normally be considered waste as potentially viable. The discourse of the potentiality of life is predicated on a woman and would-be mother, who must come literally to embody the potential life attributed to the embryos.

Just as an in-vitro fertilization (IVF) embryo—symbolic in our times of the boundaries between science and nature, science and culture, persons and non-persons—changes status dramatically in the site, so too the patient undergoes significant ontological change. A patient going through a cycle of treatment is sometimes a person juggling her work schedule to be at the clinic, sometimes a generic patient in the waiting room, sometimes ovaries and follicles on an ultrasound screen, sometimes anesthetized on a surgical table, sometimes someone with blocked tubes, and so on. It is the genius of the setting—its techniques—that it allows these ontological variations to be realized and to multiply. By passing through them a patient embodies new options for her long-term self.

Some Methodological Considerations

In this essay I look at some patient testimony in order to track these ontological variations. I am not interested here in using the testimony to develop a pro or con analysis of infertility clinics.[19] Such critical or valorizing enterprises assume the distinctness and stability of patient and technology as a starting point so as to use one to praise or debunk the other. My purpose in including patient testimony is to understand how undergoing these technologies may or may not transform the women; in how technology figures in and enables their self-making.

I am assuming that interpretive charity[20] is appropriate in assessing patient utterances. By this I mean that I am assuming that the women are broadly rational and coherent witnesses of their own treatment, and that apparent inconsistencies are to be explained not as evidence of *merely* ad hoc, post hoc, ignorant, justificatory, or self-interested verbalizations, but as revealing important elements of context that vary from one utterance and one speaker to the next. We can make sense of the process of building self-interest or of giving justifications by attending to the changes that the patients have gone through during treatment.

This use of a principle of charity in interpreting my data provides a notion of meaning that is highly context-sensitive. It is commonly accepted that context includes features of the world such as the where and when of "here" and "now," in order to resolve the reference of indexicals and demonstratives. But for my explanatory purposes in this site, context also includes changing features of the patient in order to resolve of "whom" and "what" things are predicated.

This has the following kind of implication: an utterance by a patient before she is pregnant might on the face of it be incompatible with an utterance she makes later when she is pregnant. She might say a procedure objectified her or went wrong in a cycle in which she didn't get pregnant but say very different things for an apparently identical procedure in a cycle in which she does get pregnant, for example. If the procedure did not vary, one might view this difference as a paradigm case of irrationality driven by self-interest or a need for justification. On the other hand, one can view achieving an account that is justificatory or self-interested as moving and helping to fix the identity of the patient at the time she is speaking. In this way the self-interest or justification becomes one aspect of the content of what has been said, thus removing the prima facie contradiction between the utterances. Neither a pure interest story nor a story that ignores interests or treats them as epiphenomenal is quite right. There is nothing *mere* or necessarily irrational to such things as building self-interest or giving justifications. One can say this once the interpretation of meaning is permeable to the changing lives of the patients who provide testimony at various stages of treatment.

A final methodological point involves the recoverability of the constitutive elements of the socionatural order out of which, and in maintenance of which, I am claiming purposive action arises. One can look for stable features of the way an activity is organized and try to discern the factors that influence those features, or one can look for or provoke ruptures in the normal way of going on as a means of revealing what has to be in place for normal conditions to pertain.[21] The first of these has the drawback that it misses the contingency of the organization of activity, and in this case the mechanisms of attribution and exercising of agency. The second has the drawback that there is not necessarily a good correlation between what is needed to patch together a breakdown, and what normally holds things together.

These are not, however, the only alternatives. If one considers that "stable features" are only stable at a certain level of abstraction, it becomes less compelling to think of social worlds as presenting a smooth surface that can only either be studied as such or dug up. By interrogating a setting from a different resolution, as it were, there is every reason to believe that its normal workings can yield clues as to its construction.[22] In the paragraph after the following, I draw on ethnographic data. I there attempt to vary the resolution under which the treatment setting is examined in order to see in the normal workings of the site the changing metaphysics of the clinic, the patients, the body parts, and the instruments.

This is an empiricotheoretical paper, so I do not attempt to provide an ethnography of the site that can stand on its own.[23] It is part of my argument that understanding the role of technology and objectification in the constitution of subjectivity is exemplified in infertility medicine, so talking about infertility medicine is an appropriate way of talking about subjectivity. Likewise, understanding the trails of activity through this site helps us to understand infertility clinics. I am sensitive to the contentiousness of this approach, but emboldened by my encounters with what seems to my eyes to be a new empirical philosophy: an approach adopted in some of the recent work in science studies and feminist theory.

TESTIMONY FROM WOMEN IN-VITRO FERTILIZATION PATIENTS

Why Did(n't) It Work?

This section consists of testimony from women in-vitro fertilization patients from a number of different infertility clinics.[24] The comments were offered spontaneously or elicited in response to my inquiry as to why a given procedure had or hadn't worked. The excerpts have been grouped into statements about why given treatment cycles didn't work, and statements about why given cycles did work. The comments on "failed" procedures are further subdivided into statements made by women who had subsequently become pregnant and those who had not (yet).[25]

The following are some examples of the things said about unsuccessful IVF treatment cycles by patients still in active treatment:

Everything went fine; he put back three embryos. . . . It's a numbers game . . . but maybe I didn't make enough progesterone to support a pregnancy. . . . Maybe the hormones affected my body and it wasn't ready for a pregnancy.

I had quite a few eggs: eleven; but they weren't all good and only some of them were mature . . . and then only two of the embryos looked good, so I guess something was wrong from the start.

My tubes are really damaged so I wonder if I have a lot of scar tissue on the inside of my uterus too. . . . He said it was hard doing the egg retrieval.

If it doesn't work next time, we're going to go with a mixture with donor [using sperm from a donor as well as the husband's sperm during IVF, to increase the chances of fertilization]. . . . Jake [her husband][26] didn't do well at the Ham test [a test on the sperm to see if it is motile enough to penetrate the zona pellucida of a hamster ovum]. . . . It's a lot of money and time to keep trying in-vitro when we only get one or two eggs fertilizing. . . . They do micromanipulation [microsurgical techniques in which an entrance into the egg through the surrounding zona is sometimes "drilled" to let the sperm in when "spontaneous" fertilization doesn't occur] at [another center] so we might try that if this doesn't work.

It's such a roller coaster; first you go in for the scans and blood tests and you feel on top of the world if your eggs develop OK and you get to go to surgery, then you panic, will they get any eggs? . . . The doctor tells you in the OR [operating room; or in the recovery room] how many they got and if they looked good and you don't know if you heard right because you're still half under. . . . Then there's a wait for the fertilization, and if that goes OK it's whether there are any embryos to freeze, and you get excited again if you make it to the embryo transfer — that's sort of the last step, and you definitely have a chance if you get that far. Until then everything can go fine but you don't have a chance of being pregnant. . . . Then comes the long wait [c. two weeks until the menstrual period comes or a pregnancy test can be done]. . . . If you get your period it was all for nothing. . . . That's the lowest point of all. . . . You're back to ground zero, all that expense, everything we went through.

Dr. S. said at the beginning that in the ideal world we'd be candidates for IVF but our insurance doesn't cover it so we went with the AIH [artificial insemination with the husband's sperm] and Pergonal [a drug containing LH and FSH — luteinizing hormone and follicle-stimulating hormone — that induces multiple egg maturation in a single cycle, instead of the usual one egg per month] for a few cycles but now that we're doing IVF anyway we wish we'd done that all along. . . . AIH wasn't really indicated in our case because I had an ectopic [a tubal pregnancy, where the embryo implants in a fallopian tube instead of the uterus; the embryo cannot survive, and ectopic pregnancies can be life-threatening to the woman] two years ago.

The following are some examples of the things said about "failed" cycles by women who had subsequently become pregnant as a result of in-vitro fertilization:

Last time I think the reason it didn't work was the hormones weren't right for me. . . . You know, sometimes you go through all this and it's not really you that's being treated. . . . You're just one more woman with her feet in straps getting the same drugs everyone else gets, going through all those tests. . . . This time, though, I felt more like a person. . . . I was more informed about what was happening, and Dr. S changed some things because, you know, it didn't work last time.

This time it felt like he let my body do more of the work its own way; as if my body took on the work. . . . Last time it was as if they were all just doing things to me and my body wasn't cooperating. . . . Nothing was really different in terms of the numbers of eggs they got or the fertilization rate or anything.

At [a different IVF center] it's just a production line. They see so many patients a day it's not surprising it didn't work. . . . You never know what doctor you're going to see. . . . I heard one doctor joke to another woman who was also waiting for the egg retrieval when I was, that she had no eggs. Then he laughed his seductive laugh, and patted her thigh and said he was just kidding, she had seven fine looking ones! The woman was still shaking after he went, although she managed a laugh and a smile because, you know, you have to be the doctor's friend, the best patient. . . . I don't call that humor. . . . He should have known the effect it would have on her . . . and she's not likely to get pregnant if she's treated like that, like she's at his mercy.

The following are some examples of the things said about successful IVF treatment cycles:

I guess I just got lucky—on the first time too! Now we want a sibling for her, I just hope it'll work again but you keep telling yourself it might not happen because you know it only works one in five times or whatever . . . but you don't really believe it in your own case because it's all you have experience of, you know, you think maybe there was a reason I got pregnant the first time, maybe I'm really fertile in these conditions.

Last time we had the Pergonal, but this time we moved to Metrodin [an FSH-containing drug similar to Pergonal and made by the same company but with no LH] and the nurse coordinator says she thinks Metrodin has better success rates.

I felt really good this time; Dr. S knew how my body would respond and although we got fewer eggs than last time I just had a better feeling about it; maybe we got fewer but better ones, after all, all you need is one good embryo. . . . I probably wouldn't be saying this if it hadn't worked!

They take a lot of care here; I don't think it was any one thing, but each stage is done so carefully compared to [another center]. . . . I can't really pinpoint any one thing but it all adds up.

Now it's happened I just don't want to think about it. . . . It all seems kind of irrelevant, how we got this pregnancy. . . . It's our baby now, and we're just hoping the pregnancy will go OK.

Diagnoses of Testimony

Some comments on the things said about unsuccessful IVF treatment cycles by patients still in active treatment:
When patients are still in active treatment but not yet pregnant and talking about a previous cycle that was unsuccessful, the comments about why the IVF didn't work tend to isolate a specific phase of the treatment as the or a likely faulty step in the process. For example in the testimony above, progesterone, drugs, eggs, scar tissue, and sperm motility are mentioned as causes of failure. Conception is also presented as being structured into a series of hurdles each of which must be jumped. When a specific body part or phase of treatment is isolated in this testimony it is not specific in the sense of being idiosyncratic to that patient couple. Every IVF patient couple must have eggs of sufficient maturity to fertilize and implant, sperm of sufficient motility to fertilize the eggs, and scarce enough intrauterine scar tissue for successful implantation, if in-vitro fertilization is to lead to a pregnancy. Furthermore, the faulty step of treatment that is isolated is strongly linked to the couple's diagnosis: sperm motility for male factor, scar tissue for tubal factor, egg quantity and quality for IVF patients, and so on. The diagnosis-related specific step that is picked out to try to understand why the treatment cycle was unsuccessful is, however, expressed very personally. The relevant step is suggested as the reason why this individual patient couple did not get pregnant on a previous treatment protocol.[27] When these patients mention ambiance, subjectivity, or anything personal about themselves in the causal account it is not linked to the reasons why the procedure did not work. Expense is mentioned ubiquitously, operating as an integral element in diagnostic reasoning. The interaction between insurance coverage and cost of each procedure serves as a continuous narrowing function on the possible treatment options. The practitioners are referred to simply as sources of authority.

A part of the body or phase of the treatment is singled out as the missing link in the process of getting pregnant, and surmounting it comes to represent the pregnancy and thus the woman herself in her capacity as a childbearer.

This synecdochal aspect [28] of diagnosis — the chain through which the woman's body parts come to stand in for the woman — makes these accounts characteristically mechanistic. The medical operationalization consists in its no longer being Ms. X who cannot get pregnant, but fallopian tubes that are occluded (or whatever the diagnosis is). It is not that the procedure is about the fallopian tubes rather than the woman, and nowhere do the patients make this kind of reductionist move and refer to themselves *as* fallopian tubes or whatever the diagnosis is; they are individuals who have a given diagnosis thanks to which medical treatment is appropriate for them. The promise of the site is not bypassing or fixing the fallopian tubes but Ms. X getting pregnant, much as one mends a punctured tire so as to be able to ride one's bike, and not so as to have an unpunctured tire.[29]

The patient orients to herself as an object of study and intervention, to the physician as instrument and epistemic standard bearer, and to the instruments and material setting as appropriate technology for acting on her body. This nonreductive but synecdochally operationalized ontology (the specifically targeted medical intervention doing work for the whole patient) was unquestioned in patients I talked with as long as the patient was willingly in active treatment.

Some comments on things said about "failed" cycles by patients who had subsequently become pregnant as a result of in-vitro fertilization:
Patients who have had a successful cycle are more likely to talk about previous unsuccessful cycles as having been unsuccessful because they involved lack of agency or insufficient attention to the specificity of the patient or her ability to serve as an expert witness about her own treatment ("They were all just doing things to me and my body wasn't cooperating"; "Let my body do more of the work its own way"; "The hormones weren't right for me"; "You're just one more woman with her feet in straps getting the same drugs everyone else gets"). These factors are more marked when an unsuccessful treatment was undertaken at a clinic from which the patient has now moved ("It's just a production line"; "You never know what doctor you're going to see"; "She's not likely to get pregnant if she's treated like that"). Patients who get pregnant at a given clinic tend to assimilate all their treatment cycles at that clinic to the successful one as preliminary phases of the same treatment, and are thus much less critical of them. Comments made about failed procedures at different clinics tend to be personal, critical, and denunciatory.[30] Part of this is probably a sense of loyalty to the present site, as well as a need to assert good reasons for switching allegiance.

Failed cycles that are not fully assimilated to a subsequent successful cycle provoke patient responses that portray their objectification as dehumanizing and/or against treatment interests. This makes sense if one thinks of the synecdochal relation as having failed. The relation works only if fixing the missing link really does repair the functioning whole (the bypassed tubes must refer back to a now-pregnant or potentially pregnant woman). If, however, the tubes are bypassed by in-vitro fertilization, for example, but the patient does not become pregnant, the patient is alienated from her body by the treatment. She is stranded at the phase at which she had undergone lots of procedures but had nothing to show for it. A loss of subjectivity and agency occurs after a procedure has failed or caused harm, which replaces the functioning synecdochal relation with an ontology in which there is a rift between the patient as subject and the patient as object. The objectification is indeed reductionist in these circumstances.

A case like that of the insensitivity of the doctor joking about a patient's eggs (and other examples patients report of inappropriate sexual innuendo, etc.) subvert the patient's own participation in her objectification. You have to be "the best patient," but if that involves being forced into a conversation in which the physician or someone else exploits that objectification and his/her authority, there is a deprivation of dignity and autonomy that transcends the treatment situation.[31] It is as if the physician was playing in the wrong key, misunderstanding and/or exploiting the nature of the objectifications involved in treating that patient, and it is as highly condemned by other physicians and staff as by patients.

Some comments on things said about successful IVF treatment cycles:
The accounts of successful cycles are less causal (the comment about Metrodin is causal but it is not specific to her diagnosis) and less naturalistic ("I guess I just got lucky") and less synecdochal ("I don't think it was any one thing, but each stage is done so carefully here"). Unlike the personal comments made by patients in active treatment but not yet pregnant, pregnant patients whether describing successful or unsuccessful treatment cycles tend to make a different kind of personal comment. Their personal comments tend to be highly specific to themselves rather than to their diagnosis; something quite amorphous that made the difference between a protocol on which Ms. X would get pregnant versus a generic protocol for patients with Ms. X's diagnosis.[32] The technical interventions so prevalent in the first group of quotes (Ham tests and exact numbers of eggs and embryo quality and scar tissue and micromanipulation and operating rooms and so on) drop out by becoming inevitable or invisible

or irrelevant ("Nothing was really different"; "I just a had a better feeling about it"; "I don't want to think about it. . . . It all seems kind of irrelevant").

In talking about successful cycles, the synecdochal relation has done its work. The objectifications brought about the desired transformation of the woman herself, and the cause of this success was the coordinated functioning of the whole referential chain from the desire to get pregnant through the treated body parts through the now pregnant woman. Responses are correspondingly oriented to the achieved pregnancy, and the factors affecting the whole procedure.

Patients' Active Participation in their Objectification

It is often noted that patients not only willingly accept the role of being the object of the medical gaze, but seem actively to participate in it. One of the nurses commented that almost all the women patients "flirt" with the physicians (with the female physicians, too, although to a lesser extent, apparently). When I pressed her on what she meant by this, she said that the patients want to be thought to be attractive, their bodies to be "womanly" despite their infertility, and to be compliant with and special to the physician; all of this so as to be good candidates for the procedure. The suggestion was that the circumstances of the doctor/patient relation are inherently seductive, combining the elements of intimacy and an authority the patient accepts in her active subordination to it. No patient described herself to me in this way, but several commented on how well they got on with the doctor, and the woman quoted above said, "[Y]ou have to be the doctor's friend, the best patient," when talking about another patient's compliance with the physician's stupid joke.

When a procedure has taken a large toll on a patient for no result, and when a result was extremely unlikely on statistical grounds, one wonders how the patient managed to perform with such control and civility and seeming passivity. Such a commodification of civility sounds like the very kind of thing we modern citizens should guard against. If, on the other hand, the procedure had a chance of working, it is quite reasonable to expect the patient to take an active interest in her own presentation as an object of study. The parallel with the sociological phenomenon of intentional subordination, where one subordinates one's will to the structural power of another person or organization to achieve some overarching goal, is informative.[33] The power is not something that simply resides in the physician or institution, however, as this notion tends to suggest. The physician is a point in the chain through which access to the techniques is mediated. The patients do not so much let themselves be treated like objects to comply with the physician as comply with the physician to let themselves be treated like objects.[34]

This section contains a brief description of some of the most routine elements of infertility treatments: the pelvic exam, the ultrasound, diagnostic surgery, and the manipulation of gametes and embryos in the lab. The aim is to show what is made to appear by the different equipment and procedures. Each procedure has its own physical setting and uses various methods to objectify, naturalize or bureaucratize (parts of) the patient.

The Pelvic Exam

By the time there is a woman patient entering an examination room for a pelvic exam she has already passed all the specific and generic trials required to be there (and so have the room, the instruments, and personnel of the clinic, *mutatis mutandis*). Of particular importance is what one might call her "anticipatory socionaturalization." Most infertility patients will have spent more than a year trying to get pregnant before they even approach a specialist doctor about it. During this time their thinking about their fertility will have changed dramatically. Several people reported to me that they always had in the back of their minds the possibility that they might not be able to get pregnant if and when they wanted to, but until they started "trying" the predominant fertility concerns of most of the patients had been how *not* to get pregnant.

Characteristic of the process of anticipatory socionaturalization undergone by patients prior to arriving at the clinic is to have become much more aware of the phases of the menstrual cycle and the things that can go wrong when trying to conceive. This typically involves some or all of the following: talking to other people trying to get pregnant, buying or borrowing "self-help" books on infertility, watching one's own body minutely for signs of ovulation and menstruation, timing intercourse, familiarizing oneself with the statistical arguments about the likelihood of conception in a given cycle, checking for ovulation with home test kits or by taking one's temperature every morning, going to a nonspecialist physician, getting a sperm count for the male partner, deciding for or against various support networks (who to tell about the infertility, how and where to seek help), going to infertility clinic open houses, and forming hypotheses about what might be going wrong in their own case based on personal health history and hunches.

This anticipatory socionaturalization means that when patients come to the clinic their bodies are already considerably "un-black-boxed." Where they once either tried to or tried not to get pregnant, and typically only had a vague understanding of eggs and hormones and fallopian tubes and temperatures and sperm counts and cervical mucus and endometriosis and luteal phases and so on, *they now itinerize their own bodies in these terms.* Coming to the clinic allows new access to these processes and body parts; it renders the parts visible and manipulable, and subjects them to all sorts of tests so that they yield facts on which to base diagnoses and treatment.

The pelvic exam takes place in an examination room. The patient lies on the examination table with her legs akimbo over padded leg rests, just as in a typical gynecological exam. The nurse hands the physician cleaning swabs and then the speculum and any other instruments or equipment that are needed, at the relevant times in the routine. The physician sits on a mobile stool, at the foot of the table, his/her gaze and gestures and the speculum delineating the physical zone of treatment and study. Conversation with the patient on the examining table changes character so that her internal reproductive organs become the focus of attention. This change is choreographed by the physician's, nurse's, and patient's coordinated positionings, as well as by the swabbing and gloving and placing of the speculum. These mundane steps that render the body and the instruments compatible are at the heart of objectification.

With the speculum in place, and one gloved hand examining the vagina and cervix while the other hand palpates the pelvic region from on top of the abdomen, the physician is able to establish the gross anatomical normality of the woman's body. Fibroids are distinguished from uterine walls, cysts from ovulating ovaries. Patient reactions or reports of pain are assimilated into the exam. The physician may separately feel the breasts and check the body for "unusual" amounts of secondary hair. Diagnostically unimportant differences such as the angling of the uterus or the length of the vagina are ignored. The appropriate topographic knowledge is embodied in the physician's skilled gestures and in the alignment of the instruments and the patient's self testimony. Together these elements render that which is seen or felt as something that is, in the very seeing or feeling of it, an instance of this or that probable diagnosis.

The patient is routinely called on as an expert witness in the process of rendering compatible body and instruments. She provides access to two kinds of information that wouldn't otherwise be present in the room: pain information and information about her fertility history. These are two classic sources of scepticism—first-person sensations and the past—which turn out to be fully integrated into the procedures of the examination room, and so made part of the ontology of the site by the self-witnessing of the patient. Her reactions and answers to questions during the procedure calibrate that otherwise unavailable information with the rest of the activity in the room.

An everyday metaphysics of the person dependent on, but different in kind from, her body presents the woman as dualistic: there is the desire to be pregnant and there is the body refusing to cooperate. This behind-the-scenes ontology of the body can no longer reconcile the long-term self-narrative with the physical body.[35] But once in the clinic the ontology changes.

The pelvic exam educes and classifies some of the contents of the Pandora's box that is now the patient's body.[36] For example, a cold metal speculum is as inert and blind (and often loathed) as it is possible to imagine a commonplace artifact being. But when it is incorporated in this procedure it becomes part of the trail along which the patient's uterus, ovaries, vagina, and cervix are brought into concrete being. The body parts' new concreteness consists not in their being any more real than they were all along or in the parts suddenly becoming relevant because we've had to open the body's black box, although there's something right in both these formulations. The body parts become more real only in the sense that they are enabled to display properties in their own right. And they are more relevant only in the sense that they are rendered as functional stages to which treatment can be applied.

The diagnostic and treatment setting draws out the body parts into a new metaphysical zone consisting of many perceptible functional stages where treatment can be focused. What happens during a pelvic exam is that these body parts come onto the scene of action of the patient's future chances of conception by becoming connected to new and different things.

The Ultrasound

Women patients usually undergo several ultrasounds in any given treatment cycle. This is to see if the patient is ovulating, to monitor superovulation, or to confirm the presence of a cyst, tubal pregnancy, or intrauterine pregnancy. A vaginal ultrasound probe is typically used in infertility centers. The ultrasonographer turns on the machine and the monitor, sheaths the ultrasound probe in a sterile condom, coats it with cold jelly, and inserts the probe in the woman's vagina. By rotating the probe in different directions, the ultrasonographer brings first one ovary into view on the screen, and then the other.

Follicles can be measured and compared. If, for example, the woman is undergoing a cycle of in-vitro fertilization, the ultrasonographer will be looking for several simultaneously developing follicles of roughly equal size. Once one ovary is in view, s/he measures each visibly developing follicle. A computer "mouse" is used to place first one cross on the screen on one side of a follicle, and then another cross on the other side. When a key is hit the screen distance between the crosses is computed, giving a size for the follicle, which appears on the image. Each follicle is measured in this way, and Polaroid photos of the screen are produced that record all the images and the associated follicle measurements. When the physician doesn't watch or perform the ultrasound, s/he bases the decision to continue treatment or not on the ultrasonographer's hand-collated list of numbers of ripening follicles and their sizes, plus the photos. S/he also decides whether to continue medication, whether to alter doses, and what and when the next phase of treatment should be on the basis of this information.

As in the case of the pelvic exam, the ultrasound brings out new entities in a treatment zone that is composed of trails of instruments, technicians, and objectified patient. This manifestation of actants on the screen, the ultrasonographer's list, and the Polaroid photo is how the setting produces places at which to anchor treatments. One trail moves from the ultrasound probe in the vagina, to the ovaries' appearance as images on the monitor and in the photos, to the appearance of the follicles as numbers and sizes on a list, to the ovaries' and follicles' classification in the patient's file and their travel through the physician's room where they initiate the next phase of treatment. As long as these trails of actants-in-the-setting flow back to the patient, the synecdochal relation between the body parts and the patient is maintained. This material maintenance of synecdoche ensures that the objectification of the patient that consists in the education and itinerizing of her body parts is not opposed to her subjectivity.

Diagnostic Surgery

Diagnostic surgery[37] is often justified to the patient on the grounds that it affords the physician a "proper look."[38] Most infertility surgery is done by laparoscope or hysteroscope, which enable the surgeons to visualize the peritoneum and inside of the uterus respectively (figure 1). The laparoscope is inserted through a half-inch cut at the navel. The surgeon looks through the eyepiece, then connects a camera to it and takes a number of photos of the patient's ovaries, uterus, and tubes, which will form part of the official record of the surgery. At this point the video system is hooked up to the laparoscope, and an image of everything in the line of sight of the laparoscope appears on two monitors placed on either side of the patient's body so that the surgeon and assistant can both guide their instruments without moving around. The surgeon

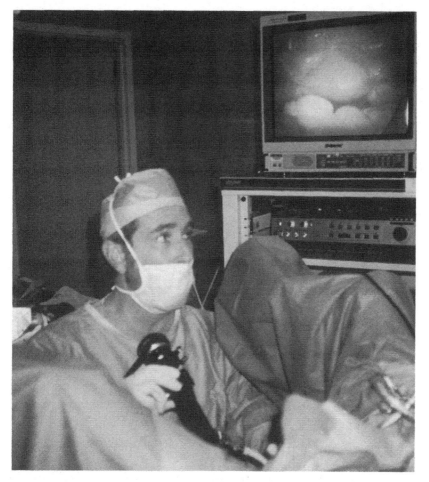

Figure 1   The patient's uterus, as shown on a "slave monitor"
during a laparoscopic/hysteroscopic procedure.

talks everyone in the room through the pictures on the screen, pointing out the
diagnosis. If all is deemed normal, the surgeon removes the laparoscope and
sews the patient back up again, once the public witnessing of her pelvic region
is complete. If something is found that is considered relevantly abnormal, and
to need treatment, two or more tiny incisions are made, through which instruments for cutting, cauterizing, or grabbing are introduced as needed. These
instruments are worked by the surgeon and either one of the scrub nurses or
an assistant surgeon.

The organs become a focus of repair and therapy with all the qualities of the classic specimen of study. The uterus and ovaries and tubes are represented *sui generis*, as it were, on the monitor, floating apart from the context of the rest of the body and the whole person.[39] The anesthesiologist and his/her instruments are crucial in this form of objectification, holding the patient's consciousness in abeyance. The surgeon does not usually need to worry about whether the patient will remain "under" or experience pain, or to question that the uterus, tubes, and ovaries are correctly "wired in" to the rest of the body so as to be able to treat them as if unto themselves.[40]

For example, left and right fallopian tubes were described as "normal" or "dye flowed through them freely," or they were "occluded," or the "fimbria were damaged or occluded," or they were "stunted and blocked" or they had "spots of endometriosis on them," or "they were stuck down with adhesions," or they could be "Novi-catheterized," or one or the other could be "missing." Sometimes the tubes contained things like an "ectopic embryo," a "reanastomosis site of tubal ligation reversal," "polyps at the cornual junction of the uterus and tubes." Adhesions on them could be "filmy" or "vascularized," and the adhesions could be lysed or left alone. Ovaries were left and right, and could be missing, and could be stuck down with adhesions, or spotted with endometriosis. They often had cysts, which were either "corpus luteum cysts" or "hemorrhagic cysts."

The patient could be "just there for us to get a look," "ginger" so in danger of lots of "bleeding," be "married to a colleague," be an employee of the clinic and so a friend or acquaintance of most of the people in the room, have been "crying in the office yesterday," have wanted her "fibroids removed only if it could be done laparoscopically," have been "referred by another physician," be "difficult," want to "go home the same day," or be in "poor health." There were also porters and three operating room nurses and one or two surgeons and the anesthesiologist; an embryologist, an ivf nurse, and an ultrasound technician for egg retrieval; and sometimes a representative of an instrument company or a medical or technical student, and me. There could be as many as eleven people in the operating room.

There were anesthesiology machinery, trays of instruments, the audiovisual system of cameras and screens, the bleeding control equipment, the cleaning and counting procedures. This range of entities and gestures, which are routine in this setting, are all required to bring out the singularity of body parts and to educe mechanistic properties in body parts so that they can be tested and fixed.

Gametes and Embryos in the Lab

The embryology laboratory is the site at which all semen is washed, spun, and separated before inseminations. The freezers containing patients' embryos and sperm, and donors' sperm are also in the lab, and eggs are brought here from the operating room for in-vitro fertilization. There are regular activities that ensure the self-reproduction of the lab, such as the making of new culture media, quality control testing of the media on mouse embryos, filling of the liquid nitrogen canister for the freezers, and the ordering and receiving of new equipment and supplies.

The lab maintains an ontology of connectedness between the body parts and patients during the time when there is a physical separation between the two. This spatial separation between patient and gametes and embryos makes possible procedures that would not otherwise be so, but also increases the work necessary to mark and maintain a potential pregnancy trajectory. The gametes become temporarily independent genetic emissaries enlisting a whole space — the lab — that enables human embryos to exist outside patients' bodies. This independence allows functional stages such as a blocked epididymus or fallopian tube to be bypassed; it allows manipulations of egg and sperm to occur; and it allows eggs and sperm alike to be derived from donors, joining in the lab a process of conception that will end up with implantation in the birth mother. These are powerful innovations.

The lab exhibits a moral economy of care, which is oriented to maintaining the ontology of educed and connected pregnancy trails. For example, work on embryos or potential embryos is carried out in semi-darkness. The care taken to protect the eggs and embryos from potentially harmful exposure to light is felt to "make sense" because it approximates in-vivo conditions.[41] This "maternal" care is exercised whenever embryos or potential embryos are around, because of the link to a possible pregnancy. These standards of care stand in contrast to the spinning and washing and freezing of sperm, and the freezing of surplus embryos, when the life potential of embryos or fragile eggs that do not form part of a pregnancy trail is on hold or not at stake.

Likewise, the use of a mobile baby isolette as the primary work station for eggs and embryos contributes to the maternal environment of care. It has an internal work space visible through an externally mounted microscope where the eggs can be counted, pipetted, and mixed with sperm, and the embryo development can be monitored (figure 2). During the fertilization and development of embryos in the lab, developmental details are recorded. These notes are used to discriminate good from bad embryos: which should be transferred

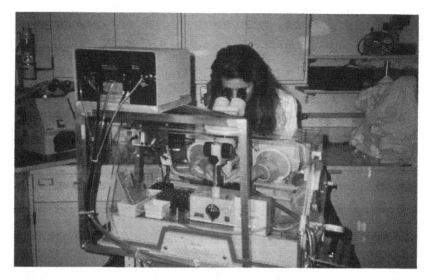

Figure 2   Working with human embryos in an isolette from the
neonatal intensive care unit.

to the patient's uterus, which should be frozen, and which can be treated as
waste. Embryos used for research are deemed to be a subset of the category
of "waste embryos." Segregating the embryos in this way is about managing
the disposal or freezing of some embryos. These developmental criteria justify
exempting certain embryos from the moral and legal standards that apply to
embryos as potential sources of life in the lab.

The gametes and embryos are tied back into trails leading to the woman,
and that this is so structures the equipment and the procedures in the lab and
the behaviour of the embryologists. The embryologists often talk about their
responsibility for the life potential of the eggs and embryos, and are always
aware of the preciousness to the primary patient couple of the eggs and embryos. Extensive legislative and bureaucratic standards penetrate the lab and
inscribe every embryo and prescribe reproducible success rates. The political
and legal registrations of the embryos when outside the body are a measure of
their precarious connectedness during this time. When the egg doesn't fertilize,
or an embryo fails to develop "normally," it is removed from the trail leading
back to the uterus and the ontological bond is severed. Leaving the trail relaxes
the legal, moral, maternal, and political registrations of the embryos.

CYCLES OF OBJECTIFICATION

Each patient features under many descriptions during the course of her treatment, and during visits to the clinic. Her subjectivity is multiply configured and her agency is consequently crafted out of different elements in the different sites. When a woman seeks a medical solution to infertility she exercises agency in her active participation in a number of different kinds of objectification: operationalization, bureaucratization, naturalization, and epistemic disciplining. This section presents a preliminary list of some respects in which the patient's agency is structured by these forms of objectification.

Objectification as Medical Operationalization

Operationalizing infertility as the education of body parts in the treatment zone is one form of objectification in this site. There is a kind of agency that is associated with this objectification. It consists in the extent to which a patient is an integrated body or person who acts as a whole over time.

Examples of objectification as medical operationalization occur during the un-black-boxing of the body in the patient's anticipatory socionaturalization, the itinerizing of a patient's body parts in the pelvic exam, the rendering visible of body parts by the ultrasound and their manipulability and public witnessing in diagnostic surgery. The woman is rendered into multiple body parts many times during a treatment cycle.

Objectification as Naturalization

Naturalization of the patient is a second form of objectification in this site. There is a kind of agency that is associated with this objectification. It consists in being a social actor. For example, during a routine visit involving a pelvic exam (see above), the woman moves from being someone who behaves in a way that carries the usual identificational weight when she is in the waiting room, to being in a place where it is appropriate to undress and wear a gown,[42] to being an object of study that can be viewed from unusual angles with the help of instruments, to being someone who gets dressed again and interacts "face to face," as we say.

Many of the woman's multiple social roles are temporarily irrelevant whilst she is being examined. This is an aspect of the synecdochal mechanism, where by making a part of her body stand in for her social role as a patient, she is signficantly naturalized.

Objectification as Bureaucratization

Bureaucratization of the patient is another form of objectification in this site. There is a kind of agency that is associated with this objectification. It consists in the extent to which the patient is interacting as a unique individual as opposed to interacting merely as a generic patient.

The woman moves from highly generic at the beginning of the appointment, to being highly specific when she is being examined, to being somewhere in between at the end of the exam. In the waiting room she is someone who has chosen to come to this appointment, but that choice is strongly constrained by available passage points in our culture for infertility,[43] and she is already being assimilated to a diagnostic form and into the normal routine of the clinic. Only her most generic properties are relevant to the clinical setting at this stage: that she arrive on time, come through when she's called or fetched, and that she behave within the normal parameters for the clinic. She is objectified in a nonspecific, bureaucratic sense, and is a token of a generic patient.

Objectification as the Epistemically Disciplined Subject

Epistemic disciplining of the patient as subject is a characteristic form of objectification in this site. There is a kind of agency that is associated with this objectification. It consists in the extent to which the patient is a rational health-care consumer who makes decisions in her own interest because she is well informed about the available options.

The clinic manages carefully what the patient is told and shown, and what things are appropriate background knowledge. Medical ethicists both within and external to the hospital administration have long been concerned with informed consent and patient access to information. The liberal principle *volenti non fit iniuria* is invoked by ethics committees to protect the clinic and physicians and to inform the patient of the risks and benefits of the treatment.[44] This informational ethic is particularly salient in medical subdisciplines like infertility medicine, which are marked by a high proportion of experimental procedures.

The clinic is saturated with information, and the epistemic capital acquired by the woman in her anticipatory socionaturalization is altered and expanded in her career as a patient. The format for advertised public sessions to attract prospective patients is a series of lectures about the prevalence and causes of infertility and the state-of-the-art treatments available at the clinic. Inside the clinic there are informational booklets for new patients, pamphlets on every aspect of infertility, newsletters, support group and counseling literature, and regular meetings on such things as how to administer subcutaneous hormone injections. The only contexts in which I heard patients expressing a lack of knowledge or understanding were over idiopathic diagnoses (no known reason why the patient was not getting pregnant), unexpected breakdowns in routines (e.g., scheduling being changed by the clinic for non-treatment-related reasons), or not really understanding what something involved until you had gone through it (a phenomenon with which we are all familiar). Much of the literature is provided by the drug and instrument companies in an exchange in which patients are educated and practitioners take on a particular line of drugs or equipment. Informational booklets authored by MDs promoting the company product are part of the infrastructural environment at these clinics.[45]

As in other circumstances where rational informed citizens are produced, participation of the educated is enhanced. Patients are better able to participate in their own care because they have been initiated into the epistemic environment of the clinic. Producing informed citizens also produces epistemic standards. Certain facts about the body, about one's own body, and about the treatment options become the things one is told or one is expected to know or one comes to know. This generation of epistemic standards in the clinic helps constitute the practitioners as experts and the procedures as reliable, and facilitates the flow of authority and accountability.[46]

Objectification and Agency as Co-constitutive or as Oppositional

Medical operationalization, naturalization, bureaucratization, and epistemic disciplining are all associated with a kind of agency, as described above. When the trails of activity lead back to the woman as pregnant, synecdoche is maintained successfully and the patient exercises agency in her active participation in each of the forms of objectification.

Medical operationalization of the woman is not necessarily opposed to her being a spatially and temporally integrated actor. Sometimes — if being pregnant is a long-range desire — a way to be an actor in this site is to undergo medical operationalization. Likewise, naturalization of the woman is not necessarily opposed to her being a social actor. Some social roles — such as being a mother — can be fulfilled by passing through this site but this requires that the patient be naturalized. Bureaucratization of the woman is not necessarily opposed to being treated as a unique individual. Being sortable by one's generic properties as a patient is a part of access to the coordinated sites of treatment honed to one's specific case. And, epistemic disciplining through, for example,

Serono's patient information booklets and through the clinic authorized protocols and statistics is not necessarily opposed to cognitive autonomy. Imbibing
the epistemic standards and culture of the clinic—why some procedures are
performed and where success projections, and so forth, come from—is essential to participating in one's own care as an informed insider. Each of these
nonoppositional ways of thinking of objectification and personhood is under-
written by what was described above as the metaphysics of the treatment zone.

However, if the synecdochal relation fails and the metaphysics of educed
trails of activity is not sustained long enough to overcome the infertility, then
the different dimensions of objectification do come apart from their associated
kinds of agency. In these cases the objectification stands in opposition to aspects of our personhood which we care about deeply and guard carefully.
The oppositional tension between objectification and agency alienates us from
technology: operationalization renders us as mechanistic discrete body parts,
naturalization turns us into objects of experimentation and manipulation, bureaucratization turns us into institutional cogs, and we are hoodwinked by
our epistemic disciplining. It is the ubiquitous possibility of this alienation resulting from synecdochal breakdown that explains our customary ambivalence
toward the benefits of technology.[47]

Retrofitting Agency and Objectification

I argued in the previous section that it is possible to discern potential gains
for the long-range self within each dimension of objectification, even when
there is a notion of agency that is commonly opposed to the dimension in
question. I also argued that the dehumanizing effects of objectification are
not mere expressions of resentment at failed procedures, but—resentment or
not—are occasioned by metaphysical ruptures between the long-range self and
the entities deployed in objectifying a patient. Because the rupture may not be
immediately apparent, or may manifest itself further down the treatment line,
seemingly contradictory things can be said about identical procedures in good
faith and with truth.

One effect of the temporal extension of metaphysical rupture is that whether
objectification and agency are oppositional or coconstitutive in a treatment
episode—and consequently the identity of the patient as subject—is revisable
retrospectively. These aspects depend on whether the cycles of objectification
in the clinic follow the dashed or the solid line in figure 3.

I do not mean by this that a patient might think at one point that she actively participated in her own objectification, and then in the light of new

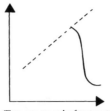

Time, over one cycle of treatment

Figure 3   The medical objectification of infertility promises the achievement of desired personal change. The dashed line represents the case where the procedures are successful; the solid line where they are not.

evidence come to think that she had in fact been alienated by her objectification — although this may sometimes happen. I also don't mean that there was a fact of the matter at time t, but that an assessment of t at t' gives different truth conditions for the state of affairs at t. The first of these would be a model of revisability based on the propensity to err displayed by the patient. The second version of revisability would be a form of epistemic presentism: an assessment of the state of affairs at time t must always be carried out from a time t', and the characteristics of time t' can have an impact on the truth conditions retrospectively of the state of affairs at time t.[48]

The problem with these models of revisability is that they take the temporal component of cycles of objectification to be essentially static, so that time is a sequence of discrete time slices. Given such an account, arguments for retrospective assignments of agency would have to maintain that an individuated time slice is porous to elements derived from a distinct individuated time slice. It is notoriously hard to argue even for the effect of one's present actions on future actions when time is seen like this, despite the high degree to which we organize our lives on the premise that the present *is* thus oriented to the future. Instead, we must view ourselves as epistemically situated in the present but not isolated in a time slice, not epistemically trapped in the present.

Viewing the semantics of time as extended and dynamic (unless rhetorical devices are used to restrict temporal reference) licenses the idea that objectification and agency inherently possess retrospective and prospective properties. It allows one to make sense of the patient testimony and their constructions of self-interest. As prefigured in the introduction to this essay, the apparent contradiction in testimony is resolved because the subject of the discourse changes depending on the stage and success of treatment. Patients still in active treatment operate with a metaphysics of educed trails in which objectification and agency are coconstitutive. Where the patient is talking about a failed treatment cycle that she doesn't assimilate to any ongoing treatment, she often expresses herself as having been alienated or dehumanized. In this case, the trails of activity have petered out without reclaiming the long-range subject, leaving a dualistic metaphysics in which objectification and agency are oppositional. When speaking about a successful cycle, the trails of activity have led back to and transformed the long-range subject and the heterogeneous ontology of the treatment zone becomes irrelevant.

ONTOLOGICAL CHOREOGRAPHY, TRAILS OF ACTIVITY AND THE *E PLURIBUS UNUM*

I argued above that a woman patient objectifies her infertility so that she passes through a number of places that promise to bring about desired changes in her identity. The rendering compatible of herself with the instruments, drugs, and material surroundings, I suggested, held the possibility of transforming her, but that it was not inevitable. She is locally and temporarily reduced to a series of bodily functions and parts, working in a mechanistic way that forge a functional zone of compatibility with the means of medical intervention. The instruments, drugs, physician, gametes, and so on, all take on some of her by standing in for the phases diagnosed as not working.

These processes of the rendering compatible of the infertile woman and infertility procedures do not of themselves guarantee a seamless and successful solution to the infertility. The objectified body must not lose its metonymic relation to the whole person, and neither must the instruments lose their acquired properties of personhood in virtue of which they fix, bypass, or stand in for stages in a woman becoming pregnant.

I call this process of forging a functional zone of compatibility that maintains referential power between things of different kinds, *ontological choreography*.[49] The choreography is the coordinated action of many ontologically heterogeneous actors in the service of a long-range self. The treatment is a series of interventions that turn "Where is it broken?" into a well-formed way of asking "Why aren't you pregnant?" (to transmute Foucault 1963).

To talk about the routes by which ontological choreography is realized, I have used the metaphor of trails.[50] I use this metaphor because I want a notion that is at once normative—there are places to go and sensible ways to get there—and yet locally constituted, contingent, informed by experience, but not laid down in advance. It is a spatiotemporal but nonrigid metaphor for capturing the cycles of objectification involved in the distribution and redistribution of activity through time and space and amongst people and things in the clinic. The movement from one to many and back again that objectification offers a patient I call the *e pluribus unum*.[51]

NOTES

I am privileged to have been able to work through the ideas in this paper with Adrian Cussins, and to have benefited from our habit of cothinking at all stages of writing. I also gratefully acknowledge the following for reading and in many cases commenting extensively on a draft: Marc Berg, Linda Derksen, Nicolas Dodier, Jerry Doppelt, Andrew Feenberg, Donna Haraway, Martha Lampland, Bruno Latour, Tanya Luhrmann, Michael Lynch, Annemarie Mol, Chandra Mukerji, Bob Pippin, Steven Shapin, Brian Cantwell Smith, and Robert Westman.

1   It is a feature of reproductive technologies that they are seen as progressing so fast that society is perpetually out of step with new developments in its legal and ethical thinking. This sentiment is almost always expressed in government legislation and ethical writings on the field. Current anxiety is focused on the extensions of the technologies to include such things as postmenopausal pregnancies with donor eggs, donor eggs from a woman of one race being used by a woman of another race, intergenerational or "grandmother" pregnancies, recovering donor eggs from aborted fetuses, selective reimplantation of biopsied and genetically screened embryos, intracytoplasmic sperm insertion, and zona drilling or thinning, cloning, and the various legal and kinship conundrums surrounding all of these. See, e.g., Strathern 1992b, which opens up a discussion of the impact of reproductive technologies on Western kinship patterns.

2   Almost every woman at the clinics I observed was a partner in a heterosexual couple hoping to have children. In this paper I consider only women patients. For interesting historical reasons, as well as pragmatic ones, women are the primary patients in infertility clinics. Treatments for male infertility are increasing, but even when the man is the "cause" of the infertility, the reinstatement of the normal pregnancy trajectory in the woman remains the treatment goal. In Cussins 1997a, I discuss some of the ways in which infertility clinics tacitly enforce heterosexuality, unlike sperm banks, which have long been associated with gay and lesbian reproductive rights.

3   See Franklin 1990 on the construction of the "desperateness" of infertility patients. "Achieving" pregnancy is an interesting formulation used a lot by practitioners of infertility medicine and counselors. It is what happens when the "most natural thing in the world"—getting pregnant—becomes work.

4   In one of the following paragraphs I distinguish different kinds of objectification in the context of infertility treatment. I work with a reconceptualization of agency that decouples any unproblematic linking between agency and the good.

5   The continental critical tradition especially has theorized technology as part and

parcel of modern industrialization, and so has tended to equate the social and personal effects of technology with the class relations mediated by the means of production of industrial capitalism. See, e.g., Marx (e.g., 1982); Weber, where the technological apparatus of bureaucracy can be thought of as the iron bars out of which the "iron cage" of increased rationalization and control of social life is forged (1958: 181–82); with recent contributions developing themes of deskilling, e.g., Braverman 1974 and Noble 1984; and increasing bureaucratization and surveillance implicated in a loss of personhood, autonomy, and agency, e.g., Foucault 1979, Garson 1988, and Zuboff 1988.

6   Examples include Foucault 1979, which argues for the historical specificity of modern medicine in enabling the individual to be "both subject and object of his own knowledge"; Horkheimer and Adorno, in the *Dialectic of Enlightenment* (1979), which argues for the possibility of an instrumental approach to objectification.

7   For examples of feminist works containing critiques of the dehumanization resulting from the objectification of women in reproductive technologies, see, e.g., Corea 1987, Spallone and Steinberg 1987, Rothman 1986, Terry 1988, Klein 1989.

8   Canonical works in the science studies literature include Bloor 1991, Latour 1987, Rudwick 1985, Shapin and Schaffer 1985, Haraway 1991.

9   E.g., Haraway 1991, Martin 1987, Clarke and Montini 1993, Rapp 1995, Franklin 1997a, Oudshoorn 1990, Singleton and Michael 1993, Suchman 1994b. Traweek (1993) gives an informative account of many of the strands tying together feminist theory, science studies, anthropology of technoscience, and cultural studies, among which the move is made to articulate politics from within technoscientific practice.

10 Franklin (1997b) in a review of Squier 1994.

11 See, e.g., Michele Martin's wonderful book (1991), which recounts the production of a new telephone exchange simultaneously with the construction of gendered and disciplined identities for its newly female workforce, including a discussion of the active role of the women operators in shaping the technologies and their own working lives (extending Foucault's later work on the possibilities for the development of self-identity and resistance around technology, e.g., 1982). See also Cockburn and Furst-Delic 1994, which argues from a fascinating array of European case studies for the coconstruction of gendered identities and technology.

12 See, e.g., Carrithers, Collins, and Lukes 1985, Ferguson et al. 1990, Kondo 1990, Gergen 1991, and Prins's 1993 exegesis of Haraway's posthumanist hybrid subject (e.g., Haraway 1992).

13 See, e.g., Kathy Charmaz's writings (e.g., 1991), which explore the identity crisis and heterogeneous and changing elements involved in the maintenance of coherent self-narratives across contexts for the chronically ill; Monica Casper (e.g., 1994b), who shows the extensions of humanness, selves, and the related notions of agency, and the politics associated with the naming of new things as persons, in the case of experimental fetal surgery; Linda Layne's account (1992) of the role of biomedicine in self-narratives about and around pregnancy loss.

14 See Shapin 1993, for an excellent discussion of the central role of assigning value in the "realization stories" that are an integral part of our sense of self: "We tell 'realization stories' about ourselves, and those who approve of us help us tell them, as a way of pouring value on those actions. Because such narratives are storehouses of value, their plausibilities are highly protected by a wide range of everyday and academic practices" (338).

15 This debate comes directly from Locke, and then Hume, where the self is seen as consisting in a bundle of experiences. Each of the elements of the bundle is constituted independently of the self. This is in contrast to the Kantian view where all experiences are irreducibly stamped with the first-person act of being experienced, and so are not dissociable from the self. See, e.g., part 3 of Parfit 1984 for an important recent statement of the Lockean and Humean tradition of work on personal identity, which covers the exotic thought experiments so characteristic of this line of inquiry.

16 See Taylor 1989 and MacIntyre 1981. Taylor criticizes Parfit for continuing in the tradition of conceiving of personal identity as an "aspiration to a disengaged subject of rational control," and therefore being unable to see the irreducibly collective, temporal and moral dimensions of identity.

17 The tension that results from deconstructing (as opposed to taking for granted, and also from constructing) the human agent is embraced as a defining contradiction for postmodernism and critical theory: agency is necessary for sustaining viable oppositional or marginal identities, but is illicit because of its historical embedding in capitalism and post-Enlightenment phallogocentrism. Haraway (1992) begins a wonderfully provocative exploration of the theme of charismatics "who might trouble our notions—all of them: classical, biblical, scientific, modernist, postmodernist, and feminist—of 'the human,' while making us remember why we cannot not want this problematic universal" (98).

18 For a summary of the aporia in medicine, see Dodier 1993b, e.g., p. 325. Unlike Dodier, I argue for agency and subjectivity under some circumstances within the objective and public aspect of the body under the medical gaze.

19 For interesting critical uses of testimony see Arditti, Klein, and Minden 1984 and especially Klein 1989. For a more valorizing account drawing on women's experiences, see Birke, Himmelweit, and Vines 1990. See, e.g., Wynne 1988 for a discourse analysis of patient testimony showing how multiple sclerosis patients ascribe scientific rationality to doctors even when the doctors have failed to come up with the correct diagnosis or to help the patient in any way.

20 The principle of charity as introduced by Quine (e.g., 1960) enjoins the analyst to interpret the utterances of those studied in such a way as to make as many of them come out true (according to one's own beliefs) as possible. The analyst for Davidson and Quine is a fixed reference point into whose interpretive schema the utterances of the other are interpreted or translated. Charity as it is used in sociology and anthropology picks up on the *verstehende* aspect of the principle in a way that requires initiation and conceptual movement of the analyst. To this ex-

tent, then, the Quinean and ethnographic principles are in conflict; my intended usage is in line with the latter.

21   These two positions correspond to the sociology criticized by Garfinkel and to his own methodology for the breaching experiments, respectively. "In accounting for the persistence and continuity of the features of concerted actions, sociologists commonly select some set of stable features of an organization of activities and ask for the variables that contribute to their stability. An alternative procedure would appear to be more economical: to start with a system with stable features and ask what can be done to make for trouble. The operations that one would have to perform in order to produce and sustain anomic features of perceived environments and disorganized interaction should tell us something about how social structures are ordinarily and routinely maintained" (Garfinkel 1963: 187).

22   Jordan and Lynch 1992 is very important for having shown this: "The social constructivists' black-box analogy places diversity and fragmentation at a preliminary stage of the narrative, whereas we see a persistent dispersion of innovations even within the frame of a highly consensual practice." The purpose of their article was not just to show that in fact all black boxes are gray, but to dispel the idea that diversity and contingency only operate at moments of uncertainty and controversy. The socionatural order displays continuous diversity and fragmentation, sometimes preserving stability across settings and other features of the black box, and sometimes not.

23   For more empirical details see Cussins 1997a and 1997b. In the first I looked at the epistemic culture of statistics, and the technical and nontechnical means by which macro effects such as who has access to a clinic, who gets a diagnosis and treatment, and what counts as a working procedure, are instantiated in the local ways of going on in the clinic. The second is an anthropological account of actual case-by-case procedures and treatment situations.

24   In-vitro fertilization, or IVF, is a method with a variety of protocols for achieving human fertilization outside the woman's body. Typically, a woman is given hormones to induce a number of eggs (instead of the usual one a month) in her ovaries to ripen during the first half of her menstrual cycle. The development of the eggs and dosage of hormones are monitored by ultrasound and blood tests, and before ovulation the mature eggs are "harvested" surgically, either via the abdomen or transvaginally. The eggs are incubated in a lab in culture medium, and mixed with sperm. (The sperm can come from the partner of the superovulated woman, from a donor, from the partner of the would-be gestational mother in the case of donor eggs, or from the partner of the would-be adoptive mother in the case of surrogacy). If fertilization occurs and embryonic development appears to be progressing according to the clinic's standards of normality, some or all of the appropriate embryos will be transferred to the woman's uterus (or, in the case of donor eggs, to the uterus of the would-be gestational mother), in an attempt to rejoin the standard pregnancy trajectory. IVF patients are only a subset of all infertility patients.

25   I am drawing on participant observation undertaken in an infertility clinic on the

West Coast of the United States, as well as visits to clinics in other parts of the United States and England, and formal and informal discussions with infertility patients. My conversations with patients in interviews were not recorded; instead I took detailed notes (in plain view). Comments offered spontaneously rather than in interview were written up with some time lag. The comments are drawn from patients at three different clinics. Some were gathered in 1988–89 and others in 1992–94. The comments were gathered shortly after the failed or successful procedure (at subsequent treatment or prenatal check-ups.) As Nicolas Dodier pointed out to me, there is no reason to think that the testimony would not change in interesting ways again at a later point as part of an evolving first-person narrative.

26   Jake wasn't in the lab when the sperm assay was performed, only his sperm was. Sperm outside bodies is normally waste, but in this context it continues to refer back to the person. The clinic only works if it is able to maintain the sperm on a trail that marks out potential pregnancy. Under these conditions body parts can be separated without losing their mereological role or being alienated from the subject. It is this double-act of part separation without alienation on which the transformative power of the clinic for the long-range self depends.

27   I have been much aided in my revisions of this discussion of the interview data by the comments of an anonymous reviewer.

28   The Shorter Oxford English Dictionary defines "synecdochism" as used in ethnology as "belief or practice in which a part of an object or person is taken as equivalent to the whole, so that anything done to, or by means of, the part is held to take effect upon, or have the effect of, the whole."

29   Some of the controversies over success rates for reproductive technologies have focused on the possible disjuncture between fixing the parts and fixing the infertility. Some clinics claim successes when the functioning of parts or stages is restored, rather than when a baby is born. See, e.g., Marcus-Steiff 1991 for a thorough exposé of the discrepancies between reported success rates by clinics that include "biochemical," ectopic, and miscarried pregnancies that are favorable for their bottom line—the higher the pregnancy rates, the more patients and other funding the clinic will draw—and the bottom line for patients—"take-home baby rate," as it gets called. (Nonetheless, many patients do report a sense of success after any kind of "result," even often in such cases as ectopic pregnancies where the patient's life might have been endangered and she will almost certainly have undergone additional surgery to remove the conceptus. The most common comment I have heard in such cases is: "At least now I know I can get pregnant.")

30   Renate Klein's important book (1984) charted the testimony of several infertility treatment "survivors" for whom the procedures didn't work. Their tales of the rigors of treatment undergone and their objectification at the hands of the medical establishment are moving, compelling, and often appalling. As an artifact of my methodology, my access was restricted almost exclusively to patients still in active treatment. The critical stance exhibited in Klein's book is a stronger version of the stance taken in my data by women who had become pregnant, and talked about a

previous failed cycle, or those who had experienced a failed procedure at another clinic.

31   Cf. Judith Lorber's discussion of the "good patient" (1975) who enacts compliance as a strategy to, amongst other things, reduce the stigma of illness for oneself and one's family.

32   A striking example of this was expressed by a non-IVF patient I talked with (she had artificial insemination using her husband's sperm, and Clomid and Pergonal). She said she is only fertile on the weekends, and that the protocol started to work once she persuaded the treating team that they had to do the insemination on a weekend day. The rationale for this was presented in terms of the regularity of her cycle, her ovulation every four weeks always at the weekend, and the tightness of the cervix hampering cannulation for insemination on all days except the very day she ovulates.

33   Cf. Goffman 1986 for a discussion of the benefits to inmates of "total institutions" in behaving with civility despite their subordinate positions. An infertility clinic is very different from a total institution, but the parallels between being a good inmate and being a good patient — managing the self to attain the privileges of the site — are striking. My account is unlike Goffman's in an important respect. Goffman uses a sociological idiom that aims to recover a coherence to the social world independently of the technoscientific world, even when he is talking about medicine. My account emphasizes the ineliminability of technical practice in creating and maintaining this coherence. The epiphenomenal character of patients' behaviors and meanings in Goffman and other sociological constructivist accounts is avoided by bringing aspects of the technoscientific world into the interests of patients and practitioners.

34   Note that each occurrence of "object" in this sentence has a different meaning. Being an object in the sense of the first occurrence is not being a subject and not having agency. Whereas being an object in the sense of the second occurrence has to do with the dynamic, myriad forms of objectification found in the treatment cycle, in which the physician is one part of the complex of procedures and instruments rather than a separate actor who stands in control of the procedures and instruments.

35   Another class of options potentially available to infertile couples in a culture with a broadly dualistic metaphysics is to seek to transform the self narrative about the desirability of having children. This can be done by addressing the collective: how society treats childless women, etc., or by addressing the individual: other ways I can express my creativity, etc. Part of our sense that one ought not to have to go to the extreme of using reproductive technologies is that it is somehow very much more dramatic and invasive than the options for changing one's self-narrative. Technologies *are* dramatic in the miscegenations they bring about between the economy, the body, social institutions, the soul and so on, and the sheer numbers and heterogeneity of entities that need to be aligned. But each of the stages is quite mundane. Whereas attempts to change self-narratives without technologies

are dramatic in the opposite sense in virtue of the power that would be required to
be concentrated in so few and homogeneous actors for them to be successful.

36   Cf. the metaphysics during the education of facts about the advance or retreat
of the forest in Bruno Latour's essay "Le 'Pédofil' de Boa Vista—montage photo-
philosophique," in Latour 1993b.

37   I refer the reader to a few superb ethnographic accounts of surgery: Goffman 1961
on role distance, Katz 1981 and Hirschauer 1991. An article by Collins (1994) and
a series of replies in *Social Studies of Science* extend some of the themes of these
accounts.

38   The fact that laparoscopy is usually at least partially covered by insurance in
America whereas IVF and many of the other "treatments" are not, means that such
surgery is much more routine here than in the United Kingdom, for example.

39   Petchesky (1987) has pointed out the dangerous side of this standard scientific way
of representing its objects of study, in the case of reproductive politics. The fact
that fetuses can be visualized on ultrasound and other screens in vivo, but as if in
splendid isolation, has been important fodder for pro-life propaganda. Hartouni
(1991) further documents this link in her analysis of the pro-life movie *The Silent
Scream.*

40   The *art/technicality* is discussed: how good the image definition is, what the image
size is, and how fast it can be translated into stills; but these are parameters that
mark the skills of the artisans involved, rather than questioning the metaphysics
enabled by these taken-for-granted representational practices.

41   Conversation with embryologist, August 1992. Both embryologists referred explicitly to these conditions of care using metaphors of motherhood. This was explained
as being good technique enabling them to control for as many variables as possible.

42   Cf. Goffman 1986: 29 on the role of putting on institutional clothing in "deface-
ment."

43   Income level, country of residence, race, and age are the best predictors of the likelihood of being an infertility patient.

44   Pippin 1996 writes "one way to allay worries stemming from a rights based political
culture, where human dignity and self-respect are essentially tied to the capacity
for self-determination, is simply to integrate such an ethical consideration much
more self-consciously and in a much more detailed way, into the transactions between patients and doctors. Thereby the fundamental liberal principle: *volenti non
fit iniuria* is preserved. No injury can be done to the willing, or here the well informed health care consumer."

45   Serono, whose laboratories manufacture Pergonal and Metrodin, have a near monopoly on infertility drugs and other aspects of infertility medicine in the West.
For example, Serono owns Bourn Hall in Cambridgeshire, England, which is the
country house site for infertility treatment set up by Edwards and Steptoe (the lab
fathers of the first test-tube baby). Given the exchange between information and
drug provision, they have a near monopoly on informational literature as well.

46   Also like other forms of education, patient education only adds to the difference

between those people with access to infertility medicine and those people whose reproductive rights do not extend to technological interventions to help them to have children, rather than hindering them from having children.

47 It is crucial to start the project of repositioning medical ethics once we have arrived at this point at which we can explain why sometimes personhood and technology stand in opposition and sometimes as partners. At this level of descriptive resolution we can see and talk about the simultaneous possibility of technological alienation and the massively generative mutual personification of technology and technologization of personhood. Instead of taking the creation of rational, informed citizen as the centerpiece, medical ethics should focus on conditions for the maintenance of synecdoche, examination of collective options created and closed by trails of activity, and examination of who and what gets to blaze which trails.

48 It is not the presentism itself that is the problem here. Undue Whiggishness, ideology, and teleology aside, presentism can be a sophisticated appreciation of the irreducible temporal situatedness of the analyst and the analysis, and the function of temporally extended narrative in creating and maintaining our collective and individual identities. The problem is cutting up time into discrete slices, so that time t is being viewed from a different frame of reference, time t'. This leads inevitably to the kinds of philosophical arguments one sees against historicism and the use of actors' categories, all of which are based on the incommensurability or inaccessibility of time t from t'. (See, e.g., Kitcher 1993: 100–101, n. 13). Historians rightly tend to react with impatience to such arguments, pointing out that they have long been deploying knowledge of states of affairs at time t from time t' with considerable effect.

49 Many writers have shown the ontological limitations of homogeneous materialist or idealist, externalist or internalist, accounts of scientific activity and progress, and have introduced heterogeneous causal elements into their accounts of the possibility of change and coordination across different communities of practice and belief. Haraway (e.g., 1991), and Latour (e.g., 1993a), Callon (e.g., 1986a) and their colleagues have developed over many years what are now canonical statements of explanatory heterogeneity.

Also of particular note are the following: Galison (1997), in his development of the metaphor of "trading zones" where the members of different communities of physicists are coordinated through forced proximity and shared materially mediated means of communication. Mol and Law (1994) show that the ontology of anemia is heterogeneous and to be decided empirically. They develop the notion of social spaces that act like fluids and are transformable without fracture. Their topology is a critique of actor-network theory and its conflation of the really there with strong and stable networks. Star and Griesemer (1989) use "boundary objects" as a means of translation between worlds, and Lynch (1991) integrates the locally realized constraints on the production and maintenance of reality with the idea of "topical contextures." Hacking (1992) details the coevolution of theory and laboratory equipment in the production of stable laboratory science by a process he calls "self-vindication."

50   A. Cussins's sensitive use of the notion "cognitive trails" (1992) is the source for this metaphor.

51   With ironic reference to the nineteen-and-a-half-foot-high bronze Statue of Freedom, atop the Capitol Dome in Washington D.C.; freedom is indeed a woman inscribed "e pluribus unum." This sense is no doubt very far from the imperialist overtones of making many into one that Thomas Crawford captured in 1863.

THE ARCHITECTURE OF DIFFERENCE: VISIBILITY, CONTROL, AND COMPARABILITY IN BUILDING A NURSING INTERVENTIONS CLASSIFICATION

Stefan Timmermans, Geoffrey C. Bowker, & Susan Leigh Star

▼

INTRODUCTION

A man and a woman sit in a kitchen. It is early in the morning. He is reading the newspaper intently; she is putting away last night's dishes and preparing breakfast. She pours a cup of coffee and puts it in front of him, carefully avoiding the angle of turning of the newspaper pages. After a moment, he takes a sip of the beverage. "Cold." From this single word, she infers the following: he is still angry over the squabble they had last night; he is feeling apprehensive about his upcoming work review; the dinner they ate together which precipitated the squabble sat heavily on his stomach, and he slept less well than usual. Correctly, she predicts that he will be a little snippy with his secretary in the office, and forget to bring his second cup of coffee in the car with him on the way to work, a practice he has recently adopted. This omission will result in a late-morning headache.

Psychologist Gail Hornstein[1] analyzes this snippet of conversation as a means to understanding the relationship between intimacy and language; the more intimate the relationship, the more seemingly telegraphic may language become with no loss of meaning. Contrast it with the following anecdote told by literary critic Alice Deck:

In the 1930s, an African American woman travels to South Africa. In the Capetown airport, she looks around for a toilet. She finds four, labeled: "White Women," "Colored Women," "White Men," and "Colored Men." (Colored in this context means Asian.) She is uncertain what to do; there are no toilets for "Black Women" or "Black Men," since black Africans under the apartheid regime are not expected to travel, and she is among the first African Americans to visit South Africa. She is forced to make a decision that will cause her embarrassment or even police harassment.[2]

The movie *A Few Good Men* hinges on an anecdote about several soldiers who perform a "code red" on another soldier, during which he dies. A "code red" is an illegal informal punishment/harassment in the manner of a rough fraternity joke. The death of the soldier causes an investigation; the commanding officer is suspected of deliberately ordering the code. The harassing soldiers defend themselves by saying that they could not have been ordered to perform a code red because that was forbidden by the manual of conduct. The denouement of the film has the prosecuting attorney closely questioning one defendant in a truly ethnomethodological moment:

"Does he do *everything* by the book?"

"Yes."

"Does the book contain *all* knowledge about how to conduct oneself in military life?"

"Yes."

"Did he have breakfast this morning?"

"Yes."

"Does the manual specify how to get to the mess hall, or where it is located?"

"No."

"Q.E.D. — the manual does not contain all knowledge."

These three anecdotes illustrate three central issues in the architecture of differentiation and dedifferentiation — that is, how one makes a successful, practically workable classification scheme. Dedifferentiation means that existing differences are covered up, blurred, merged, or removed altogether, while differentiation refers to the construction of new distinctions or reinforcement of existing differences. This mutual process of constructing and shaping differences through classification systems is crucial in our conceptualization of any reality. The case studies in Douglas and Hull 1992 point to the ways in which a category can be nonexistent (distributed out of existence) until socially created. Thus Hacking 1986 talks about the creation of "child abuse" this century: it is not that there was nothing in the nineteenth century that we call child abuse, but rather that that category did not exist then and so tended to go by a disaggregated host of other names. Once the category was declared a legal and moral one at a particular historical juncture, then people who abused children could learn socially how to be a child abuser; reports in the press and so on would teach them what was expected of the abuse personality (see also Becker 1963 on how to become a marijuana user). The result is a shifting of balances of differences, a change in the architectural relationships. For every newly constructed difference, or every new dedifferentiation merger, changes the workability of the classification in the ecology of the places of its use. As with all tools and all knowledge, such classification schemes are entities with consequences, to be managed, negotiated, and experienced all at once (see Clarke and Casper 1992 for an excellent exposition of this in the relationship between cancer, classification, and laboratory techniques).

"Difference" is the prime negotiated entity in the construction of a classification system, and it enters the workstream in a subtle and complex fashion. The work to be classified doesn't go away with new classification schemes, but the work of classifying causes shifts in ways that present challenges to both the designers of the scheme (faced with decisions about how fine-grained it should be) and to users (filling out forms and encoding diagnoses). Work is neither created nor destroyed in this process—but is shaped to fit into the emerging matrix. Commonly, the larger contexts within which these classification shifts occur include professionalization, automation, and informatization, and the creation of international research and record-keeping procedures.

There are three main areas of challenge in crafting a classification scheme that will fit the workstream and agendas created by these larger contexts:

1. *Comparability.* A major purpose of a classification system is to provide good comparability across sites, to ensure that there is a regularity in semantics and objects from one to the other, thus enhancing communication. If "injection" means giving medication by needle in one country and enema in another, there is no use trying to count the number of injections given worldwide until some equivalence is reached by negotiation. The more intimate the communication setting, the less necessary are such negotiations for a variety of reasons, including that they may already exist historically, or by convention; or that they are more private and less subject to regulatory scrutiny.

2. *Visibility.* How does one differentiate areas of work which are invisible? While they are invisible, they are by definition unclassifiable except as a residual category: other. As for the African American traveler, there is no choice to be made. Invisibility can come from intimacy, too, though, as with the cup of coffee that carries so many messages invisible to the ordinary listener, who lacks intimate context and history.

3. *Control.* No classification system, any more than any representation, may specify completely the wildness and complexity of what is represented. Therefore any prescription leaves some amount of discretionary space to the user, be it as small as in the most Taylorist factory or prison, or as large as the most privileged artists' retreat. Control, like visibility, has good and bad elements, depending on one's perspective. Freedom trades off against structurelessness; being able to exercise a wide range of judgment is only worthwhile if one has

the power and resources to do so safely and effectively. Too much freedom for a novice or a child may be confusing, or lead to breakdowns in comparability across setting, thus impairing communication. Judgment about how differentiated to make the classification must revolve in due consideration of this factor. The answer to the unspecified knowledge in *A Few Good Men* is not to spell out where every mess hall is in every marine base in the world, and include instructions about how to walk there putting one foot in front of the other — but rather to measure the degree of control required to get the job done well, for most people, most of the time.

From the point of view of design, the creation of a perfect classification scheme ideally preserves commonsense control, enhances comparability in the right places, and makes visible what is wrongly invisible, leaving justly invisible discretionary judgment. It has, simultaneously, intimacy, immutability/standardization, and is manageable. A *manageable* classification system works in practice, is not too fine-grained or arcane in its distinctions, and fits with the way work is organized. *Standardization/immutability* means that the classification system appears the same in every setting, and is stable over time as well.[3] A classification system that preserves *intimacy* acknowledges common understandings that have evolved among members of the community.

However, such a perfect scheme does not really exist, since these areas trade off against each other in real world setting. Maximizing visibility and high levels of external control threaten intimacy; comparability and visibility pull against the manageability of the system; comparability and control work against immutability/standardization. In order for a classification system to be standardized, it needs to be comparable across sites and leave a margin of control for its users. However both requirements are difficult to fulfill. A manageable classification system (for whomever) doesn't only require that the system classifies the same things across sites and times but also that it uncovers invisible work that impacts recording. Finally, to keep a level of intimacy in the classification system control is traded off against the requirement to make everything visible. These characteristics become the areas of negotiation, sometimes conflict.

Because one cannot optimize all three characteristics at once to produce simultaneously perfect degrees of intimacy, manageability, and immutability/standardization, a classification scheme encompasses a thorough, pragmatic understanding of these tradeoffs in their historical context. It places them, as we have said above, in the workstream. In the next part of this essay, we situate this architecture in our observations of the building of a classification system in progress, the Nursing Interventions Classification.

The Nursing Interventions Classification (NIC) aims to depict the range of activities that nurses carry out in their daily routines. The classification system consists of a list of 336 interventions each comprised of a label, a definition, a set of activities, and a short list of background readings. Each of those interventions is in turn classified within a taxonomy of six domains and twenty-six classes. For example, one of the tasks nurses commonly perform is getting a patient emotionally ready for a risky or painful treatment. The nursing intervention "preparatory sensory information"[4] is defined as describing "both the subjective and objective physical sensations associated with an upcoming stressful health care procedure/treatment" (McCloskey and Bulechek 1992: 253) (see table 1). This intervention is followed by a list of activities that are related to the assessment of patients, situations, and care provision. The intervention is then further classified in the class of "Coping Assistance" which in turn is classified under the domain of "Behavioral" (see table 2).

This classification system is being developed at the University of Iowa, with Joanne McCloskey and Gloria Bulechek, experienced and well-respected nursing scientists, as principal investigators. The NIC group built up their system of nursing interventions inductively. They surveyed compilations of discrete nursing activities and created a preliminary list that distinguished between nursing interventions and activities. Expert surveys of nurses with master's degrees and focus groups narrowed the preliminary list of interventions to the original 336 published in Nursing Interventions Classification (McCloskey and Bulechek 1992). These interventions were further validated via surveys sent to specialist nursing organizations. Based on hierarchical cluster and similarity analyses, the different interventions were grouped and reviewed to assure clinical relevance and significance (Iowa Intervention Project 1993). The taxonomy was then validated through surveys with nurse experts in theory development and a coding scheme was developed (Iowa Intervention Project 1995). The classification system is thus growing slowly through a wide-scale cooperative process, with nurses in field sites trying out categories, and suggesting new ones and refinements in a series of regional and specialist meetings. Since 1992, the group of nursing researchers have added over fifty interventions to their original list.

The nursing investigators modeled NIC after the classification system of NANDA (North American Nursing Diagnosis Association) which was established in the early seventies (Gebbie and Lavin 1975). NANDA brought about a major change in the nursing profession by establishing nursing-specific diag-

Table 1   Example of one intervention from
the Nursing Intervention Classification

Preparatory Sensory Information

Definition: Describing both the subjective and objective physical sensations associated with an upcoming stressful health care procedure/treatment

---

Activities:

Identify the sensations surrounding the procedure/treatment

Describe the sensations in objective terms

Indicate the cause of a sensation

Present the sensations in the sequence that they are most likely to be experienced

Include information about the timing of events

Include information about the spatial characteristics of the environment in which the procedure/treatment takes place

Focus on the typical sensory experiences described by the majority of patients

Include typical sensations related to seeing, touching, smelling, tasting, and hearing, as appropriate to the procedure/treatment

Choose several words to describe each sensation, because one or the other of the descriptors should strike the patient as accurate

Use lay terms to describe the sensations

Use the word "pain" sparingly, but include it if it is typical

Personalize the information by using personal pronouns

Focus on the sensations to be experienced, but also include procedural information

Provide an opportunity for the patient to ask questions and clarify misunderstandings

---

Background Readings:

Christman, N.J., & Kirchhoff, K.T. (1985). Preparatory sensory information. In G.M. Bulechek & J.C. McCloskey (Eds.), Nursing Interventions: Treatments for Nursing Diagnoses (pp. 259–276). Philadelphia: W.B. Saunders.

Christman, N.J., Kirchhoff, K.T. and Oakley, M.G. (1992). Concrete objective information. In G.M. Bulechek & J.C. McCloskey (Eds.), Nursing Interventions: Essential Nursing Treatments (2nd ed.) (pp. 140–150). Philadelphia: W.B. Saunders.

CURN Project. (1981). Preoperative sensory preparation to promote recovery. New York: Grune & Stratton.

Sime, A.M. (1992). Sensation information. In M. Snyder (Ed.), Independent Nursing Interventions (2nd ed.) (pp. 165–170). Albany: Delmar Publishers.

Source: McCloskey and Bulechek 1992: 394.

Table 2   Domains and Classes
Nursing Intervention Classification Taxonomy

	Domain 1	Domain 2	Domain 3
Level 1 Domains	1. *Physiological: Basic* Care that supports physical functioning	2. *Physiological: Complex* Care that supports homeostatic regulation	3. *Behavioral* Care that supports psychosocial functioning and facilitates life-style changes
Level 2 Classes	A *Activity and Exercise Management:* Interventions to organize or assist with physical activity and energy conservation and expenditure B *Elimination Management:* Interventions to establish and maintain regular bowel and urinary elimination patterns and manage complications due to altered patterns C *Immobility Management:* Interventions to manage restricted body movement and the sequelae D *Nutrition Support:* Interventions to modify or maintain nutritional status E *Physical Comfort Promotion:* Interventions to promote comfort	G *Electrolyte and Acid-Base Management:* Interventions to regulate electrolyte/acid base balance and prevent complications H *Drug Management:* Interventions to facilitate desired effects of pharmacological agents I *Neurologic Management:* Interventions to optimize neurologic functions J *Perioperative Care:* Interventions to provide care before, during, and immediately after surgery K *Respiratory Management:* Interventions to promote airway patency and gas exchange L *Skin/Wound Management:*	O *Behavior Therapy:* Interventions to reinforce or promote desirable behaviors or alter undesirable behaviors P *Cognitive Therapy:* Interventions to reinforce or promote desirable cognitive functioning or alter undesirable cognitive functioning Q *Communication Enhancement:* Interventions to facilitate delivering and receiving verbal and nonverbal messages R *Coping Assistance:* Interventions to assist another to build on own strengths, to adapt to a change in function, or to achieve a higher level of function S *Patient Education:* Interventions to facilitate learning

Domain 1	Domain 2	Domain 3
using physical techniques F *Self-Care Facilitation:* Interventions to provide or assist with routine activities of daily living	Interventions to maintain or restore tissue integrity M *Thermoregulation:* Interventions to maintain body temperature within a normal range N *Tissue Perfusion Management:* Interventions to optimize circulation of blood and fluids to the tissue	T *Psychological Comfort Promotion:* Interventions to promote comfort using psychological techniques

Domain 4	Domain 5	Domain 6
4. *Safety* Care that supports protection against harm	5. *Family* Care that supports the family unit	6. *Health System* Care that supports effective use of the health care delivery system
U *Crisis Management:* Interventions to provide immediate short-term help in both psychological and physiological crises V *Risk Management:* Interventions to initiate risk-reduction activities and continue monitoring risks over time	W *Childbearing Care:* Interventions to assist in understanding and coping with the psychological and physiological changes during the childbearing period X *Lifespan Care:* Interventions to facilitate family unit functioning and promote the health and welfare of family members throughout the lifespan	Y *Health System Mediation:* Interventions to facilitate the interface between patient/family and the health care system a *Health System Management:* Interventions to provide and enhance support services for the delivery of care b *Information Management:* Interventions to facilitate communication among health care providers

Source: Iowa Intervention Project 1992.

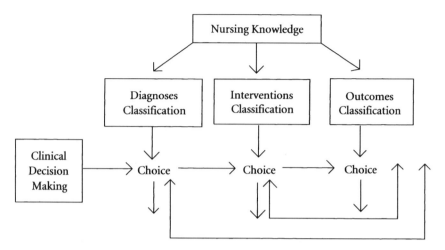

Figure 1   Relationship of nursing knowledge classifications to nurse's clinical decision-making. *Source:* McCloskey and Bulechek (1992: 7).

noses. The nursing profession used the diagnosis classification system to promote the claim that nurses diagnose patients in certain domains of care. They are thus not solely dependent on physician's orders. Along similar lines, the NIC investigators want to further the professional struggle for autonomy by creating a list of all nursing interventions. As one respondent stated: "It's very hard to be autonomous and independent unless you can say what it is you treat and what it is you do." The list is intended to make the invisible work of nursing visible via a detailed representation of the range of nursing tasks. NIC makes a historical connection between diagnoses and outcomes. Having listed nursing interventions, another group of researchers will make a list of possible nursing outcomes to measure the impact of nursing interventions. This will provide classification systems for the full range of nursing work and responsibility (see figure 1).

The Nursing Interventions Classification system, although still relatively young, promises to be a major rallying point for nurses in the decades to come. Since its first workable version in 1992, NIC has been taken up by a major medical publisher, formally used to organize nursing training, endorsed by the major hospital accrediting agency, adopted by two main nursing reference indexes, added to the National Library of Medicine's Metathesaurus for the Unified Medical Language System, sold its translation rights in different languages, and it is currently being tested in five field sites across the United States.

So, what is NIC? As a set of interventions it provides a list of what nurses do and therefore what nursing is. Although NIC might look like a straightforward organizational tool, it is much more than that. It merges scientific knowledge, practice, bureaucracy, and information systems. NIC coordinates bodies, impairments, charts, reimbursement systems, vocabularies, patients, and health care professionals. Ultimately, it provides a manifesto for an organized occupation: a domain of living scientific knowledge, a highly specialized practice, and an important element of cost and cost-containment in health care.

Creating and establishing NIC means balancing the architecture of differentiation and dedifferentiation, against an ongoing backdrop of struggle and change in the domain of nursing autonomy. The past few decades have seen the emergence of nursing science, and the general processes of professionalization. It also occurs against the backdrop of a changing classification arena in the American state.[5] In the following sections we explore how the NIC researchers negotiated the different requirements of the architecture in the construction of the classification. We evaluate the intentions and rhetoric of the NIC researchers as a process of defining the characteristics of their object and the world in which it functions. With Akrich (1992a) and Latour (Akrich and Latour 1992), we see this process as "inscribing" their vision of what nursing is and should be in the technical content of the classification system. A close analysis of the negotiations permits one to evaluate the process of balancing out differentiation and dedifferentiation. The empirical material for this analysis consists of all the minutes of NIC team meetings and publications of the NIC group since 1987, eighteen open ended in-depth interviews with principal investigators, co-investigators, and research associates, and observations of team meetings.

DIFFERENTIATION AND DEDIFFERENTIATION: COMPARABILITY

The construction of a classification system for nursing interventions implies a drive to abstract away from the local, the particular — to make "nursing" the same entity wherever it may appear. Ideally, local language, the idiosyncrasies of each ward and each staff nurse should change immediately through an adoption of NIC in hospital administration. Those making the classification examine variability in order to either eliminate or translate it across settings. This is the strategy of moving toward universality: rendering things comparable, so that each actor may fit their allotted position in a standardized system, and comparisons may be communicated across sites. Julius Roth has described this process for the operation of tuberculosis sanatoria (rendering patients equivalent) (1963); Marc Berg for the development of medical protocols (rendering treatment equivalent) (this volume); Geoffrey Bowker and Leigh Star for the development of the International Classification of Diseases (rendering statistics equivalent) (1991; 1994); and Stefan Timmermans for resuscitation techniques (rendering life saving equivalent) (1995).

For the Nursing Interventions Classification, the urge to erase the particular and communicate equivalents is apparent in several strategies the group adopts to further their cause. The developers consider NIC a basis for curriculum development: they reason that only with a complete classification system can one guarantee thorough, standardized, and cross-site comparability in professional training. The Nursing Interventions Classification system is being integrated into model course development efforts at Iowa and elsewhere. The basic interventions are part of undergraduate nursing curricula, while the more advanced interventions will be taught to master's students. But NIC is ultimately as well a standardized language for comparability. A respondent stated: "The classification is an aspect that makes it a tool, more usable, but it is the standardized language that is really critical." According to the NIC researchers "a standardized language for nursing treatments is a classification about nursing practice that names what nurses do relative to certain human needs to produce certain outcomes" (McCloskey and Bulechek 1994a: 57). In the eyes of the NIC creators, the classification system provides such a standardized language for nursing treatments that can be used across units, across health care settings, and across health care disciplines. A classification alone would be useful for costing, recordkeeping, and teaching, but the linguistic aspect is necessary for research and comparability. This was clearly expressed in several interviews:

Certainly we are aiming at standardizing nursing languages. So that when we talk among other nurses and other health professionals we all know what we talk about. Because what one nurse might be talking about is very different [from another nurse]. What is the difference between therapeutic play and play therapy? And then we need to communicate with parents, consumers, patients, physicians, and other health professionals and knowing that they are talking the same language. It is really important that we talk in a language that is not foreign to other groups. Maybe we like to be unique, but sometimes we need to bend so that we talk the same language as families, consumers, and medical professionals.

A hospital administrator told me a couple of years ago: "If nursing could just tell us what they do?" You can't say "the nursing process" because everyone does nursing assessment, intervention. That is a model that everyone can apply. Physical therapy can say what they do: muscles and bones. Respiratory therapy can define their tasks. But nurses do all that. Nursing is so broad. The only thing that they know is that they can't work without us. NIC is extremely helpful because it provides a language to communicate what we do with a firm scientific base.

The Unified Medical Language System, among others, is indicative of the drive for a standardized langauge in new developments of health care information systems. To study the effectiveness of nursing care, the nursing profession proposed the uniform and routine collection of essential nursing information: the Nursing Minimum Data Set (NMDS) (Werley and Lang 1988; Werley, Lang, and Westlake 1986). "The purpose of the NMDS is to foster comparability of nursing care across patient populations, with the ultimate goal the improvement of health care" (McCloskey and Bulechek 1994a: 56). This data set consists of sixteen data elements including four nursing care elements: nursing diagnoses, nursing interventions, nursing outcomes, and nursing intensity. NIC is promoted by its creators as providing the nursing intervention variable for the NMDS. A standardized language is also necessary to communicate with extant information systems.

Ironically, NIC's biggest critics come from the same information systems world. Criticism has been directed against NIC's standardized language ambitions. Susan Grobe, a nurse and information scientist at the University of Texas, Houston, criticizes the attempts at creating an universal standardized system as scientifically outmoded and inflexible. Instead Grobe proposes her own nursing intervention system, the Nursing Intervention Lexicon and Taxonomy (NILT), which consists of eight broad categories of nursing interventions. According to Grobe, in NILT "the burden of standardized language is resident in the automated systems and not dictated to practicing professionals for their memorization and adoption" (Grobe 1993: 94). Where NIC expects nurses to learn and use a standardized terminology, Grobe believes that nurses should keep their natural language and computers should be used to standardize language. She argues that having computers decide how terms will be standardized is inevitable and cites researchers who are working on this in health care documentation.

NIC researchers defend themselves against Grobe's criticism by specifying how a standardized language increases comparability. They note that although the advent of computers was an impetus for standardized languages, different organizations and agencies developed their own system "with the result that we cannot collect comparable data from multiple agencies, or even within agencies from one unit to the next." They further quote Sherrer, Cote, and Mandill 1989: "[I]ntelligent documentation systems cannot totally discard classifications. Moreover, the availability of at least one classification is a necessary condition for a good documentation system. Classifications are not a necessary evil but a very effective way of representing knowledge about the domain of discourse" (quoted in McCloskey and Bulechek 1994a: 59; see also Bulechek and McCloskey 1993). Thus since a "natural language" is at this moment lacking in nursing, the NIC researchers claim that their classification system fills the void and at the same time achieves the goal of comparability.

In their newsletter, the NIC investigators summarize their vision about a standardized language to achieve comparability across sites and professions: "Norma Lang has often been quoted as saying, 'If we cannot name it, we cannot control it, finance it, teach it, research it, or put it into public policy . . .' We would like to be quoted as saying: 'Now that we have named it, we can control it, finance it, teach it, research it, and put it into public policy' " (NIC Newsletter 1994).

The strive for comparability in a standardized language across settings conflicts with the need for manageability within local settings. The nursing intervention architects want their entire system to be adopted by health care institutions. As a language, its entire vocabulary needs to be available to nursing professionals. However, certain institutions will most likely only need part of the NIC taxonomy. For example, nurses in a geriatric hospital will probably not require "newborn care" as an intervention. The results of validation studies with different nursing specialties suggests that between 20 and 80 percent of the terminology would be routinely used by several nursing specialties. This raises the issue of how to limit each institution's modifications. Too much flexibility would obviously undermine the birth of a standard language, but too much external control makes a system user-unfriendly, especially in such a safety-critical and busy line of work. The NIC designers were aware of this dilemma:

> We are having to work out the tension between the ivory tower academic approach and the real practice world. We think probably that the big hospitals should have it totally on their systems so that all the interventions are available but units may decide not to put all 336 on, they may only take certain classes. We talk about that and as soon as we start zeroing in, we find that most institutions are going to use at least two-thirds or three-fourths of the classes. . . . The thing about nursing is that nursing is holistic, it is very hard for people to break it up.

As a rule of thumb, the NIC group decided that an institution should adopt the whole classification system at the level of the copyrighted interventions, definitions, and labels but that activity-level descriptions could be modestly changed. However, control and enforcement of this rule ultimately rests with the publisher and with the goodwill of institutions adopting NIC to follow the policy set out by the Iowa NIC group. Again pragmatics abound:

That was probably one of the major reasons that pushed us into going with the major publisher for the classification rather than holding it in Iowa and doing it our selves. We're not so naive to think that if a little rural hospital in Iowa violates the copyright agreement that our publisher's going to come dashing in and do something about it. They will only pick the situations where it's in their financial best interests to do it. But at least they're handling all the licensing agreements.

DIFFERENTIATION AND DEDIFFERENTIATION: VISIBILITY

Comparability rests on the management and mobility of differences and equivalences across sites. The issue becomes: what is local and particular or what do all nurses have in common that can be rendered equivalent across settings and nursing specialties? The nursing classification designers employ a definition of nursing interventions as guideline. "A nursing intervention is any direct care treatment that a nurse performs on behalf of a client. These treatments include nurse-initiated treatments resulting from nursing diagnoses, physician-initiated treatments resulting from medical diagnoses, and performance of the daily essential functions for the client who cannot do these" (Bulechek and McCloskey 1989). Here, the emphasis is on direct care: that which nurses do to increase the well-being of a patient at the bedside. Direct care is separated from care that only indirectly benefits the patient—e.g. coordinating treatment schedules, discharge planning, and patient supervision. One step further removed from the bedside is administrative care, activities for creating an environment for direct and indirect care. This includes coordinating administrative units and supervising nurses. Initially, the NIC group concentrated on direct care interventions. The researchers deliberately supported an image in the classification of nursing as a clinical discipline. This was a political decision, as several NIC team members noted in interviews: "Nurses think that laying hands on patients is nursing. We would not have had the attention of the nursing community if we had not begun there."

However, questions arose in the course of the project about the distinction between direct and indirect care.

The indirect care are things that staff nurses do but they are not on the patients' behalf. It includes all the coordinating, amassing the resources, and discharge planning. For instance, we make sure that the emergency cart is ready and available for when a patient is at risk of coding. Nurses do all of this stuff and if it is not in NIC it will not be reimbursed. Some people say that nurses are the glue that hold the system together, and that's the indirect part of it.

Time spent on these tasks will be invisible if they are not included in NIC, and thus fiscally wasted. Over the course of the project, indirect interventions grew in importance and will be included in the second edition of the NIC book. The researchers even adapted their initial definition of a nursing intervention to include the indirect interventions.

However, nurses themselves are somewhat ambivalent about how to account for indirect care time. Statistical analyses based upon different validation studies reveal that several of the indirect care interventions are indeed considered in a different category by nurses responding to the surveys.

Administrative care is even more controversial. In interviews, some of the NIC collaborators, whose main tasks are administrative, expected that NIC would eventually also contain those kind of interventions: "Nursing is very different in that when you make changes, it involves many people. The need for managers, supervisors and coordinators of planned change is a central part of nursing. I think anything that reflects nursing, needs to reflect those work aspects."

However, a majority of the design team and consulting group was not sure whether administrative care was typical for nurses and thus whether it belonged in a nursing classification. "The administrators are not actually nursing. When they are not there the nursing continues without them." Or, in the words of Gloria Bulechek, "Management science is a different discipline; all managers have to manage people and it is not unique to nursing." For the latter group, the need to make administrative care visible is not as urgent as the need to differentiate nursing as a hands-on discipline. Although the nursing researchers are aware that the boundaries between direct, indirect, and administrative care are not firm, administrative care is not part of NIC nor is it scheduled to be part of the revised edition of NIC. This dilemma about the encoding of administrative work points to a practical limit on the visibility-discretion axis. In order to fully abstract from the local, everything must be spelled out; in order to avoid resistance from nurses and nursing administrators, some work must be left implicit. What is left implicit becomes doubly invisible: it is the residue left over when other sorts of invisible work has been made visible (Strauss et al. 1985; Star 1991a). That is, where claims are made for the completeness of an accounting system, that which is not accounted for may be twice overlooked. We are noting this here as both a formal and a practical challenge for the classification designers and users.

The tension between visibility on the one hand and control and intimacy on the other became apparent when several group members noted that the classification is strong, and maybe too strong, within the nursing specialties of the system's developers, such as the complex physiological domain. However, it is still underdeveloped in other nursing areas such as community health and social-psychological nursing. Social-psychological caregiving is one of the areas where the control/visibility dilemma is very difficult to grasp. For example, NIC lists as one nursing intervention "humor." How can one capture humor as a deliberate nursing intervention? Does sarcasm, irony, or laughter count as a nursing intervention? How to reimburse humor, how to measure this kind of care? No one would dispute its importance, but it is *by its nature* a situated and subjective action. Since NIC does not contain protocols and procedures for each intervention, a gray area of common sense remains for the individual staff nurse to define whether some of the nursing activities can be called nursing interventions or are worth charting. Of course, this same gray area remains for more clinical interventions such as "cerebral edema management" or "acid-base monitoring."[6] But because the classification is modeled after a clinical model of nursing, the team felt it easier to define and include those more clinical interventions.

Not only in the interventions themselves but also in the decisions underlying NIC, the borderland between professional control and the urge to make nursing visible is fraught with difficult choices and balances. Team members recalled discussions where interventions were so singular and demarcated as to warrant inclusion, but they ended up not being included. For example, one will not find "leech therapy" as an intervention in the classification, although there was enough research literature to support this intervention as typical nursing in many parts of the world[7] (Neumann 1995). Also, the advanced statistical analysis of the validation studies was located in what the design team members typified as "common sense." One could have a coefficient of .73, but if it didn't respond to a visible or controllable enough nursing reality, it became an outlier, a nonresult, or resulted in a residual category. As with all statistical analyses, a link with theory and practice must precede testing or the results are meaningless.

In other cases, the criteria for inclusion and control are themselves contested. One research member confided in an interview that her intervention was rejected because it was not supported with research evidence. Her plan was to first publish a paper about the intervention in a research journal and then resubmit the intervention for consideration with her own reference as research evidence. In these examples, the goal of making as much visible as possible clashes with what should remain taken for granted. The nursing researchers temper their quest to make nursing visible with the image of what nursing is or should be about. Again, there is no final answer or algorithm but a complex balance of experience and rules. Visibility is tempered by common practice, contingency, and legitimacy.

DIFFERENTIATION AND DEDIFFERENTIATION: CONTROL

There is a continuing tension within NIC, as we have noted, between abstracting away from the local and rendering "invisible work" visible. Nurses' work is often quintessentially invisible for a combination of good and bad reasons. Nurses have to ask mundane questions, rearrange bedcovers, move a patient's hand so that it is closer to a button, and sympathize about the suffering involved in illness (Olesen and Whittaker 1968). Bringing this work out into the open and differentiating its components has encountered problems from the nurses themselves. In naming and differentiating someone's work, there is a fine line between being too obvious and being too vague, once one has decided to take on naming as a central task. If the task that is brought under the glare of Enlightenment science is too obvious and mundane, then some nurses who are testing the system find it insulting. To tell a veteran nurse to shake down a thermometer after taking a temperature puts him or her into a childlike position. Some experienced nurses, encountering interventions they felt were too obvious, have called them a NSS or "No Shit, Sherlock" intervention. That is, it really doesn't take a Sherlock Holmes to realize that nurses have to do this! The same incongruity plays in the difference between the learned and the daily practice. As one interviewee expressed: "I don't know how many times nurses have said to me 'I know this isn't the way you were taught, but this is the way we do it here.'" Creating difference by cutting up the continuum of duties that make up "looking after the patient's welfare" is thus sociologically, as well as phenomenologically and philosophically, very difficult. One must be explicit enough for the novices, and not insulting to the veterans, include the textbook knowledge without bypassing the daily tricks of the trade. Reading the NIC minutes, one is frequently reminded of ethnomethodological texts: just how much "common sense" can be taken for granted is a perpetually open question, and to whom it is in fact common sense is not always so obvious (e.g., Sacks 1975). But ethnomethodology alone will not solve the political and organizational controversies and dilemmas of standardization.

One of the battlefields where comparability and control appear as opposing factors is in linking NIC to costing. NIC researchers assert that the classification of nursing interventions will allow a determination of the costs of services provided by nurses and planning for resources needed in nursing practice settings. In our interviews with them, team members noted that although nurses fill in for physical therapists during weekends, the nursing department is not always reimbursed for this service. Sometimes the money flows back to the hospital at large, to the physical therapy department, or these treatments are simply not reimbursed.

> [Nursing activities] are not a part of the patient's bill and nursing does not get credit for those dollars. My goal is to get nursing credit for those dollars and to have nursing seen as a revenue-generating part of the hospital system. Nursing care has always been a part of the room charge, and the room charge might change if we do these things. Some interventions that therapists charge for and nurses do as well, I think nurses should charge for, and that may show up on the patient's bill.

According to the NIC researchers, NIC will allow hospital administrators to determine nursing costs and resource allocation and stop such apparent "freeloading." Until it is made explicit exactly what nurses do on a daily basis, administrators have trouble rationally allocating tasks. Similarly, NIC is used in the development of nursing health care systems and communication with the classification systems of other health care providers. This coordination provides a safety net and planning vehicle for untraced costs. In order to reach the administration, the NIC team members hoped to interest medical vendors in their project: "Vendors are a very important group. There are about 130 vendors in health care and nursing, each of them with a very small market share, very competitive. I believe that we have to work more with these vendors. They are moving toward computerization of patient records. We've only had two of those vendors ask for computer licenses."

The horizon is not fully clear, however. Wagner and Robinson have studied the implementation of similar measures in Europe.[8] While they have the effect of making nursing work visible and differentiated, they may also become a target for social control and surveillance of nursing work, working *against* control in the sense of discretionary judgment and common sense. Wagner notes that "Nurses' striving for a higher degree of professionalization contains a contradictory message. Nurses might gain greater recognition for their work and more control over the definition of patients' problems while finding out that their practice is increasingly shaped by the necessity to comply with regulators' and employers' definitions of 'billable categories'" (1993). She states that while computerization of care plans in French and Austrian hospitals is partly designed to give nurses greater scope of responsibility, and legitimize their care giving in some detail, it also has another side:

> The idea of computerized care-plans, as put forward in nursing research, is to strengthen the focus on nurses' own pre-planned nursing "projects." Like "the autonomous profession," nurses are seen as setting apart time for specialized activities, irrespective of ad-hoc-demands. . . . The reality of computerized care plans—even when nurses themselves have a voice in their development—may lag far behind this idea, given the authority structures in hospitals. With management focusing on case plans as instruments that may help them with their legal and accreditation issues, and nurses having to continue documenting their work on the KARDEX and other forms as well, care plans cannot unfold their potential. (Wagner 1993: 302–3)

Once designed, a classification system is then not a "black box" before it becomes part of nursing practice. The balancing act of the designer team needs to continue on every ward of every hospital (Timmermans and Berg 1997).

PROFESSIONALIZATION, CLASSIFICATION SYSTEMS, AND NURSING AUTONOMY

Since the focus of the Nursing Interventions Classification is on making nursing visible, along with balancing out control and comparability, it is interesting to compare the strategies chosen by the NIC researchers in order to fully professionalize nursing to the range of strategies discussed by Abbott in *The System of Professions* (1988). Abbott puts the struggle for jurisdiction in central place, and his model of "the cultural machinery of jurisdiction" (ibid., 59) characterizes professional work in terms of diagnosis, treatment, inference, and academic work. The very words are drawn from the medical profession. Staking out a jurisdictional claim within that profession is particularly difficult—what is specific in a "nursing diagnosis" that differentiates it from "medical diagnosis"? He does not describe any other case where a central tool has been the creation of a classification system. Yet within the medical system as a whole, having access to one's own classification has long been a control strategy. Kirk and Kutchins (1992), for example, discuss jurisdictional disputes between the *International Classification of Diseases* and the *Diagnostic and Statistical Manual of Mental Disorders*, and show convincingly that the *Diagnostic and Statistical Manual of Mental Disorders* became a tool for a particular theory of psychiatry, empowering more physiologically based models at the expense of psychological models. There is such a "Tower of Babel" of classification systems within medicine[9] that a major thrust now is the creation of a unified medical language system (UMLS), which will allow cross-translation among the various classifications. NIC has been recognized by the UMLS as a valid nursing classification; and this is a major victory for the development group.

In order to gain equity with the medical profession (where they have often been seen as subordinate), nursing research is an important aspect of legitimation. In turn, classification of work is a cornerstone of research. Nursing classification creates the possibility of equivalence on the research end. Because nursing had long been defined as the undifferentiated other (everything that doctors don't do with respect to the treatment of patients), it was impossible to create precise arguments for professionalization based on research results.

But as nursing differentiates and becomes more autonomous, it too creates its own undifferentiated other. In what sense? As Abbott emphasized, professionalization depends upon the scope of the professions' jurisdiction. For NIC this implies that if nurses define a number of activities as specifically nursing activities, they also claim *only* these activities. Although the researchers mean to include all the activities that nurses do, it is impossible to be totally inclusive, as we have demonstrated. Regional variations, and those activities which cut across professional domains, cannot be articulated in an interventions classification system. Some may be left in residual categories, or left for other health care groups such as licensed vocational nurses and technicians. Implicit in the physician's classification systems was the assumption that *nurses* would perform any unaccounted work that would allow the fit between the doctors' prescription and the patients' health.[10] Now that nurses are creating their own classification system, they too might rely in a changed fashion on the invisible and unaccounted work of others.

The NIC group hopes that their classification system will sensitize the entire health care sphere to the contribution that nurses make to the well-being of patients. But the road to such an outcome is a difficult (and potentially even dangerous) one for nurses as a group, as Wagner has shown for the European example. For instance, it is possible that NIC might be used against nursing professionalization in some computerization and surveillance scenarios. Imagine a hospital administrator who has implemented NIC and evaluates what the nurses are doing. In an effort to curtail costs and adequately allocate resources, the administrator might prescribe nursing activities that are more cost-efficient. When asked about this issue, one of the principal investigators, Joanne McCloskey, emphasized that is more important that nurses deal with those questions instead of leaving them tacit. "It may create some problems, but it forces nursing into the mainstream and forces nurses to be responsible, accountable health care providers. Then, of course, you have to deal with the questions that physicians have had to deal with for a long time. And we ought to be able to deal with that and find a good new solution" (see also McCloskey and Bulechek 1994b).

A classification system is an important tool in the struggle for professional recognition. When the tensions between visibility, comparability, and control are skillfully managed in the construction of the classification system itself, the same processes need to be balanced at the level of users and policy makers. NIC's goal is to promote the work of nurses by communicating newly visible (in the sense of inscribed and legitimated) work practices and by leaving enough space for controllable action. But even if the designers succeed in creating an equilibrium at the information system level, there are potential utilization problems in the political arena. Professionalization through visibility alone may have latent consequences: constant surveillance in the name of the panopticon of cost containment (Foucault 1979). In this era of information infrastructure shifts, the gravity of this scenario is enormous.

CONCLUSION

The Nursing Interventions Classification constitutes an attempt to produce a classification scheme that can subtend the creation of nursing knowledge (by creating differences between nursing practices — not leaving nursing as the undifferentiated other represented in the phrase that nurses do "everything to do with the patient"). At the same time NIC has to respond to a variety of needs for information of all sorts, from all sides: each user has his or her own unique spin on the world of what constitutes relevant information. And it has to juggle the strategy of professionalization by visibility with that of professionalization by defending an autonomous region. What, in Bateson's terms, is the difference that makes a difference? Some developers of the system want to specify and standardize down to the level of activities; others claim that only the intervention level can be made fully explicit.

In general, classification schemes provide both a living organizational memory (Walsh and Ungsen 1991) and a means for bureaucratic control. Suchman says: "Categorization device are devices of social control involving contests between others' claims to the territories inhabited by persons or activities and their own, internally administered forms of organization" (1994a: 188). The ramified lists of concepts that build up a classification system reflect an attempt, at the larger scale, to create a displacement of interests—the genesis of the state or a discipline. A classification system is then a political actor in the attempts to establish power on broad institutional and historical levels. When a classification system intends to promote a professional group, the challenges are geared toward their ability to enhance professionalization. In the best case, classification systems hold a memory of work which has been done (laboratory, organizational, epidemiological, sociological) and so permit the recommendation of a reasonable due process for future work (Star and Gerson 1986).

It is difficult to retrace these processes after the classification is black-boxed. We have been fortunate to observe an effort to classify work in its early days, coordinated by a group of American nursing researchers, which is beginning to spread to other locations as well. Their work exemplifies a profoundly skilled "balancing act" revolving around managing the tradeoffs outlined above. The NIC project team has a global strategy of balanced classification through a series of sophisticated moves of differentiation and dedifferentiation. This strategy assumes that the work of producing equivalence (making other things equal) will reduce the overall amount of effort: retraining when a nurse needs to move into a new situation, introducing the nurse to the medical information system in a new hospital, and so on. It is linked with the strategy of the creation of a single information infrastructure to facilitate hospital operation. As such, NIC is embedded in and interacting with numerous structures and institutions. As a standardized language, NIC links the vernacular of every practicing nurse, the terminologies of nursing curricula, nursing research, even the basic thinking about nursing. As a classification system, NIC connects with NANDA, the outcome classification systems, the Unified Medical Language System and other national and international medical classification systems. When used for cost containment, NIC enters the world of computerization with vendors, hospital administrators, insurance companies, and health care reform. Finally, NIC becomes a tool for the American Nursing Association in its struggle for autonomy and professionalization.

A favorite metaphor of NIC proponents to describe their task is "to make the invisible work visible." As the layers of complexity involved in its architecture reveal, however, a light shining in the dark illuminates certain areas of nursing work, but may cast shadows elsewhere. The whole picture is a very complex one. The Nursing Interventions Classification is at once an attempt at a universal standardized tool, with a common language; at the same time, its development and application proceeds by managing and articulating local and particulars. It is in that sense a boundary object between communities of practice, with a delicate cooperative structure (Star and Griesemer 1989); at the same time, it is balanced in a work flow and historical period which makes it a potential target for control. The fact that NIC researchers are carefully involving a huge web of nurses and nursing researchers, building slowly over time, with revisions, is central to this. The conservation of work inscribed in the static list of concepts and activities that form a classification system will be inserted in a field of ongoing practices, negotiations, and professional autonomy disputes. These practices, at the political field in which they occur, form the architecture of intimacy, manageability, and standardization. The local and macro contexts of the classification system and its attendant practices (Berg 1997) determine in final instance the extent of the displacement of nursing work. In classification systems, differentiation and dedifferentiation emerge as a continuous and negotiated accomplishment over time. It is not a question of map or territory, but map *in* territory.

NOTES

We are very much indebted to the members of the Nursing Interventions Project at the University of Iowa. In particular, Joanne McCloskey and Gloria Bulechek provided many helpful suggestions during conversations. We would further like to thank the following Iowa team members who have graciously allowed us to interview them: Laurie Ackerman, Sally Blackman, Gloria Bulechek, Joan Carter, Jeanette Daly, Janice Denehy, Bill Donahue, Chris Forcucci, Orpha Glick, Mary Kanak, Vicki Kraus, Tom Kruckeberg, Meridean Maas, Joanne McCloskey, Barbara Rakel, Marita Titler, Bonnie Wakefield, and Huibin Yue. We would also like to thank our colleagues on the Classification Project, University of Illinois: Theresa Chi Lin, Merrie Ritter, Niranjan Karnik, and Laura Neumann for ongoing discussions and insight; the Advanced Information Technologies Group; and the Department of Sociology at the University of Illinois for support. Comments by Annemarie Mol, Marc Berg, Isabelle Baszanger, Pauline Cochran, and anonymous reviewers were most helpful.

1 Personal communication.
2 From a talk given at the Program for Cultural Values and Ethics, University of Illinois, December 1993.
3 Although it may seem at first sight that comparability and standardization are the same thing, we see an important difference between the two concepts. An example might explain this. Two things can be comparable but not standardized: thus you can compare an education at Harvard with an education at Southern Illinois, because you know that in general a lot more resources are pumped into Harvard and outcomes tend to be different because of the homogeneity of backgrounds. In that case, one would be high on the "comparability" side of standardization but low on the "visibility" side: no one spells out exactly what the difference is. If you then

subject all students to a single standardized test, then you have to match comparability with visibility to provide standardization.

4   Incidentally, this is what sociologists have called "sentimental work" (Strauss et al.
1982).

5   This was made more urgent by changes to the national health care system proposed
under the Clinton administration, and by the widespread increase in medical infor-
matics and multimedia electronic imaging systems for remote medical diagnosis
and testing.

6   See Michael Lynch's work on "turning up signs" for an example of the inexhaust-
ible discretion and improvisation in every human activity—the study of which has
been the major contribution of ethnomethodology and phenomenology.

7   This was the situation during our interview round. According to Joanne McCloskey, leech therapy probably will be included in the next edition of the NIC book.

8   See Wagner 1993, in press; Egger and Wagner 1993; Gray, Elkan, and Robinson 1991;
and Strong and Robinson 1990.

9   Including occupational classifications, disability, geographical and regional, and
specialty-based systems, among others. Also looming on the horizon is a map
dispute between allopathic and complementary ("alternative" or traditional) approaches to medicine, which both the WHO and the NIH have acknowledged in the
establishment of directives and committees to study the problem.

10 Strauss et al. (1985) call this activity articulation work.

ORDER(S) AND DISORDER(S):
OF PROTOCOLS AND
MEDICAL PRACTICES

Marc Berg

▼

[O]ne of the basic assumptions underlying the practice of medicine is being challenged. This assumption concerns the intellectual foundation of medical care. Simply put, the assumption is that whatever a physician decides is, by definition, correct. The challenge says that while many decisions no doubt are correct, many are not, and elaborate mechanisms are needed to determine which are which. . . . [T]he challenge can be justified solely by a concern for quality. The plain fact is that many decisions made by physicians appear to be arbitrary—highly variable, with no obvious explanation. The very disturbing implication is that this arbitrariness represents, for at least some patients, suboptimal or even harmful care. — D. M. Eddy, "The Challenge"

In the last two decades, many editorials and articles in medical journals have uttered warnings similar to Eddy's statement quoted here. Medical practice, it is argued, is in trouble. Enormous variations in physicians' decision-making behavior have become apparent. The numbers of operations between regions, for example, shows variations which are in the order of three- to twentyfold (Wennberg 1984). Similarly, when having to decide on the appropriateness of indications for coronary angiography or coronary artery bypass graft, United Kingdom physicians appeared to judge wholly differently from United States doctors (Brook et al. 1988). Apparently, physicians' decision making is a highly capricious affair, well in need of some support.

According to these authors, the problems are not surprising. The "ingredients needed for accurate decisions are simply missing for many medical practices." There is often no evidence available as to what should be the action of choice; thus, physicians "turn to their own experiences [which] are notoriously misleading" (Eddy 1990b). The physician also often lacks uniform procedures to deal with medical problems. As yet, it is argued, he cannot articulate "the logic of his rational pathway"; he or she suffers "scientific aphasia" and thus dwells in a state of "amorphous judgment" (Feinstein 1974; 1987b). Moreover, many authors argue that the problems modern doctors face are often too complex for ordinary humans to grasp comprehensively. As Eddy states: "Even if good evidence were available, it is unrealistic, even unfair, to expect people to be able to sort through it all in their heads. . . . We are trying to solve in our heads problems that far exceed the capacity of the unaided human mind. There are tools, already in use in many other domains, to help us" (1990b).

What are these tools? The authors quoted here refer to *protocols;* or, as they call them, "algorithms," or "practice policies," which can "improve the capacity of physician to make better decisions" (ibid.). Protocols are "preformed recommendations issued for the purpose of influencing decisions about health interventions." By analyzing "decisions before the fact," they prevent the "mental paralysis or chaos" that would otherwise result from having to rationally decide every time again from scratch. A protocol can be an "intellectual vehicle," which can have immense leverage and be very detailed at the same time (Eddy 1990c). A protocol is a set of instructions; it informs the user what to do in a specified situation. Through the branching structure of the protocol, "a clinician can now, at long last, specify the flow of logic in his reasoning, [so that he] can begin to achieve the reproducibility and standardization required for science" (Feinstein 1974).

Tools like these are nothing new to the practice of medicine. In its simplest form, a protocol is nothing but a written instruction; and, of course, the idea of regulating action through a recipe is an ancient one (cf. Goody 1977). As a tool that could solve some of medical practice's problems, however, protocols first came into full view in the late 1960s and 1970s. The success of medical science during and after World War II had shown the merits of strengthening the collective effort through the coordination and linking of individual actions. Protocols were part and parcel of this enterprise: in the booming field of clinical research, the protocol was essential to assure that the actions and interpretations of outcomes would be similar in all participating institutions (cf. Marks 1988; 1997). Riding the wave of these developments, several authors argued that the particular science of medical *practice* could be enhanced in a similar fashion. Protocols, these authors argued, can "describe good clinical reasoning" in such a way that it becomes transferable, evaluable—and scientific (Margolis 1983; Eddy 1990a). It is a vehicle through which order can be brought to all those practices where messiness reigns. If we want to bring "physician practices into greater compliance with standards based on current biomedical research"

(Kanouse et al. 1989), we call upon a protocol in which these standards are embedded. If practice X does conform to these standards and Y does not, we can import the protocol containing the essence of X into Y and thus attempt to turn practice Y into a practice resembling X. For example, if in practice X breast cancer is treated in a way deemed optimal by a group of surgeons and oncologists, they can attempt to write the essentials of this approach in a protocol and distribute the protocol to other practices where this method of treatment is not yet, or not optimally, followed.

The protocol is thus seen as an optimal solution to the "unscientific" state of current medical practice. It would be a mistake, however, to interpret its current ubiquity (ranging from broadly phrased consensus-based statements via ad hoc, institutional arrangements to detailed research protocols)[1] as due to the profession's own desire to rationalize medical work. Judicial, economic, and administrative pressure for uniformity and reproducibility (cf. Dodier this volume; Löwy 1995a; Good 1995), the drive to better oversee and intervene in physician's work—all this is of the utmost importance for an understanding of the protocol's current (and contested) position in medical practice. In this paper, however, I will only address the protocol's promise to bring order where there was disorder; to replace the messiness of Y with the orderliness of X. I will investigate its claim to introduce homogeneity where there was variation. Is the protocol indeed the perfect and "inert" medium, the optimal homogenizing device it is depicted to be?[2]

To answer these questions, I recreate a small segment of the story of the construction of a Dutch, multi-institutional research protocol. Through this story, I elaborate what it is the protocol *does* in medical practices.[3] Homogenizing medical practices through protocols, I demonstrate, is not simply replacing manifold messiness with the orderliness of a "good" medical practice X. In *getting* the protocol to work, the relationships between the "order" embedded in the protocol and the "messiness" of medical practices become much more complex. First, the order embedded in the end-product inevitably contains much of the messiness it set out to erase. In addition, the order of X is not merely polluted in the process of construction and implementation of a protocol: it is also distinctively *transformed*. A protocol is not an inert tool: its specific, *formal* structure transforms the order it transports in distinctive ways.

As will become apparent, focusing on a research protocol inevitably raises issues that would not be at stake in other types of protocols, such as the representability of choices made for future scientific publications, and so forth. These issues do not affect the arguments set out here, however. Highlighting research protocols has the advantage of focusing on tools that are generally very detailed and precise. In comparison to for instance consensus statements, they are also generally more stringently adhered to. The issues involved in implementing and working with a protocol, thus, come out most clearly in these cases.

During a multiinstitutional research meeting of oncologists, a suggestion of one of the institutions is discussed.[4] This center is currently treating patients with locally advanced breast cancer (i.e., with involved local lymph nodes but no apparent distant metastases) in a new way, and its oncologists have suggested that their approach should be turned into an multiinstitutional research protocol. This protocol would treat these patients with an experimental therapy called "peripheral stem cell transplantation," and compare these cases with similar patients treated with "conventional" chemotherapy. In this experimental treatment, blood stem cells are filtered ("leukapheresis") from the patient's bloodstream, and deep-frozen.[5] Subsequently, the patient is treated with massive ("ablative") doses of chemotherapy, hopefully eradicating all tumor cells. These doses are so high that they would ordinarily also kill the bone marrow cells, responsible for the production of the blood cells. Without these cells, the patient would be depleted of vital parts of her immune system and die of infection. Also, the lack of platelets, crucial for hemostasis, could cause lethal internal and external bleedings. In this treatment, however, the unfrozen blood stem cells are given back to the patient after the highly toxic chemotherapy.

A first, rough agreement on the desirability of this project has already been reached. Paula, chairing the meeting, asks the group how many lymph nodes they want to settle upon. (This number stands for the amount of axillary nodes in which, after the first surgical resection of the tumor, cancer cells were found. On the whole, it is assumed that the more lymph nodes are involved, the poorer the prognosis. Settling on ten would imply that only patients with ten or more involved lymph nodes would be eligible. The number chosen is dependent on a host of different considerations. These oncologists want to reserve an experimental, intense treatment as this only for patients with a poor prognosis. Some people will probably die from this treatment, so they do not want to include patients who have a reasonable chance of survival anyway. On the other hand, the poorer the overall prognosis and condition of their patients, the less effect their therapy will have.)

"If we set the limit to ten," one oncologist says, "we might get too few patients. After all, the category of 'more than ten positive nodes' contains only some 10 percent of our patients. We might have too few cases for our study." "How many patients are we talking about?" somebody else intervenes. Some numbers are mentioned, but nobody is really sure. "But we can ask the national registration office," Paula says. "Although I'm actually not even sure that our pathologists do not stop counting at some point. They might not even reach ten; they might get bored beforehand, and just make a rough guess. I'm not sure." Some doctors laugh, and a fourth oncologist asks: "How many patients would have more than seven nodes?" Paula shakes her head: "The registration does not register that. 'Five' or 'ten' they will know. But that will be too much; we'll be flooded in patients. We cannot do more than so many of these treatments per year." "Not if we set the eligibility age lower," the same oncologist counters. "That clears away much."

Another oncologist joins the discussion: "If you would set the number of nodes lower than, say, ten, our center would get in trouble. We've already got some local trials running for these categories; this protocol would interfere." John, the main author of the protocol, interrupts: "That's no problem. You can enter all patients you want. We will deal with the differences in entry between centers. And about the expected number: if you realize that some 20 percent will drop out, and that we've got a control group [receiving the conventional treatment], and that we need quite some number of patients to show the small difference in survival we expect, then I would argue for going for, say, four nodes. Which is also a cutoff point often used in the scientific literature — where we want to be, right? If we settle on seven, for example, we cannot compare ourselves to other studies. Finally, if we have more eligible patients, we can finish our study sooner. This is good news both for our financiers and for our publication plans — and it also supports the choice for a low number of nodes."

Building upon recent social studies of science and technology, I study the construction and implementation of a protocol as a *technique*.[6] I focus on the *script* the tool embodies: how it delineates the roles and tasks of the nurses, physicians, lymph nodes, patients, and financiers in the practices in which it is supposed to be implemented (Akrich 1992a; Akrich and Latour 1992). This script includes the written text of the protocol, but extends beyond that. Many roles and tasks are to alter in ways not explicitly elaborated in the protocol's lines: the way the nurses work is affected, for example, or the way the patient's body is redefined often only becomes clear to the observer once the tool actually touches the practice involved.

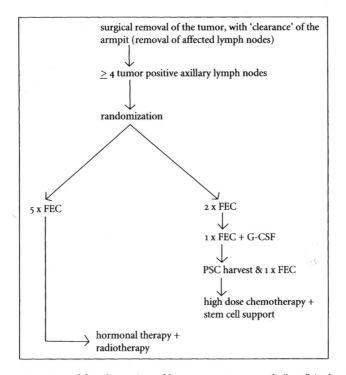

Figure 1   Overview of fourth version of breast cancer protocol. "FEC" is the abbreviation for the combination of three chemotherapeutic agents used. "PSC" stands for "peripheral stem cell." See text for further explanation.

As a first step, it is important to get a better picture of what a protocol is. The protocol discussed in the fragment above contains detailed, sequenced prescriptions as to how to act given such-and-such a situation. It tells exactly what diagnostics to pursue, what the entry criteria and the exact treatment steps are, when to ask for informed consent, what laboratory tests to order, and so on. The lymph nodes are only one of the "eligibility criteria": the patient should also, for example, be fifty-five or younger, her "performance status" (a measure for the overall condition of the patient) and renal and hepatic (liver) function should be adequate, and the breast cancer should be of a specific kind. As figure 1 shows, once the patient is eligible, a randomization procedure determines in which arm of the protocol the patient will fall. In the standard treatment (control) arm, the patient receives five courses of a regularly used combination of chemotherapeutic agents. The experimental treatment arm starts with the same medications, but G-CSF is added (a so-called growth factor, which stimulates the recovery of blood stem cells from the chemotherapy treatment).[7] Subsequently, stem cells are harvested and high-dose chemotherapy starts. All throughout this path, the protocol contains explicit criteria on whether and when the next step can be taken, and what to do when side effects occur. The dosages and timings are precisely prescribed, as is, for instance, the time of leukapheresis: "when CD34-positive [blood] cells are detectable in the peripheral blood." (CD34 stands for a group of immunological markers which, according to the protocol's authors, constitute a standardized way of checking the presence of the blood stem cells. When a certain level of CD34-positive cells show up in the blood, the chances of gathering sufficient blood stem cells are high).

The protocol requires that medical personnel delegate some of their coordinating activities to it, while, in turn, the protocol delegates specific tasks to them. It is there to create (a new) order, to realign the heterogeneous elements of the medical practice so as to reproduce the first oncology center's mode of treatment into a whole series of practices. The protocol *articulates* activities over different sites and times. The nurses know when to do which laboratory tests, and when to shift from one chemotherapeutic drug to another. Likewise, the radiotherapist knows when what is expected of her, and how her actions fit the overall picture. Through the making of detailed lists, actions in different spaces and times are brought together and coordinated (Goody 1977; Star 1989a; Callon 1991). The protocol functions as a focal point of reference to which different staff members refer, can orient themselves, and can find instructions on what to do next. In this way, through taking coordination tasks out of the hands of the medical staff, the protocol makes the administration of highly complex treatment schedules *possible* in the first place.[8]

How does the protocol fulfill this coordinating role? It does more than merely standardizing procedures or terminologies between practices — although that is both a prerequisite and a consequence of its functioning. It also *guides* the medical personnel through sequenced paths of action, geared toward features of the patient or situation at hand. At any important moment, given, for example, certain laboratory results, the tool will tell the staff what to do. So, FEC is administered in one day, once every twenty-one days. When, however, at day 21 the number of white blood cells is below a given threshold (indicating poor recovery), the protocol instructs to "delay one week." At day 28, the white blood cells are measured again; given the results, the patient is either given the full dose of FEC, or a 25 percent reduced dosage, or sent "off study." The guiding function of the tool is thus achieved through its structuring as a series of "if . . . then" statements: in the case of A, the protocol instructs to do B. A protocol is a *formalism:* it operates using a collection of specific, explicit rules, which turn input data into output. Given, for example, the number of lymph nodes (input), the protocol, according to its (branching) logic, delivers the judgment on eligibility (output).

Formal tools contain some specific requirements, which must be elaborated since they play an important role in the rest of this chapter. First, formalisms require a well-defined set of clear-cut, elementary bits of information as *input:* input items must at all times match a possible, discrete starting point contained in the rules. All eligibility criteria, for example, are made exact through laboratory tests and specific checklists. The cancer should be "histologically confirmed stage IIA, IIB, or IIIA adenocarcinoma of the breast," the performance status should be "ECOG-ZUBROD 0 or 1" (appendixes of the protocol tell you what these codes mean), the "creatinine clearance" should be "$\geq$ 60 ml/min." (a measure for renal function), and so on. There is no room for "the kidneys look alright," or "this patient is in between stage IIA and B": the protocol has no rules to deal with such vague or undetermined statements.

Second, the *output* of formal systems is defined within the rules. The protocol often merely says either yes or no; sometimes, specific branches might make intermediate options possible (as when, in the case of a reduced white blood cell count, the FEC dosage is reduced by 25 percent). A seemingly innocent consequence of this feature is that at all times, all possible output must be feasible in the practice in which the tool is implemented. If, for example, one of the output statements requires the performance of a laboratory test not available in that particular setting, the system is useless. Similarly, the users have to be disciplined to act upon the advice — and to do so in the way intended by the protocol (cf. Collins 1990).

The protocol thus continually requires test results as input, and gives "next steps to take" as output. It meticulously describes *when to do what.* It cannot deal with input that does not conform to this prescribed precision and, likewise, its equally precise output statements make high demands on the practices involved. Therapeutic techniques have to be available, and staff members need to have the time, skills, and discipline to follow all steps through.

In addition to these requirements on in- and output, a certain stability in the relations between the data items input and the content of the output statements is also necessary. For the tool to work, the links between the input items and output statements have to match the rigidity of the protocol itself. If not, the protocol will mechanically process output statements that may be totally out of place. Obviously, for instance, the usage of CD34-positive cells as a criterion for leukapheresis is senseless if their presence in the blood is not related in any clear-cut way to the chances of obtaining a good sample of blood stem cells. Similarly, this criterion can only be used if all institutions measure these cells with the same techniques, and if the different immunological markers used function identically—something that was questioned by some of the oncologists. If not, centers might be harvesting stem cells at completely different times—which might have all kinds of unanticipated effects on the success of the harvest and the outcomes of the trial. In such a situation, a data item would not behave predictably enough: an unequivocal (chain of) rule(s) has to be feasible linking the item with one of the possible outcome statements.

All in all, the protocol, as a formal system, embodies a script that requires many of the diverse elements constituting the medical practices to behave in a uniform, stable, and predictable way. In the script, these heterogeneous elements are thoroughly intertwined: ensuring the proper execution of the CD34 test is just as much a problem of getting the laboratory staff to act in similar ways as a problem of ensuring that different immunological markers behave identically. Similarly, administering the FEC cycles requires both the patients and the hospital organization to adhere to this "rigorous three-week schedule"—and to be ready for a one-week delay when the blood cell counts so indicate. It is a whole, hybrid practice that must be made sufficiently docile—including nurses, physicians, data items, and organizational routines.

Moreover, whether a practice is disciplined enough for the tool to work is not a fixed, given fact. In the active redescription of the medical practices, many heterogeneous elements are *transformed* to make their behavior definite, uniform, and predictable enough for the protocol to work. The networks of elements constituting the medical practices involved have to be made sufficiently "tight" for the protocol to function (Callon 1991).[9] A sufficiently disciplined practice is an actively achieved accomplishment: the pathologists will have to be instructed to count precisely, the CD34 will have to be measured in a similar way in all centers, and the medical personnel involved will have to be trained to meticulously measure and document "side effects" (cf. Latour 1987; O'Connell 1993; Bowker 1994).

OF LYMPH NODES, ONCOLOGISTS, AND NEGOTIATIONS

Every protocol is a political compromise. — Dr. Fred Harrison, oncologist

In the implementation of the breast cancer protocol, the practices are being restructured so as to fit the requirements of this formal tool.[10] To achieve all this, however, the diverse elements must indeed subscribe to the protocol's script.

They need to make room, create a niche, for an additional, dominant element that will transform them all: the protocol. Some centers would have to sacrifice their own local trials, for example. Patients would have to comply with the often severe treatment, and all centers would need the expensive machinery required for peripheral stem cell transplantation. As is clear from the excerpt of the discussion constructing of the breast cancer protocol, a protocol is not simply imposed on the diverse practices. Rather, the construction (and implementation) of a protocol is a process of ongoing, continuing *negotiations.* In these negotiations, the practices are transformed *and* the tool itself acquires its final shape — the two are inextricably linked.[11]

The excerpt above dealt solely with the number of lymph nodes to be used as a cutoff point. Already in this small slice, however, it is again clear how thoroughly the details of the protocol are interwoven with a wide, heterogeneous specter of elements. This pathological-anatomical criterion is related to the statistical power of the trial, the workload of the centers, the habits of the registration office, the position of other local protocols, the financial situation of the whole group, their alignment with the scientific literature, the fate of individual patients, and the (not explicitly discussed) question of which patients can be asked to "suffer" this therapy. All these issues had to be aligned with each other for the protocol to become feasible; all these issues are affected by the seemingly simple choice of four versus ten nodes.

When in the end the protocol settled on four positive nodes, the upper age limit was cut down from sixty to fifty-five to reduce the number of eligible patients. The centers would get their extra share of work, and the oncologists would have to renegotiate, within their own departments, how this protocol would interact with other, already existent protocols. Similarly, everybody had to agree to administering this treatment to the larger group of (relatively) less ill patients. If all went well, the participating centers would receive financial support, with which some could buy the equipment necessary to perform the peripheral stem cell transplantation. Also, the group might succeed sooner, and more convincingly, in showing that this treatment is beneficial.

In the end result of this process, in the protocol as it is finally accepted, the traces of these negotiations are readily apparent. The protocol's final state is the highly *contingent* outcome of all the struggles that were fought. So, the originating center had set a maximum time of fourteen days between the surgical removal of the tumor and the start of chemotherapy; a trade-off between the time required for the patient's recovery of surgery and the need to prevent potentially remaining cancer cells from proliferating. Other centers, however, objected to this, by arguing that this time span would be too short for obtaining patients from regional hospitals. As one oncologist argued: "If we want their patients as well, and I think we do need them in order to reach our quota, then fourteen days is too short. I mean, you'd have to wait for the regional oncology meetings; that's how it goes. And we have these meetings twice a month." Finally, they settled for six weeks.

Similarly, the protocol authors first included all patients with surgically re-moved breast cancer—whether they had undergone a radical mastectomy (re-moval of the whole breast) or a breast-conserving procedure (where the tumor is excised but the breast is not removed). However, the radiologists of one of the participating centers did not agree with this. These physicians felt that patients who had had the breast-conserving procedure required immediate radiother-apy to kill tumor cells possibly remaining in the breast. In the proposed proto-col, the radiotherapy would come at the end, delaying the radiotherapy some sixteen to eighteen weeks (see figure 1). Although not all radiotherapists felt that this radiation of the breast was so urgent, the authors of the protocol felt obliged to give in in order to retain the cooperation of these radiologists. Con-sequently, in the next version, the protocol excluded patients treated with a breast-conserving procedure. In addition, it appeared to be in general very dif-ficult to get the different radiologists to agree on a given therapeutic regimen. So, although the protocol did contain recommendations for radiotherapeutic treatment, the oncologists included the statement that "modifications of the radiotherapy according to local views are permitted." They succumbed to their conviction that they would never be able to get the radiologists in the different centers to agree on one set of prescriptions.[12]

All the transformations described are closely intertwined: in taking from physicians (who use rules of thumb, blood cell curves, and so forth) the deci-sion to harvest peripheral stem cells and delegating it to CD34-positive cells, re-sponsibilities are redistributed, and the method of timing the harvest changes. Likewise, as the treatment of choice shifts from radiotherapy to chemotherapy, the patient flow is redirected: patients are channeled out of the clinics of the radiotherapists and into the oncologists' offices. Just as the "inside" and the "outside" of the technology, through the mutual redescriptions, are intimately connected, the medical knowledge embedded in the protocol is inextricably interwoven with its "context" (cf. Akrich 1992a).

One corollary of the scope and depth of this interrelatedness is that proto-cols are, and are perceived to be by the personnel affected, thoroughly *political* tools.[13] Protocols' scripts inevitably embed prescriptions as to who is in charge; who, in the case of a research protocol, is the research director; and who gets to use the expensive technologies (and gets the status that goes with that: cf.

Löwy 1995a).[14] In prescribing, for example, expensive drugs and tests, the tools define where and what costs are made, and who gets to make these decisions. Similarly, the tool redefines which laboratory tests are important and which medications are used—and whose labs are thus passed, and whose offices are filled. Physicians working with research protocols are often "wielders of hope": in their hands lie new drugs that might help where other medications have failed. Furthermore, the tool determines which patient is eligible and which patient is not; how much risk and suffering is tolerable; and who gets "a last chance" and who does not. Setting the number of lymph nodes to ten settles these issues very differently than setting the cutoff point at four. In the latter case, (relatively) less ill patients, who might otherwise live some years free of symptoms, receive the intense chemotherapy—including the suffering and health risks that go with that. Simultaneously, a larger group of patients is denied access to what might also be a last straw of hope.

How does all this relate back to the promises of the protocol? First, the protracted, ongoing process of negotiations is incorporated in the core of the tool itself. Trying to create niches for a protocol is a process of making ad hoc compromises, going back to the tool, and tinkering to get the medical practice's elements in line. The number of lymph nodes is juggled so as to articulate the heterogeneous issues involved, and the pathologists have to be asked to count accurately. The tool makers take whatever opportunities they perceive in order to adequately constrain the links between the diverse, constituent elements of the medical practices. Moreover, the required control is never complete: in adjusting a practice to a protocol, the protocol itself is also inevitably transformed. Its final script can be read as reflecting the continual need to "give in" to resistances coming from the different practices in which the tool is incorporated. Radiologists were given their way, entry criteria were modified, and so forth. Continually, contingencies erode the adjustments accomplished; continually, idiosyncracity seeps in from all sides. This unending, ad hoc compromising leads to a tool nobody had planned beforehand.

And because we are talking about protocol, we are talking about embedded decision criteria that nobody had planned beforehand. We are talking about transformations in the criteria to enroll patients in an intense treatment schedule, and to exclude others, and about changes in the treatment given—about, therefore, what "untreatable" breast cancer *means,* and what proper therapy *is.* There is no direct, straight line between the first blueprints of the tool and the tool the practice ends up with. There is, similarly, no simple "ironing out" of idiosyncratic variations. Instead of changing practice Y to X we end up with a hybrid that contains traces of X, Y, and all the struggles that have been fought.

Instead of the transparent, optimal, unified clinical rationality hoped for, we end up with opaque, impure, *additional* rationalities. Instead, thus, of imposing order where there was disorder, a new order is achieved that *incorporates* the very messiness it started out to erase.[15]

THE SPECIFIC EXIGENCIES OF A FORMAL TOOL

> Writing a good protocol is not so difficult. What is hard is getting and
> keeping it in place. — Dr. Fred Howard, oncologist

There is, moreover, a second complication in the relation between the "order" of the good medical practice X, transmitted by the protocol, and the "messiness" of many other medical practices. Not only do the protocols inevitably *contain* much of the messiness they wanted to get rid of, they also distinctively alter the order of X as transported through the tool. Tool builders continually attempt to weed out possible contingencies that might threaten their carefully recrafted order. In order to satisfy the tool's demands on the input data items, output statements, and the links between these, they continually attempt to ensure the stability and predictability of the involved elements. In preparing the practices for the protocol, in laying the "infrastructure" for the tool (Bowker 1994), some reappearing motifs can be discerned.

These reoccurring patterns point at how the formal structure of the protocol *itself* tends to transform medical practices in distinctive, recognizable ways. A protocol is not an inert, perfect medium that simply and faultlessly transports a "perfect approach," or X's order to practices Y and Z. The specific demands of a formal tool reconfigure the practices in a highly specific manner. Medical criteria, and the position of medical personnel and patients with regards to these, are distinctively and importantly reshaped.

Building Simple, Robust Worlds. I point at three related ways through which the formal tool's requirements are often produced: reinforcing bureaucratic hierarchies, materializing the tool's demands, and shifting decision power to the most uniform and predictable elements.

Reinforcing bureaucratic hierarchies. A first way through which protocol builders often attempt to prevent a practice's potential obstinacy is through the implementation of specific rules and the installment or reinforcement of specific hierarchies. In the case of the breast cancer protocol, eligible patients have to be registered at a national trial office. Here the randomization takes place, and the name, age, diagnosis, and number of positive lymph nodes are registered. Also, it is checked whether informed consent has been obtained.

The patient's therapy is thus determined nationally; the local physicians do not even get to do the randomization. Moreover, the registration ensures that, from that moment on, the patient is "entered": the physician will now have to justify every nonprescribed action. For every "protocol violation," the study coordinator will have to be contacted.

Hierarchical relations can also be installed or reinforced *within* institutions (cf. Kling 1991). The following account from one of the participating centers illustrates how supervising relations among physicians can often be enforced in order to ensure meticulous compliance:

> In a discussion between oncologists and residents in a university hospital, one of the residents asks whether they should not be given the freedom to modify chemotherapeutic dosages in the case of side effects. This resident works at the oncological outpatient-clinic, where she is responsible for the administration of these medications. One of the oncologists disagrees: "I feel that we cannot give that responsibility to you. If we write a prescription, you have to be able to follow that blindly. Often some protocol is involved, which you might not be aware of; in these cases different rules apply for whether or not you can continue treatment in the light of side effects. So, I would say that you just call us when you're not sure. Don't go changing things on your own."

Materializing the tool's demands. Embedding the tool's exigencies in material arrangements as instruments and other artifacts is another often attempted means of ensuring obedience. Having the tool's demands materialized prestructures the medical personnel's work environment so that the protocol becomes an unavoidable (and often unnoticed) part of daily practice (cf. Fujimura 1988; Suchman 1993). In the next example, such a materialization is already in place:

> When nurses change the Hickman catheter [a catheter inserted in the subclavian artery, just below the collar bone, through which chemotherapy and blood cells can be easily administered], they always use what they call the "Hickman set." Usage of this set is prescribed by the protocol on Hickman catheter replacement. The set is a sterile, preassembled package containing the material required for changing the catheter according to the protocol, such as bandages, small trays for the disinfectant, tweezers, and so on.

Similarly, in research protocols, medications can be centrally distributed. Participating centers obtain the (expensive) drugs free of charge, in a prepackaged form, with dosages adjusted to the protocol at hand. Finally, forms are an often used method to ensure, for example, the complete and adequately detailed gathering of data. By requiring the usage of protocol-specific forms, medical personnel can be directly guided in the taking of a history or the sequencing of a therapy.

Materializing a tool's demands is often intertwined with the implementation of bureaucracies. After all, bureaucracies can be, and often are, materialized as well. Forms requiring signatures from superiors, prepackaged chemotherapy that can only be modified through consultation with the study coordinator: all these materializations embed hierarchical relations.

Reshuffling spokesmanship: shifting decision power amongst the elements. A third recurring pattern in the disciplining of a practice to the tool concerns the decision power encoded in the protocol: which input items matter most when a protocol chooses between branches or opts for a specific output statement. Here we see that tool builders have a preference for "trustworthy" elements: those elements which, from the perspective of the tool builder, exhibit the most predictable and unequivocal behavior. "Trustworthy" does *not* imply "better" or "more true," but points at the tool builders' preference to delegate deci-sion power to those signs, symptoms, and tests which best, or most easily, fit the formal tool's prerequisites. As a result, spokesmanship is often delegated from staff and patients to laboratory tests or machines. Rather than letting local physicians decide when to harvest peripheral stem cells, CD34-positive cells settle the matter. The protocol builders deemed the criteria used by the local physicians to be overly idiosyncratic, and saw the CD34 cells as a test that would yield identical results in all centers. Rather than allow clinical judg-ment to have its way, also, the number of lymph nodes and other quantitative, laboratory-derived values determine eligibility for this protocol.

Likewise, the patients' abilities to control the specific course of events is often limited. Patients can always step out of a protocol—but that is the only active role they can take. Besides that, they have little room for influence. In the breast cancer protocol, the patient signs an informed consent form asking her to participate in the trial. She is told that "she has the right to withdraw co-operation at any moment." But in the tight network required for the protocol to work, there is again no room for additional desires such as "a somewhat less intense second course of chemotherapy." If the laboratory tests do not register side effects, the second course will be as the first; and if they do, the dose modi-fications are already precisely prescribed.

In addition to a shift away from patients' and medical personnel's voices and toward cells and chemical reactions, there is also a selection of the most trustworthy element *among* the physical signs and laboratory tests. Laboratory tests and physical signs are not more trustworthy per se: as many studies have shown, their robustness is *itself* the result of much work.[16] So, the CD34 test is debated among the oncologists exactly *because* its trustworthiness is debatable. Since the centers might use different techniques to measure these cells, a critic remarked, "center [A] might be looking at something quite different than [B]." Similarly, the data item should speak in a clear voice. As "the general condition of the patient" is an item that is notoriously difficult to assess unequivocally, the protocol uses elaborate coding systems spelled out in its appendixes.

A Different Order

Through a plethora of means, thus, practices are disciplined. Whether through reinforcing bureaucratic hierarchies, through materializing the protocol's demands, or through delegating decision power to stable and uniform elements, potential obstinacy or unpredictability is averted. Through these recurring patterns, threats to the straightforwardness required by the tool can be checked.

These patterns, however, do create a tension with the protocol's ideal typed promises. We do not simply see an imposition of order X in Y. Nor is the resulting order, embedded in the protocol, merely a polluted version of X. Rather, the tool's formal structure predisposes the generation of an order in which the roles of medical personnel and patients are *specifically* altered and, simultaneously, medical criteria are *specifically* changed.

To ensure the successful functioning of this formal tool, to make the distributed and highly complex deliverance of this treatment scheme possible, individual nurses, physicians, and patients tend to lose direct influence on the course of events. Physicians now have to hand the judgment as to whether a patient should enter the protocol over to an interplay of laboratory values and lymph node counts. Similarly, bringing the patient's own voice back to either yes or no brings about the unequivocality needed for protocols to work. In the order contained in the protocol, these actors are repositioned: inevitably, the requirement for stable and predictable elements predisposes the taming, or even silencing of these potential sources of contingency (cf. Star 1989a).

Closely linked with this tendency to restrain medical personnel's and patients' input are specific changes in medical decision criteria. In a nonprotocolized situation, medical personnel can allow a myriad of more or less precise laboratory tests, historical data, psychosocial circumstances, and so forth to shape the course of action undertaken. The protocol, however, will strive to anchor decision moments precisely and concisely — and redelegate spokesmanship to a few unambiguous and stable items.

For example, counting the number of lymph nodes is an easily performed test, which will yield similar results in different centers — that is, if the pathologists do their counting properly. As a criterion for suitability for treatment, however, it is a rather rough and blunt means to distinguish between patients. In medical practices most such tests are rough and blunt: there are no simple ways to precisely determine how far cancer cells have spread. However, when not working according to a protocol, physicians will often try to construct some image of the extent of the spread through physical examination (can small tumors be felt elsewhere?), clues in the history (pain may indicate spread), different imaging techniques (are the bones affected?), and so forth. In this way, some more specific idea of whether and to what extent cancer cells have actually disseminated to distant organs may be generated. This plethora of methods, however, is much less clear-cut, much harder to define and much more difficult to standardize than counting the number of nodes.

Similarly, the age limit in the breast cancer protocol was set at fifty-five — a straightforward decision criterion for inclusion or exclusion. In a nonprotocolized situation, such a strict cutoff point would not have been regarded as meaningful. As one oncologist remarked, it might have been better to differentiate between pre- and postmenopausal women. "Biologically spoken, it's a different disease," he remarked. Determining the menopausal status, however, is "tricky," as another oncologist stated. It is time-consuming, and it has none of the simplicity and clearness of simply setting an age limit. It would thus endanger the smoothness and tightness built up which is so crucial for the optimal functioning of the protocol.

These examples do not show that the protocol is inhumane or wrong. In the new configuration created in and through the protocol, new possibilities are opened too: nurses may get to do tasks that they were not allowed to do before, residents get to handle new, promising drugs they would otherwise not even have heard of, and some patients might willingly give up some right of voice in exchange for a straw of hope.[17] I am not arguing that the protocol misses a crucial point. Rather, these examples illustrate how the protocol constructs its own, *specific* order, which is *different* from the order contained in a nonprotocolized "good medical practice." The changes described go beyond "importing good medical practice X into Y," and are not discussed as such by authors such as Eddy and Feinstein. If anything, these authors stress that the protocol *strengthens* "good clinical reasoning," that it would open up a space for patients' and staff input, rather than repositioning them in a secondary position (cf. Komaroff 1982; Feinstein 1987a: 370-79). The tool itself is regarded as merely mirroring the reflection of a good practice to wherever it is needed; it is supposed to merely explicate that what was already implicit in the practice it derives from (Grimm et al. 1975).

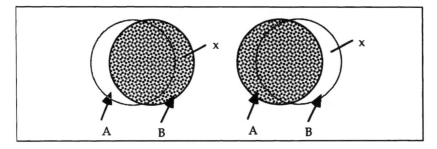

Figure 2   This diagram (after Wulff 1981: 106) illustrates the subtle shift in the medical criteria for "treatable breast cancer." (a) is before and (b) after the implementation of the protocol. The shaded areas indicate the group of patients to whom the diagnostic label is applied; the shift from A to B indicates the subtle, often unnoticed change in the use of this diagnostic label. Patient X would be treated in (a), but not in (b).

As has become clear, however, this mirror transforms the reflection by merging it with the exigencies coming from its own structure. The introduction of a protocol generates a propensity to refocus medical criteria on those elements which behave in predictable and easily traceable ways. The tool contains a predisposition to build *simple, robust worlds*, without too many interdependencies or weak spots where contingencies can leak back in.[18] In doing so, in selecting those measurements and indications whose behavior mirrors its structure, the protocol *redefines* what eligibility for bone marrow transplantation treatment *denotes* — what, thus, "potentially curable disseminated breast cancer" *is*.

Settling on a minimum of four lymph nodes as the inclusion criterion selects a different group of patients than using inclusion criteria based on extensive testing for dissemination: the lymph nodes have now become the salient sign determining the patient's fate. A patient with three positive lymph nodes but a large, fixed lump in the breast, for example, might be deemed a good candidate for this bone marrow treatment by some physicians — but the protocol would rule her out.

Likewise, opting for the CD34 test above the physician's judgment transforms what it means to be suitable for stem cell harvest: the two methods will yield different results in many patients. The age limit, also, carves out significantly different cutoff lines than a measurement of menopausal status: different criteria are invoked, which will create different groups of included and excluded patients, and rewrite the significance of particular signs and symptoms (see figure 2 for a graphical representation of this argument).

The muting of the nurses', patients', and residents' voices, and the changes in medical criteria I described, are tied up with the *structure* of the tool and have nothing particular to do with whatever happened in practice X.[19] Although the tool builders remain silent on this issue, the tool does not simply transport the "profound clinical experience and thought" of X; it *transforms* it. In their transmission through a protocol, medical decision criteria are changed; they are increasingly tied up to a limited set of simple, clear-cut variables. Instead of spreading the "proper practice of X," instead of strengthening a "clinical rationality," the protocol silently creates a *new* order that is as yet waiting to be explored.

NOTES

I would like to thank Annemarie Mol, Antoinette de Bont, Geof Bowker, Monica Casper, Nicolas Dodier, Ilana Löwy, Leigh Star, Stefan Timmermans, Gerard de Vries, and Dick Willems for their help, their many suggestions, and their support.

1 Eddy distinguishes three different types of practice policies, varying in the range of flexibility they accomodate. *Guidelines* are protocols which "*should* be followed in *most* cases, but there is an understanding that, depending on the patient, the setting, the circumstances, or other factors, guidelines can and should be tailored to fit individual needs." Second, *standards* "are intended to be inflexible. They define correct practice, and should be followed, not tailored." Finally, an *option* merely says that "some practitioners use the intervention, while others do not, and there is little basis for determining which choice is correct" (Eddy 1990c). In my empirical research, I have focused primarily on the construction and use of research protocols. There were several reasons for this choice. First, investigating the implementation and functioning of protocols requires a setting where these tools are frequently used. The oncology ward, always a site of numerous research protocols, was such a location. Moreover, through contacts made at this department, I was able to become an observer in the construction of several oncological research (and nonresearch) protocols. See Eddy 1992 for an inside story on the construction of a guideline in which many of the issues discussed in this chapter return.

2 For a more elaborated account of the protocol's background and present status (and of other decision support techniques), see Berg 1997.

3 This is necessarily a very *partial* image of what protocols do. See Whalen 1993, Berg 1997, and Timmermans and Berg 1997 for an analysis of personnel at work with protocols. Cf. Suchman (1987) and Star (1992) whose theoretical accomplishments informs much of this work.

4 All names in this story have been changed. The account is transcripted from meeting in June 1992.

5 This therapy is a recent alternative for bone marrow transplantation, where bone marrow cells are harvested from the patient's pelvic bone. The advantages of this new technique are claimed to be more convenience for the patient and a more rapid restoration of normal blood cell levels.

6   See, e.g., Bijker and Law 1992, Latour 1987, and Pickering 1992. The work of Bowker, Star, and others on classification has also been influential—cf. Bowker and Star 1994 and Timmermans et al. (this volume).

7   Stem cells are not harvested *before* the treatment since it is hoped that the chemotherapy will kill potential tumor cells in the blood. These tumor cells might otherwise be accidentally transplanted with the stem cells.

8   The highly differentiated diagnostic and therapeutic schemes characterizing oncology, I would argue, would not have been possible without the mediating and structuring role of the protocol, which has been a ubiquitous element of oncology since its early days (Marks 1988; Löwy 1995a).

9   Oncology practices, partially through their historical tie with research protocols, are already heavily structured in ways congenial to new protocols. Medical personnel are used to these intervening instruments, data items, or criteria are often taken over from earlier protocols, and central registration agencies are already in existence (as was alluded to in the excerpt). In fact, these links to interinstitutional and international protocols partially explain why, e.g., oncology wards look so alike all over the Western world—much more alike, often, than different wards within one and the same hospital (Fujimura 1987).

10   For a discussion of the counterpart of the disciplining of the practice (the *localization* of the *tool*), see Berg 1997.

11   Often, these tools do not survive the negotiations. The fact that the implementation of protocols is frequently unsuccessful is not often reported in the literature, but was frequently alluded to in interviews. See, on the troubles to get physicians to work with protocols, Grimm et al. 1975; Eisenberg 1986; Wachtel et al. 1986. On the limited effect of consensus reports, see Greer 1987; Kosekoff et al. 1987; Kanouse et al. 1989.

12   Similarly, precision is often sacrificed when laboratory tests cannot be disciplined sufficiently. The designers of a pulmonary cancer protocol I studied, for example, found themselves not being able to define precisely how "sufficient pulmonary function" would be measured without either losing too many or too few potential patients in their research protocol. So, they decided to leave this issue up to the physicians' discretion.

13   By using the word "political" here, I do not imply that the consequences mentioned were necessarily intentional (see further). Likewise, there is no immediate judgment attached to saying this; I want to point out that the tool is highly consequential in many domains which would ordinarily be dubbed "political."

14   As pointed out, joining the breast cancer protocol group had a distinctive advantage for oncological centers: they would get additional funds with which they could buy "shiny," state-of-the-art technology.

15   For a similar tale vis-à-vis a different decision support technique (decision analysis), see Ashmore, Mulkay, and Pinch 1989. In an excellent article, Jordan and Lynch (1992) show how a standardized, preparatory procedure in molecular biology takes on a different shape in each and every different laboratory. Due to a host of con-

tingent factors, each lab "develops its own procedural dialect" (86). In analogy, the *appropriation* of a protocol in a series of different medical practices would result in an equally large amount of different interpretations and effectuations of the "same" tool. In trying to get the "order" of the protocol to actually *work*, thus, it inevitably becomes swamped with more and more disorder. See also note 3.

16   See, e.g., Fujimura 1992 and Latour and Woolgar 1986. See also Horstman on the construction of reliability in the case of the urine test in insurance medicine (1997). A beautiful attempt to come to terms with the way matter is *not* regularly tamed, is Haraway's discussion of nature as "coyote/trickster" (1991: 198–201).

17   The protocol opens up some worlds and closes others — and global judgments as to which worlds are preferable are hard to make. Cf. Kling 1991 and Berg 1997.

Stating that the protocol is either more wrong or more right also bypasses the issue that there is no way in which either judgment can be grounded. There is no way to determine what is the "more *truly* indicative" set of data items, for example. There is no solid, independent ground from which to make some ultimate judgment on a new selection of indicants. Lynch (1985) shows this point beautifully in his research of laboratory science. See also Latour 1988; Hirschauer 1991; Pasveer 1992.

18   This simplicity, it should be clear, is partly a *consequence* of the work performed to achieve this robustness — what O'Connell, after Latour, calls "metrological practices" (O'Connell 1993).

19   Of course, it can be argued that these effects are part and parcel of the rationalization of medical work: the process through which medical practice becomes a science. In this view, the protocol's propensity for predictable and stable elements is a sign of its scientific nature. This argument, however, is *itself* a product of the historical processes through which the protocol became prominent in medicine. Only *with* the coming of the protocol has medical practice been (re)described as a scientific process, as the logical and sequential execution of the steps of the scientific method (Berg 1995).

REFERENCES

Abbott, A. 1988. *The System of Professions: An Essay on the Division of Expert Labor.* Chicago: University of Chicago Press.

Adamsons, K., Jr., V. J. Freda, L. S. James, and M. E. Towell. 1965. Prenatal Treatment of Erythroblastosis Fetalis Following Hysterotomy. *Pediatrics* 35:848–55.

Akrich, M. 1992a. The De-Scription of Technical Objects. In *Shaping Technology/Building Society: Studies in Sociotechnical Change,* edited by W. E. Bijker and J. Law. Cambridge, Mass.: MIT Press.

———. 1992b. Beyond Social Construction of Technology: The Shaping of People and Things in the Innovation Process. In *New Technology at the Outset,* edited by M. Dierkes and U. Hoffmann. New York: Westview Press.

———. 1993. Les Objets techniques et leurs utilisateurs. In *Les Objets dans l'action: De la maison au laboratoire.* Collection Raisons Pratiques, edited by B. Conein, N. Dodier, and L. Thévenot. Paris: Editions de l'Ecole des Hautes Etudes en Sciences Sociales.

Akrich, M., and B. Latour. 1992. A Summary of a Convenient Vocabulary for the Semiotics of Human and Non-Human Assemblies. In *Shaping Technology/Building Society: Studies in Sociotechnical Change,* edited by W. E. Bijker and J. Law. Cambridge, Mass.: MIT Press.

Andersen, Tavs Folmer, and Gavin Mooney, eds. 1990. *The Challenges of Medical Practice Variations.* Houndsmills, England: Macmillan Press.

Anspach, Renée R. 1993. *Deciding Who Lives: Fateful Choices in the Intensive Care Nursery.* Berkeley: University of California Press.

Arditti, R., R. Klein, and S. Minden, eds. 1984. *Test-Tube Women: What Future for Motherhood?* London: Pandora Press.

Armstrong, David. 1983. *Political Anatomy of the Body: Medical Knowledge in Britain in the Twentieth Century.* Cambridge: Cambridge University Press.

———. 1984. The Patient's View. *Social Science and Medicine* 18 (9): 737–44.

Arney, William R., and Bernard J. Bergen. 1984. *Medicine and the Management of Living: Taming the Last Great Beast.* Chicago: University of Chicago Press.

Ashmore, M., M. Mulkay, and T. Pinch. 1989. *Health and Efficiency: A Sociology of Health Economics*. Milton Keynes, England: Open University Press.

Ashmore, M., R. Wooffitt, and S. Harding, eds. 1994. *Humans and Others: The Concept of "Agency" and Its Attribution*. Special issue of *American Behavioral Scientist* 37 (6).

Association of Community Health Councils for England and Wales. 1989. *Cervical Cytology Screening: Getting It Right*. Health News Briefing. London: Association of Community Health Councils for England and Wales.

Astin, L., and V. Wehbi. 1991. L'Aptitude réglementaire en médecine du travail dans les transports routiers. *Actes des XXIèmes journées nationales de médecine du travail* (Rouen, June 12–15, 1990). Paris: Masson.

Atkinson, Paul. 1995. *Medical Talk and Medical Work*. London: Sage.

Atkinson, P., and C. Heath, eds. 1981. *Medical Work: Realities and Routines*. Westmead, England: Gower.

Austin, J. L. 1970. *Quand dire c'est faire*. Paris: Seuil.

Bariety, M., et al. 1981. *Sémiologie médicale*. Paris: Masson.

Barnett, R., and R. Fox. 1986. *A Feminist Approach to Pap Tests*. Vancouver: Vancouver Women's Health Collective.

Baszanger, Isabelle. 1986. Les Maladies chroniques et leur ordre négocié. *Revue Française de Sociologie* 27 (4): 3–27.

———. 1987. *Entre comprendre et soigner: Les Débuts des centres de la douleur en France*. Report for A.T.P. Santé, Maladie, Société, C.N.R.S./Ministère des Affaires Sociales (M.I.R.E.).

———. 1990. Emergence d'un groupe professionnel et travail de légitimation: Le Cas des médecins de la douleur. *Revue Française de Sociologie* 31 (2): 257–82.

———. 1992. Deciphering Chronic Pain. *Sociology of Health and Illness* 14 (2): 181–215.

———. 1993. From Pain to Person: A New Object for Medicine. In *Medicine and Change—Innovation, Continuity and Recurrence: Historical and Sociological Perspectives*, edited by I. Löwy. Paris: John Libbey Eurotext.

———. 1995. *Douleur et médicine, la fin d'un oubli*. Paris: Seuil. Translated as *Inventing Pain Medicine: From the Laboratory to the Clinic* (New Brunswick, N.J.: Rutgers University Press, 1988).

Bates, B. 1985. *Guide de l'examen clinique*, 2d ed. Paris: MEDSI (original English version: 1983).

Becker, H. 1963. *Outsiders: Studies in the Sociology of Deviance*. New York: Free Press.

———. 1986. *Doing Things Together*. Evanston, Ill.: Northwestern University Press.

Berg, M. 1992. The Construction of Medical Disposals: Medical Sociology and Medical Problem Solving in Clinical Practice. *Sociology of Health and Illness* 14 (2): 151–80.

———. 1995. Turning a Practice into a Science: Reconceptualizing Postwar Medical Practice. *Social Studies of Science* 25:437–76.

———. 1997. *Rationalizing Medical Work: Decision Support Techniques and Medical Practices*. Cambridge, Mass.: MIT Press.

Berg, Marc, and Monica Casper, eds. 1995. *Constructivist Perspectives and Medical Work:*

Medical Practices and Science and Technology Studies. Special issue of *Science, Technology and Human Values* 20 (4).

Bijker, W. E., and J. Law, ed. 1992. *Shaping Technology—Building Society: Studies in Sociotechnical Change.* Cambridge, Mass.: MIT Press.

Billings, D., and T. Urban. 1982. The Socio-Medical Construction of Transsexualism. *Social Problems* 29:266–82.

Birke, L., S. Himmelweit, and G. Vines. 1990. *Tomorrow's Child: Reproductive Technologies in the 90s.* London: Virago Press.

Blank, R. H. 1992. *Mother and Fetus: Changing Notions of Maternal Responsibility.* Westport, Conn.: Greenwood Press.

Bloor, Michael. 1978. On the Routinised Nature of Work in People-Processing Agencies: The Case of Adenotonsillectomy Assessments in ENT Out-Patient Clinics. In *Relationships between Doctors and Patients,* edited by A. Davis. Farnborough, England: Gower.

Bloor, D. 1991. *Knowledge and Social Imagery.* Chicago: University of Chicago Press.

Blumer, H. 1969. *Symbolic Interactionism: Perspective and Method.* Englewood Cliffs, N.J.: Prentice-Hall.

Böhme, Gernot. 1980. Politische Medizin. 1848 und die Nicht-Entstehung der Sozialmedizin. *Alternativen der Wissenschaft.* Frankfurt: Suhrkamp.

Boltanski, L., and L. Thévenot. 1991. *De la justification: Les Économies de la grandeur.* Paris: Gallimard.

Bonica, J. J. 1953. *The Management of Pain.* Philadelphia: Lea and Fabiger.

Bosk, Charles L. 1979. *Forgive and Remember: Managing Medical Failure.* Chicago: University of Chicago Press.

Bourdieu, P. 1979. *La Distinction: Critique sociale du jugement.* Paris: Les Editions de Minuit.

Boureau, F., M. Luu, and A.-S. Koskas. 1985. Approche cognitive-comportementale des douleurs chroniques. *Actualités psychiatriques* 2:57–66.

Bowker, G. 1994. *Science on the Run: Information Management and Industrial Geophysics at Schlumberger, 1920–1940.* Cambridge, Mass.: MIT Press.

Bowker, G., and S. L. Star. 1991. Situations vs. Standards in Long-Term, Wide-Scale Decision-Making: The Case of the International Classification of Diseases. In *Proceedings of the 24th Hawaiian International Conference on Systems Sciences in Washington,* 73–81. IEEE Computer Society Press.

———. 1994. Knowledge and Infrastructure in International Information Management: Problems of Classification and Coding. In *Information Acumen: The Understanding and Use of Knowledge in Modern Business,* edited by L. Bud. London: Routledge.

Braverman, H. 1974. *Labor and Monopoly Capital.* New York: Monthly Review.

British Thoracic Society. 1991. Guidelines for the Management of Asthma in Adults, vol. I: Chronic Persistent Asthma. *British Medical Journal* 301:651–53.

Brook, R. H., et al. 1988. Diagnosis and Treatment of Coronary Disease: Comparison of Doctors' Attitudes in the USA and the UK. *Lancet,* April 2, pp. 750–53.

Bucher, R. 1988. On the Natural History of Health Care Occupations. *Work and Occupations* 15 (2): 131–47.

Bucher, R., and A. Strauss. 1961. Professions in Process. *American Journal of Sociology,* 66:325–34. Reprinted in Anselm L. Strauss, 1991, *Creating Sociological Awareness* (New Brunswick, N.J.: Transaction).

Bulechek, G. M., and J. C. McCloskey. 1989. Nursing Interventions: Treatments for Potential Diagnoses. In *Proceedings of the Eighth NANDA Conference,* edited by R. M. Carroll-Johnson. Philadelphia: J. B. Lippincott.

———. 1993. Response to Grobe. In *Canadian Nurses Association, Papers from the Nursing Minimum Data Set Conference,* 158–60. Edmonton, Canada: Canadian Nurses Association.

Butler, J. 1990. *Gender Trouble: Feminism and the Subversion of Identity.* New York: Routledge.

Callon, M. 1986a. Some Elements of a Sociology of Translation: Domestication of the Scallops and the Fishermen of St Brieuc Bay. In *Power, Action and Belief—A New Sociology of Knowledge?* edited by J. Law. London: Routledge.

———. 1986b. The Sociology of an Actor-Network: The Case of the Electric Vehicle. In *Mapping the Dynamics of Science and Technology,* edited by M. Callon et al. London: Macmillan.

———. 1987. Society in the Making: The Study of Technology as a Tool for Sociological Analysis. In *The Social Construction of Technological Systems,* edited by W. E. Bijker et al. Cambridge, Mass.: MIT Press.

———. 1991. Techno-Economic Networks and Irreversibility. In *A Sociology of Monsters: Essays on Power, Technology and Domination,* edited by J. Law. London: Routledge.

Callon, M., Law, J. and Rip, A., eds. 1986. *Mapping the Dynamics of Science and Technology.* London: Macmillan.

Canguilhem, G. 1966. *Le Normal et le pathologique.* Paris: Presses Universitaires de France.

Carrithers, M., S. Collins, and S. Lukes, eds. 1985. *The Category of the Person: Anthropology, Philosophy, History.* Cambridge: Cambridge University Press.

Cartwright, L. 1992. Women, X-Rays, and the Public Culture of Prophylactic Imaging. *Camera Obscura* 29:19–56.

Casper, M. J. 1994a. At the Margins of Humanity: Fetal Positions in Science and Medicine. *Science, Technology, and Human Values* 19 (3): 307–23.

———. 1994b. Reframing and Grounding "Non-Human" Agency: What Makes a Fetus an Agent? *American Behavioral Scientist* 37 (6).

———. 1998. *The Making of the Unborn Patient: A Social Anatomy of Fetal Surgery.* New Brunswick, N.J.: Rutgers University Press.

Cassel, E. J. 1982. The Nature of Suffering and the Goals of Medicine. *New England Journal of Medicine* 306:639–45.

Castel, R. 1981. *La Gestion des risques: De l'anti-psychiatrie à l'après-psychanalyse.* Paris: Minuit.

Chapman-Walsh, D. 1987. *Corporate Physicians: Between Medicine and Management.* New Haven: Yale University Press.

Charmaz, K. 1991. *Good Days, Bad Days: The Self in Chronic Illness and Time.* New Brunswick, N.J.: Rutgers University Press.

Chomet, J., and J. Chomet. 1989. *Cervical Cancer, All You and Your Partner Need to Know about Its Prevention, Detection and Treatment.* Wellingborough, England: Grapevine.

Cicourel, A. 1975. Discourse and Text: Cognitive and Linguistic Processes in Studies of Social Structure. *Versus* 12 (2): 33–83.

———. 1985. Raisonnement et diagnostic: Le Rôle du discours et de la compréhension clinique en médecine. *Actes de la recherche en sciences sociales,* no. 60: 79–89.

Clarke, A. E. 1987. Research Materials and Reproductive Science in the United States, 1910–1940. In *Physiology in the American Context, 1845–1940,* edited by G. L. Geison. Bethesda: American Physiological Society.

———. 1990a. A social world research adventure: the case of reproductive science. In *Theories of Science and Society,* edited by S. Cozzens and T. Gieryn. Bloomington: Indiana University Press.

———. 1990b. Controversy and the Development of Reproductive Sciences. *Social Problems* 37 (1): 18–37.

———. 1991. Social Worlds/Arenas Theory as Organization Theory. In *Social Organization and Social Process: Essays in Honor of Anselm Strauss,* edited by D. Maines. Hawthorne, N.Y.: Aldine de Gruyter.

Clarke, A. E., and M. Casper. 1992. *From Simple Technology to Complex Arena: Classification of Pap Smears, 1917–1990.* Working paper. San Francisco: University of California.

Clarke, A. E., and J. H. Fujimura. 1992. What Tools? Which Jobs? Why Right? In *The Right Tools for the Job: At Work in Twentieth-Century Life Sciences,* edited by A. E. Clarke and J. H. Fujimura. Princeton: Princeton University Press.

Clarke, A. E., and T. Montini. 1993. The Many Faces of RU486: Tales of Situated Knowledges and Technological Contestations. *Science, Technology and Human Values* 18:42–78.

Clavreul, Jean. 1978. *L'Ordre médical.* Paris: Editions du Seuil.

Cockburn, C., and R. Furst-Dilic. 1994. *Bringing Technology Home: Gender and Technology in a Changing Europe.* Milton Keynes, England: Open University Press.

Collins, Harry M. 1985. *Changing Order: Replication and Induction in Scientific Practice.* London: Sage.

———. 1990. *Artificial Experts: Social Knowledge and Intelligent Machines.* Cambridge, Mass.: MIT Press.

———. 1994. Dissecting Surgery: Forms of Life Depersonalized. *Social Studies of Science* 24:311–89.

Collins, H. M., and S. Yearley. 1993. Epistemological Chicken. In *Science as Practice and Culture,* edited by A. Pickering. Chicago: University of Chicago Press.

Corbett, K. K. 1986. *Adding Insult to Injury: Cultural Dimensions of Frustrations in the Management of Chronic Back Pain.* Ph.d. diss. Berkeley: University of California.

Corea, G. 1987. *Man-Made Women: How the New Reproductive Technologies Affect Women.* Bloomington: Indiana University Press.

Creasy, R. K., and R. Resnick, eds. 1994. *Maternal-Fetal Medicine: Principles and Practice.* Philadelphia: W. B. Saunders.

Csordas, T., and J. Clark. 1992. Ends of the Line: Diversity among Chronic Pain Centers. *Social Science and Medicine* 34 (4): 383–94.

Cussins, A. 1992. Content, Embodiment and Objectivity: The Theory of Cognitive Trails. *Mind* 101:651–88.

Cussins, C. 1997a. Reproducing Reproduction: Techniques of Normalization and Naturalization in Infertility Clinics. In *Reproducing Reproduction,* edited by S. Franklin and H. Ragone. Philadelphia: University of Pennsylvania Press.

———. 1997b. Quit Snivelling, Cryo-Baby; We'll Decide Which One's Your Mama. In *Cyborg Babies: From Techno Tots to Techno Toys,* edited by J. Dumit and R. Floyd-Davis. London: Routledge.

Daniels, C. R. 1993. *At Women's Expense: State Power and the Politics of Fetal Rights.* Cambridge, Mass.: Harvard University Press.

Dejours, C. 1993. *Travail: Usure mentale: De la psychopathologie à la psychodynamique du travail.* Paris: Bayard Editions.

Desrosières, A. 1993, *La Politique des grands nombres: Histoire de la raison statistique.* Paris: La Découverte.

Dirksen, W. J., et al. 1992. NHG-Standaard astma bij Kinderen. *Huisarts en Wetenschap* 35 (9): 355–62.

Dodier, N. 1993a. Les Appuis conventionnels de l'action: Eléments de pragmatique sociologique. *Réseaux* no. 62: 63–85.

———. 1993b. *L'Expertise médicale: Essai de sociologie sur l'exercice du jugement.* Paris: Métailié.

———. 1994. Expert Medical Decisions in Occupational Medicine: A Sociological Analysis of Medical Judgement. *Sociology of Health and Illness* 16 (4): 489–514.

Dompeling, E., et al. 1992. Treatment with Inhaled Steroids in Asthma and Chronic Bronchitis: Long-Term Compliance and Inhaler Technique. *Family Practice* 9 (2): 161–66.

Douglas, M. 1985. *Risk Acceptability According to the Social Sciences.* New York: Russell Sage Foundation.

Douglas, M., and D. L. Hull. 1992. *How Classification Works: Nelson Goodman among the Social Sciences.* Edinburgh: Edinburgh University Press.

Douglas, M., and A. Wildavski. 1982. *Risk and Culture: An Essay on the Selection of Technological and Environmental Dangers.* Berkeley: University of California Press.

Duden, B. 1987 [1991]. *Geschichte unter der Haut: Ein Eisenacher Arzt und seine Patientinnen um 1730.* Stuttgart: Klett-Cotta. Translated as *The Woman beneath the Skin: A Doctor's Patients in Eighteenth-Century Germany* (Cambridge, Mass.: Harvard University Press, 1991).

―――. 1993. *Disembodying Women: Perspectives on Pregnancy and the Unborn.* Cambridge, Mass.: Harvard University Press.

Duka, W., and A. DeCherney. 1994. *From the Beginning: A History of the American Fertility Society, 1944–1994.* Alabama: American Fertility Society.

Durand, H., and P. Biclet. 1991. *Dictionnaire des examens biologiques et investigations paracliniques,* 3d ed. Paris: Doin Editeurs.

Eddy, D. M. 1990a. Anatomy of a Decision. *Journal of the American Medical Association* 263:441–43.

―――. 1990b. The Challenge. *Journal of the American Medical Association* 263:287–90.

―――. 1990c. Practice Policies – What Are They? *Journal of the American Medical Association* 263:877–78, 880.

―――. 1992. Applying Cost-Effectiveness Analysis: The Inside Story. *Journal of the American Medical Association* 268:2575–82.

Egger, E., and I. Wagner. 1993. Negotiating Temporal Orders: The Case of Collaborative Time Management in a Surgery Clinic. *Computer Supported Cooperative Work* 1:255–75.

Ehrenreich, B., and D. English. 1978. *For Her Own Good.* New York: Anchor Press.

Eicher, W. 1984. *Transsexualismus: Möglichkeiten und Grenzen der Geschlechtsumwandlung.* New York: Fischer.

Eisenberg, J. M. 1986. *Doctors' Decisions and the Cost of Medical Care.* Ann Arbor: Health Administration Press.

Eisenberg, L., and A. Kleinman. 1981. Clinical Social Science. In *The Relevance of Social Science for Medicine,* edited by L. Eisenberg and A. Kleinman. Dordrecht: Reidel.

Ewald, F. 1986. *L'État-providence.* Paris: Grasset.

Fagot, A. 1982. Calcul des chances et diagnostic médical. *Traverses,* no. 24: 85–102.

Fattorusso, V., and O. Ritter. 1984. *Vademecum clinique du médecin practicien, du symptome à l'ordonnance,* 9th ed. Paris: Masson.

Feinstein, A. R. 1974. An Analysis of Diagnostic Reasoning, pt. 3: The Construction of Clinical Algorithms. *Yale Journal of Biology and Medicine* 1:5–32.

―――. 1987a. *Clinimetrics.* New Haven: Yale University Press.

―――. 1987b. The Intellectual Crisis in Clinical Science: Medaled Models and Muddled Mettle. *Perspectives in Biology and Medicine* 30:215–30.

Ferguson, R., M. Gever, T. Minh-ha, and C. West. 1990. *Out There: Marginalization and Contemporary Cultures.* Cambridge, Mass.: MIT Press.

Fleck, L. 1980 [1935]. *Entstehung und Entwicklung einer wissenschaftlichen Tatsache.* Frankfurt: Suhrkamp.

Foucault, M. 1963 [1975]. *La Naissance de la clinique: Une Archéologie du regard médical.* Paris: Presses Universitaires de France. Translated by A. M. Sheridan Smith as *The Birth of the Clinic: An Archaeology of Medical Perception* (New York: Vintage, 1975).

―――. 1979. *Discipline and Punish: The Birth of the Prison.* Translated by Alan Sheridan. New York: Vintage Books.

―――. 1982. Subject of Power. *Critical Inquiry* 8:777–95.

Fox, Renée C., and Judith P. Swazey. 1978. *The Courage to Fail: A Social View of Organ Transplants and Dialysis*. Chicago: University of Chicago Press.

Frankenberg, R., ed. 1992. *Time, Health and Medicine*. London: Sage.

Franklin, S. 1990. Deconstructing 'Desperateness': The Social Construction of Infertility in Popular Representations of New Reproductive Technologies. In *The New Reproductive Technologies*, edited by M. McNeil, I. Varcoe, and S. Yearley. London: Macmillan.

————. 1991. Fetal Fascinations: New Dimensions to the Medical-Scientific Construction of Personhood. In *Off-Centre: Feminism and Cultural Studies*, edited by S. Franklin, C. Lury, and J. Stacey. London: HarperCollins.

————. 1995. No Stranger Than Fiction—Babies in Bottles: Twentieth-Century Visions of Reproductive Technology by Susan Merrill Squier. *Women's Review of Books* 12:27–28.

————. 1997. *Embodied Progress: A Cultural Account of Assisted Conception*. London: Routledge.

Freidson, Eliot. 1970. *The Profession of Medicine: a Study of the Sociology of Applied Knowledge*. New York: Harper and Row.

Fujimura, J. H. 1987. Constructing "Do-Able" Problems in Cancer Research: Articulating Alignment. *Social Studies of Science* 17:257–93.

————. 1988. The Molecular Biological Bandwagon in Cancer Research: Where Social Worlds Meet. *Social Problems* 35 (3): 261–83.

————. 1992. Crafting Science: Standardized Packages, Boundary Objects, and "Translation." In *Science as Practice and Culture*, edited by A. Pickering. Chicago: University of Chicago Press.

Fujimura, Joan, and D. Y. Chou. 1994. Dissent in Science: Styles of Scientific Practice and the Controversy over the Cause of AIDS. *Social Science and Medicine* 38:1017–36.

Galison, P. 1997. *Image and Logic: The Material Culture of Modern Physics*. Chicago: University of Chicago Press.

Garfinkel, H. 1963. A Conception of, and Experiments with, "Trust" as a Condition of Stable Concerted Actions. In *Motivation and Social Interaction*, edited by O. Harvey. New York: Ronald Press.

————. 1967. *Studies in Ethnomethodology*. Englewood Cliffs, N.J.: Prentice Hall.

Garson, B. 1988. *The Electronic Sweatshop*. New York: Simon and Schuster.

Gebbie, K. M., and M. A. Lavin. 1975. *Classification of Nursing Diagnoses: Proceedings of First National Conference*. St. Louis: Mosby.

Gergen, K. 1991. *The Saturated Self: Dilemmas of Identity in Contemporary Life*. New York: Basic Books.

Gerhardt, Uta. 1989. *Ideas about Illness: An Intellectual and Political History of Medical Sociology*. Houndsmills, England: Macmillan Education.

Goffman, E. 1961. *Encounters: Two Studies in the Sociology of Interaction*. Harmondsworth, England: Penguin Books.

————. 1974. *Frame Analysis: An Essay on the Organization of Experience*. New York: Harper & Row.

————. 1976. *Gender Advertisements*. Cambridge, Mass.: Harvard University Press.

————. 1977. The Arrangement between the Sexes. *Theory and Society* 4:301–31.

————. 1986 [1961]. *Asylums: Essays on the Social Situation of Mental Patients and Other Inmates*. Harmondsworth, England: Pelican Books.

Good, Byron J., and Mary-Jo Delvecchio Good. 1980. The Meaning of Symptoms: A Cultural Hermeneutic Model for Medical Practice. In *The Relevance of Social Science for Medicine*, edited by L. Eisenberg and A. Kleinman. Dordrecht: Reidel.

Good, Marie-Jo Delvecchio. 1995. *American Medicine, The Quest for Competence*. Berkeley: University of California Press.

Goodman, N. 1978. *Ways of Worldmaking*. Indianapolis: Hackett Publishing.

Goody, J. 1977. *The Domestication of the Savage Mind*. New York: Cambridge University Press.

Gordon, Deborah. 1988. Tenacious Assumptions in Western Medicine. In *Biomedicine Examined*, edited by Margaret Lock and Deborah Gordon. Dordrecht: Kluwer.

Gray, A., R. Elkan, and J. Robinson. 1991. *Policy Issues in Nursing*. Milton Keynes, England: Open University Press.

Great Britain, Ministry of Health. 1996. *Population Screening for Cancer of the Cervix*. Health Memorandum HM(66)76. London: Ministry of Health.

Great Britain, Department of Health and Social Security. 1984 *Screening for Cervical Cancer*. Health Circular HC(84)17. London: Department of Health and Social Security.

————. 1988. Health Services Management: Cervical Cancer Screening. Health Circular HC(88)1. London: Department of Health and Social Security.

Green, R., and J. Money. 1969. *Transsexualism and Sex Reassignment*. Baltimore: John Hopkins University Press.

Greer, A. 1987. The Two Cultures of Biomedicine: Can There Be Consensus? *Journal of the American Medical Association* 258:2739–40.

Grimm, R. H., K. Shimoni, W. R. Harlan, and E. H. Estes. 1975. Evaluation of Patient-Care Protocol Use by Various Providers. *New England Journal of Medicine* 292:507–11.

Grobe, S. J. 1993. Response to J. C. McCloskey's and G. M. Bulechek's Paper on Nursing Intervention Schemes. In *Papers from the Nursing Minimum Data Set Conference*. Edmonton, Canada: Canadian Nursing Association.

Hacking, I. 1986. Making Up People. In *Reconstructing Individualism*, edited by T. C. Heller et al. Stanford: Stanford University Press.

————. 1992. The Self-vindication of the Laboratory Sciences. In *Science as Practice and Culture*, edited by A. Pickering. Chicago: University of Chicago Press.

Hahn, Robert, and Atwood Gaines, eds. 1985. *Physicians of Western Medicine*. Dordrecht: Kluwer.

Haraway, D. 1991. *Simians, Cyborgs and Women: The Reinvention of Nature*. New York: Routledge.

————. 1992. Ecce Homo, Ain't (Ar'n't) I a Woman, and Inappropriate/d Others: The

Human in a Post-Humanist Landscape. In *Feminists Theorize the Political,* edited by J. Butler and J. Scott. New York: Routledge.

Harrison, M. R. 1991. Professional Considerations in Fetal Treatment. In *The Unborn Patient: Prenatal Diagnosis and Treatment,* edited by M. R. Harrison, M. S. Golbus, and R. A. Filly. Philadelphia: W. B. Saunders.

Harrison, M. R., N. S. Adzick, and A. W. Flake. 1993. Congenital Diaphragmatic Hernia: An Unsolved Problem. *Seminars in Pediatric Surgery* 2 (2): 109–12.

Harrison, M. R., M. S. Golbus, and R. A. Filly, eds. 1991. *The Unborn Patient: Prenatal Diagnosis and Treatment.* Philadelphia: W. B. Saunders.

Harrison, M. R., and M. T. Longaker. 1991. Maternal Risk and the Development of Fetal Surgery. In *The Unborn Patient: Prenatal Diagnosis and Treatment,* edited by M. R. Harrison, M. S. Golbus, and R. A. Filly. Philadelphia: W. B. Saunders.

Hart, H. 1961. *The Concept of Law.* Oxford: Oxford University Press.

Hartouni, V. 1991. Containing Women: Reproductive Discourse in the 1980s. In *Technoculture,* edited by C. Penley and A. Ross. Minneapolis: University of Minnesota Press.

Heath, C. 1988. *Body Movement and Speech in Medical Interaction.* Cambridge: Cambridge University Press.

Heath, Deborah, and Paul Rabinow. 1993. *Bio-Politics: The Anthropology of the New Genetics and Immunology.* Special issue of *Culture, Medicine and Psychiatry* 17 (1).

Helman, Cecil G. 1978. "Feed a Cold, Starve a Fever" — Folk Models of Infection in an English Suburban Community, and Their Relation to Medical Treatment. *Culture, Medicine and Psychiatry* 2:107–39.

———. *Culture, Health and Illness,* 2d ed. London: Butterworth-Heinemann.

Herzlich, C. 1984. Médecine moderne et quête de sens. In *Le Sens du mal — anthropologie, histoire, sociologie de la maladie,* edited by M. Augé and C. Herzlich. Paris: Editions des Archives Contemporaines.

Hilbert, R. 1984. The Accultural Dimension of Chronic Pain: Flawed Reality Construction and the Problem of Meaning. *Social Problems* 31 (4): 365–78.

Hirschauer, Stefan. 1991. The Manufacture of Bodies in Surgery. *Social Studies of Science* 21:217–319.

———. 1992. The Meanings of Transsexuality. In *The Social Construction of Illness,* edited by J. Lachmund and G. Stollberg. Stuttgart: Steiner.

———. 1993. *Die soziale Konstruktion der Transsexualität: Über die Medizin und den Geschlechtswechsel.* Frankfurt: Suhrkamp.

Hohlfeld, Rainer. 1978. Praxisbezüge wissenschaftlicher Disziplenen: Das Beispiel der Krebsforschung. In *Die gesellschaftliche Orientierung des wissenschaftlichen Fortschritts.* Starnberger Studien I. Frankfurt: Suhrkamp.

Hopkins, L. 1991. *I'm Alive.* Liverpool, England: Changing Places Publications.

Horkheimer, M., and T. Adorno. 1979. *Dialectic of Enlightenment.* New York: Seabury Press.

Horstman, K. 1997. Chemical Analysis of Urine for Life Insurance: The Construction of Reliability. *Science, Technology and Human Values* 22:57–78.

Howell, L. J., N. S. Adzick, and M. R. Harrison. 1993. The Fetal Treatment Center. *Seminars in Pediatric Surgery* 2 (2): 143–46.

Hughes, E. C. 1971. *The Sociological Eye: Selected Papers.* New Brunswick, N.J.: Transaction Press.

Hurst, J. 1987. *Médecine clinique pour le médecin praticien.* Paris: Masson.

Imbernon, E., et al. 1992. *Les Pratiques professionnelles des médecins du travail à EDF-GDF: Résultats d'une enquête par questionnaire.* Rapport. Paris: Electricité de France.

Iowa Intervention Project. 1992. *Taxonomy of Nursing Interventions.* Iowa City: IIP, University of Iowa.

———. 1993. The NIC Taxonomy Structure. *Image: Journal of Nursing Scholarship* 25 (3): 187–92.

———. 1995. Validation and Coding of the NIC Taxonomy Structure. *Image: Journal of Nursing Scholarship* 27 (1): 43–49.

Jackson, J. E. 1992. 'After a While No One Believes You': Real and Unreal Pain. In *Pain as Human Experience: An Anthropological Perspective,* edited by M. J. Delvecchio Good, P. Brodwin, B. Good, and A. Kleinman. Berkeley: University of California Press.

Johnston, K. 1989. *Screening for Cervical Cancer: A Review of the Literature.* Health Economics Research Unit Discussion Paper 04/89. Aberdeen, Scotland: University of Aberdeen.

Jordan, Kathleen, and Michael Lynch. 1992. The Sociology of a Genetic Engineering Technique: Ritual and Rationality in the Performance of the "Plasmid Prep." In *The Right Tools for the Job: At Work in Twentieth-Century Life Sciences,* edited by Adele E. Clark, and Joan H. Fujimura. Princeton: Princeton University Press.

Kanouse, D. E., et al. 1989. *Changing Medical Practice through Technology Assessment: An Evaluation of the NIH Consensus Development Program.* Ann Arbor: Health Administration Press.

Katz, P. 1981. Ritual in the Operating Room. *Ethnology* 20:335–50.

Kessler, S., and W. McKenna. 1978. *Gender: An Ethnomethodological Approach.* New York: Wiley.

King, D. 1987. Social Constructionism and Medical Knowledge: The Case of Transsexualism. *Sociology of Health and Illness* 9:351–77.

Kirk, S. A., and H. Kutchins. 1992. *The Selling of the DSM: The Rhetoric of Science in Psychiatry.* New York: Aldine de Gruyter.

Kitcher, P. 1993. *The Advancement of Science: Science without Legend, Objectivity without Illusions.* Oxford: Oxford University Press.

Klein, R. 1989. *Infertility: Women Speak Out about Their Experiences of Reproductive Technologies.* London: Pandora Press.

Klein, R., and R. Rowland. 1988. Women as Test Sites for Fertility Drugs: Clomiphene Citrate and Hormonal Cocktails. *Reproductive and Genetic Engineering* 1:251–374.

Kleinman, A. 1980. *Patients and Healers in the Context of Culture.* Berkeley: University of California Press.

Kling, R. 1991. Computerization and Social Transformations. *Science, Technology, and Human Values* 16:342–67.

Knorr-Cetina, K. D. 1981. *The Manufacture of Knowledge*. Oxford: Pergamon Press.

Kohrman A. F. 1994. Chimeras and Odysseys: Toward Understanding the Technology-Dependent Child. Special supplement to *Hastings Center Report* 24 (5): S4–S6.

Komaroff, A. L. 1982. Algorithms and the "Art" of Medicine. *American Journal of Public Health* 72:10–12.

Kondo, D. 1990. *Crafting Selves: Power, Gender and Discourses of Identity in a Japanese Workplace*. Chicago: University of Chicago Press.

Koop, C. E. E. 1986. Editorial. *Fetal Therapy* 1:1–2.

Kosekoff, J., et al. 1987. Effects of the National Institutes of Health Consensus Development Program on Physician Practice. *Journal of the American Medical Association* 258:2708–13.

Kotarba, J. A. 1977. The Chronic Pain Experience. In *Existential Sociology*, edited by J. D. Douglas and J. M. Johnson. New York: Cambridge University Press.

Laplantine, François. 1986. *Anthropologie de la maladie*. Paris: Payot.

Latour, Bruno. 1984 [1988]. *Les Microbes: Guerre et paix / irréductions*. Paris: Métailié. Translated as *The Pasteurization of France* (Cambridge, Mass.: Harvard University Press 1988).

———. 1986. The Powers of Association. In *Power, Action and Belief*, edited by J. Law. London: Routledge.

———. 1987. *Science in Action: How to Follow Scientists and Engineers Through Society*. Cambridge, Mass.: Harvard University Press.

———. 1993a [1991]. *We Have Never Been Modern*. Cambridge, Mass.: Harvard University Press.

———. 1993b. *La Clef de Berlin et autres leçons d'un amateur de sciences*. Paris: Editions la Découverte.

Latour, B., and M. Callon. 1993. Don't Throw the Baby Out with the Bath School! In *Science as Practice and Culture*, edited by A. Pickering. Chicago: University of Chicago Press.

Latour, B., and S. Woolgar. 1986 [1st ed. 1979]. *Laboratory Life: The Construction of Scientific Facts*. Princeton: Princeton University Press.

Law, J. 1986. On the Methods of Long-Distance Control: Vessels, Navigation and the Portuguese Route to India. In *Power, Action and Belief: A New Sociology of Knowledge?* edited by J. Law. London: Routledge.

———. 1987. Technology and Heterogeneous Engineering: The Case of Portuguese Expansion. In *The Social Construction of Technological Systems*, edited by W. E. Bijker et al. Cambridge, Mass.: MIT Press.

———. 1995. Organization and Semiotics: Technology, Agency and Representation. In *Accountability, Power and Ethos*, edited by J. Mouritsen and R. Munro. London: Chapman Hill.

———, ed. 1991. *A Sociology of Monsters: Essays on Power, Technology and Domination*. London: Routledge.

Law, J., and A. Mol. 1994. *On Hidden Heterogeneities: The Design of an Aircraft.* Unpublished manuscript.

Layne, L. 1992. Of Fetuses and Angels: Fragmentation and Integration in Narratives of Pregnancy Loss. *Knowledge and Society: The Anthropology of Science and Technology* 9:29–58.

Leslie, Charles, and Allan Young, eds. 1992. *Paths to Asian Medical Knowledge.* Berkeley: University of California Press.

Liley, A. W. 1963. Intrauterine Transfusion of Fetus in Hemolytic Disease. *British Medical Journal* 2:1107–9.

Lindenbaum, S., and M. Lock, eds. 1993. *Knowledge, Power, and Practice: The Anthropology of Medicine and Everyday Life.* Berkeley: University of California Press.

Lock, Margaret, and Deborah Gordon, eds. 1988. *Biomedicine Examined.* Dordrecht: Kluwer.

Longino, H. 1995. Knowledge, Bodies, and Values: Reproductive Technologies and Their Scientific Context. In *Technology and the Politics of Knowledge,* edited by A. Feenberg and A. Hannay. Bloomington: Indiana University Press.

Lorber, J. 1975. Good Patients and Bad Patients. *Journal of Health and Social Behavior* 16:213–25.

Löwy, I. 1992. The Strength of Loose Concepts—Boundary Concepts, Federative Experimental Strategies and Disciplinary Growth: The Case of Immunology. *History of Science* 30:371–96.

———. 1995a. Nothing More to Do: Palliative Care versus Experimental Therapy in Advanced Cancer. *Science in Context* 8:209–30.

———. 1995b. La Standardisation de l'inconnu: Les Protocoles thérapeutiques en cancérologie. *Techniques et Culture* 25–26:263–84.

Lynch, M. 1984. Turning Up Signs in Neurobehavioral Diagnosis. *Symbolic Interaction* 7 (1): 67–86.

———. 1985. *Art and Artifact in Laboratory Science: A Study of Shop Work and Shop Talk in a Research Laboratory.* London: Routledge and Kegan Paul.

———. 1991. Laboratory Space and the Technological Complex: An Investigation of Topical Contextures. *Science in Context* 4:51–78.

———. 1993. *Scientific Practice and Ordinary Action: Ethnomethodology and Social Studies of Science.* New York: Cambridge University Press.

McCloskey, J. C., and G. M. Bulechek. 1992. *Nursing Interventions Classification.* St. Louis: Mosby Year Book.

———. 1994a. Standardizing the Language for Nursing Treatments: An Overview of the Issues. *Nursing Outlook* 42 (2): 56–63.

———. 1994b. Response to Edward Halloran. *Image: Journal of Nursing Scholarship* 26 (2): 93.

McCormick, J. S. 1989. Cervical Smears: A Questionable Practice? *Lancet,* July, pp. 207–9.

MacIntyre, A. 1981. *After Virtue.* London: Duckworth.

Macklin, R. 1990. Maternal-Fetal Conflict: An Ethical Analysis. *Women's Health Issues* 1 (1): 28–30.

McRae, F. B., and G. E. Markle. 1984. The Estrogen Replacement Controversy in the USA and UK: Different Answers to the Same Question? *Social Studies of Science* 14:1–26.

Marcus-Steiff, J. 1991. Les Taux de 'succès' de FIV — Fausses transparences et vrais mensonges. *La Recherche*, no. 225, special 20th anniversary issue, 1300–12.

Margolis, C. Z. 1983. Uses of Clinical Algorithms. *Journal of the American Medical Association* 249:627–32.

Marks, Harry M. 1988. Notes from the Underground: The Social Organization of Therapeutic Research. In *Grand Rounds: 100 Years of Internal Medicine,* edited by R. C. Maulitz, and D. E. Long. Philadelphia: University of Pennsylvania Press.

———. 1997. *The Progress of Experiment: Science and Therapeutic Reform in the United States, 1900–1990.* Cambridge: Cambridge University Press.

Martin, E. 1987. *The Woman in the Body: A Cultural Analysis of Reproduction.* Boston: Beacon Press.

———. 1994. *Flexible Bodies.* Boston: Beacon Press.

Martin, M. 1991. *"Hello, Central?": Gender, Technology and Culture in the Formation of Telephone Systems.* McGill, Canada: Queen's University Press.

Marx, K. 1982. The Economic and Philosophical Manuscripts. In *Classes, Power and Conflict: Classical and Contemporary Debates,* edited by A. Giddens and D. Held. Berkeley: University of California Press.

Mead, G. H. 1934. *Mind, Self, and Society.* Chicago: University of Chicago Press.

Melzack, R., and P. Wall. 1965. Pain Mechanisms: A New Theory. *Science* 150:971–79.

Mol, A. 1993. What Is New? Doppler and Its Others: An Empirical Philosophy of Innovations. In *Medicine and Change: Historical and Sociological Studies of Medical Innovation,* edited by I. Löwy. Paris: INSERM.

———. Forthcoming. Cutting Surgeons, Walking Patients. In *Complexities in Science, Technology and Medicine,* edited by John Law and Annemarie Mol.

Mol, A., and M. Berg, 1994. Principles and Practices of Medicine. *Culture, Medicine and Psychiatry* 18:247–65.

Mol, A., and J. Law. 1994. Regions, Networks and Fluids: Anaemia and Social Topology. *Social Studies of Science* 24:641–71.

Mol, A., and A. Lettinga. 1991. Bodies, Impairments and the Social Constructed: The Case of Hemiplegia. In *The Social Construction of Illness: Illness and Medical Knowledge in Past and Present,* edited by J. Jachmund and G. Stollberg. Stuttgart: Verlag.

Mol, Annemarie, and Peter van Lieshout. 1989. *Ziek is het woord niet.* Nijmegen: SUN.

Montmolin, M. de. 1986. *L'Ergonomie.* Paris: La Découverte.

National Association of Cytologists. 1990. *Scan.* Newsletter 1, January.

National Co-ordinating Network. 1991. *First Annual Report: NHSCSP.* Oxford: Redcliffe Hospital, National Co-ordinating Network.

Nelkin, D., ed. 1985. *The Language of Risk: Conflicting Perspectives on Occupational Health.* Beverly Hills: Sage.

Neumann, L. J. 1995. *What about Leech Treatment? Classification Systems and the Profes-sionalization of Nursing.* Paper presented at the American Sociological Association annual meeting, Washington, D.C.

Newman, S. P., D. Pavia, and S. W. Clarke. 1989. How Should a Pressurized β-Adrenergic Bronchodilator Be Inhaled? *European Journal of Respiratory Diseases* 62:3–21.

Noble, D. 1984. *Forces of Production.* New York: Oxford University Press.

O'Connell, J. 1993. Metrology: The Creation of Universality by the Circulation of Par-ticulars. *Social Studies of Science* 23:129–73.

Olesen, V. L. and E. W. Whittaker. 1968. *The Silent Dialogue: A Study in the Social Psy-chology of Professional Socialization.* San Francisco: Jossey-Bass.

O'Neill, A. 1994. Danger and Safety in Medicines. *Social Science and Medicine* 38:497–509.

Oudshoorn, N. 1990. On the Making of Sex Hormones: Research Materials and the Pro-duction of Knowledge. *Social Studies of Science* 20:5–33.

Parfit, D. 1984. *Reasons and Persons.* Oxford: Oxford University Press.

Pasveer, Bernike. 1992. *Shadows of Knowledge: Making a Representing Practice in Medi-cine: X-ray Pictures and Pulmonary Tuberculosis, 1895–1930.* Ph.D. diss. University of Amsterdam.

Payer, Lynn. 1989. *Medicine and Culture. Notions of Health and Sickness in Britain, the U.S., France and West Germany.* London: Victor Gollancz.

Peräkylä, A. 1989. Appealing to the "Experience" of the Patient in the Care of the Dying. *Sociology of Health and Illness* 11 (2): 117–34.

Petchesky, R. P. 1987. Fetal Images: The Power of Visual Culture in the Politics of Repro-duction. In *Reproductive Technologies: Gender, Motherhood, and Medicine,* edited by M. Stanworth. Minneapolis: University of Minnesota Press.

Pickering, A., ed. 1992. *Science as Practice and Culture.* Chicago: University of Chicago Press.

Pippin, R. 1996. Medical Practice and Social Authority. *Journal of Medicine and Philoso-phy* 21:357–73.

Pool, R. 1994. *Dialogue and the Interpretation of Illness: Conversations in a Cameroon Village.* Oxford: Berg.

Posner, T. 1987. *An Abnormal Smear: What Does That Mean?* London: Women's Health and Reproductive Rights Information Centre.

Posner, T., and M. Vessey. 1988. *Prevention of Cervical Cancer: The Patient's View.* Lon-don: King Edward's Hospital Fund for London.

Prins, Baukje. 1995. The Ethics of Hybrid Subjects: Feminist Constructivism According to Donna Haraway. *Science, Technology and Human Values* 20:352–67.

Purdy, L. M. 1990. Are Pregnant Women Fetal Containers? *Bioethics* 4 (4): 273–91.

Quilliam, S. 1989. *Positive Smear.* London: Penguin Books.

Quine, W. 1960. *Word and Object.* Cambridge, Mass.: MIT Press.

Rapp, Rayna. 1993. Accounting for Amniocentesis. In *Knowledge, Power and Practice. The Anthropology of Medicine and Everyday Life,* edited by Shirley Lindenbaum and Margaret Lock. Berkeley: University of California Press.

———. 1994. Women's Responses to Prenatal Diagnosis: A Sociocultural Perspective on Diversity. In *Women and Prenatal Testing: Facing the Challenges of Genetic Technology*, edited by K. Rothenberg and E. Thompson. Columbus: University of Ohio Press.

———. 1995. Real Time Fetus: The Role of the Sonogram in the Age of Monitored Reproduction. In *Cyborgs and Citadels*, edited by G. Downey, J. Dumit, and S. Traweek. Seattle: University of Washington Press.

Reed, C. 1991. Aerosol Steroids as Primary Treatment of Mild Asthma. *New England Journal of Medicine* 325:425–26.

Reiser, Stanley Joel. 1978. *Medicine and the Reign of Technology*. Cambridge: Cambridge University Press.

Rey, R., and L. E. Wallace. *History of Pain*. Cambridge, Mass.: Harvard University Press.

Roberts, A. 1982. Cervical Cytology in England and Wales, 1965–1980. *Health Trends* 14:41–43.

Roth, Julius A. 1979 [1963]. *Timetables: Structuring the Passage of Time in Hospital Treatment and Other Careers*. Indianapolis: Bobbs-Merrill.

Rothman, B. K. 1986. *The Tentative Pregnancy: Prenatal Diagnosis and the Future of Motherhood*. New York: Penguin Books.

Rothshuh, Karl. 1978. *Konzepte der Medizin in Vergangenheit und Gegenwart*. Stuttgart: Hippokrates Verlag.

Rudwick, M. 1985. *The Great Devonian Controversy: The Shaping of Scientific Knowledge among Gentlemanly Specialists*. Chicago: University of Chicago Press.

Sacks, H. 1975. Everyone Has to Lie. In *Sociocultural Dimensions of Language Use*, edited by M. Sanches and B. G. Bount. New York: Academic Press.

Saffron, L. 1987. Cervical Cancer—The Politics of Prevention. In *Women's Health: A Spare Rib Reader*, edited by S. O'Sullivan. New York: Pandora.

Schaffner, K., ed. 1985. *Logic of Discovery and Diagnosis in Medicine*. Berkeley: University of California Press.

Shapin, S. 1993. Essay Review: Personal Development and Intellectual Biography: The Case of Robert Boyle. *British Journal for the History of Science* 26:335–45.

Shapin, S., and S. Schaffer. 1985. *Leviathan and the Air-Pump: Hobbes, Boyle and the Experimental Life*. Princeton: Princeton University Press.

Sherrer, J. R., R. A. Cote, and S. H. Mandell. 1989. *Computerized Natural Medical Language Processing for Knowledge Representation*. New York: Elsevier.

Sicard, D. 1987. *L'Approche clinique*. Paris: Maloine.

Silverman, D. 1987. *Communication and Medical Practice: Social Relations in the Clinic*. London: Sage.

Singer, A., and A. Szarewski. 1988. *Cervical Smear Test: What Every Woman Should Know*. London: Macdonald Optima.

Singleton, V. 1992. *Science, Women and Ambivalence: An Actor-Network Analysis of the Cervical Screening Programme*. Ph.D. diss. Lancaster University, England.

Singleton, Vicky, and Mike Michael. 1993. Actor-Networks and Ambivalence: General

Practitioners in the UK Cervical Screening Programme. *Social Studies of Science* 23:227–64.

Smith, Barbara. 1981. Black Lung: The Social Production of a Disease. *International Journal of Health Services* 11:3343–359.

Souhami, R. L., and J. Moxham, eds. 1990. *Textbook of Medicine.* Edinburgh: Churchill Livingstone.

Spallone, P., and D. Steinberg, eds. 1987. *Made to Order: The Myth of Reproductive and Genetic Progress.* New York: Pergamon Press.

Squier, S. 1994. *Babies in Bottles: Twentieth-Century Visions of Reproductive Technologies.* New Brunswick, N.J.: Rutgers University Press.

Star, S. L. 1983. Simplification in Scientific Work: An Example from Neuroscience Research. *Social Studies of Science* 13:208–26.

———. 1989a. Layered Space, Formal Representations and Long-Distance Control: The Politics of Information. *Fundamenta Scientiae* 10:125–54.

———. 1989b. *Regions of the Mind: Brain Research and the Quest for Scientific Certainty.* Stanford: Stanford University Press.

———. 1991a. Invisible Work and Silenced Dialogues in Representing Knowledge. In *Women, Work and Computerization: Understanding and Overcoming Bias in Work and Education,* edited by I. V. Eriksson, B. A. Kitchenham, and K. G. Tijdens. Amsterdam: Elsevier–North Holland.

———. 1991b. Power, Technologies and the Phenomenology of Conventions: On Being Allergic to Onions. In *A Sociology of Monsters,* edited by J. Law. London: Routledge.

———. 1991c. The Sociology of the Invisible: The Primacy of Work in the Writings of Anselm Strauss. In *Social Organization and Social Process: Essays in Honor of Anselm Strauss,* edited by D. R. Maines. Hawthorne, N.Y.: Aldine de Gruyter.

———. 1992. Craft vs. Commodity, Mess vs. Transcendence: How the Right Tool Became the Wrong One in the Case of Taxidermy and Natural History. In *The Right Tools for the Job: At Work in Twentieth-Century Life Sciences,* edited by A. E. Clarke and J. H. Fujimura. Princeton: Princeton University Press.

———, ed. 1994. *Ecologies of Knowledge: New Directions in Sociology of Science and Technology.* Albany: State University of New York Press.

Star, Susan Leigh, and Geoffrey C. Bowker. 1997. Of Lungs and Lungers: The Classified Story of Tuberculosis. In *Mind, Culture and Activity,* in press. Reprinted in Anselm Strauss and Juliet Corbin, eds. (Thousand Oaks, Calif.: Sage, 1997).

Star, S. L., and E. M. Gerson. 1986. Analyzing Due Process in the Workplace. ACM *Transactions on Office Information Systems* 4:257–70.

Star, S. L., and J. Griesemer. 1989. Institutional Ecology, "Translations" and Boundary Objects: Amateurs and Professionals in Berkeley's Museum of Vertebrate Zoology, 1907–39. *Social Studies of Science* 19:387–420.

Starr, Paul. 1982. *The Social Transformation of American Medicine.* New York: Basic Books.

Stein, Howard. 1990. *American Medicine as Culture*. Boulder, Colo.: Westview Press.

Stoller, R. 1968. *Sex and Gender*. London: Hogarth.

———. 1975. *The Transsexual Experiment*. London: Hogarth.

Stone, S. 1991. The Empire Strikes Back: A Posttranssexual Manifesto. In *Body Guards: The Cultural Politics of Gender Ambiguity*, edited by J. Epstein and K. Straub. New York: Routledge.

Strathern, Marilyn. 1991. *Partial Connections*. Savage, Rowman and Littlefield.

———. 1992a. *After Nature: English Kinship in the Late Twentieth Century*. Cambridge: Cambridge University Press.

———. 1992b. *Reproducing the Future: Anthropology and the New Reproductive Technologies*. Manchester, England: Manchester University Press.

Strauss, A. 1975. *Chronic Illness and the Quality of Life*. St. Louis: C. V. Mosby.

———. 1978a. A Social World Perspective. In *Studies in Symbolic Interaction*, vol. 1, edited by N. Denzin. Greenwich, Conn.: JAI Press.

———. 1978b. *Negotiations: Varieties, Contexts, Processes, and Social Order*. San Francisco: Jossey-Bass.

———. 1982. Social Worlds and Legitimation Processes. In *Studies in Symbolic Interaction*, vol. 4, edited by N. Denzin. Greenwich, Conn.: JAI Press.

———. 1984. Social Worlds and Their Segmentation Processes. In *Studies in Symbolic Interaction*, vol. 5, edited by N. Denzin. Greenwich, Conn.: JAI Press.

———. 1993. *Continual Permutations of Action*. New York: Aldine de Gruyter.

Strauss, A., S. Fagerhaugh, B. Suczek, and C. Wiener. 1985. *Social Organization of Medical Work*. Chicago: University of Chicago Press.

Strauss, A., L. Schatzman, R. Bucher, D. Erlich, and M. Sabshin. 1964. *Psychiatric Ideologies and Institutions*. Glencoe, Ill.: Free Press.

Strong, P. M. 1979. *The Ceremonial Order of the Clinic: Parents, Doctors and Medical Bureaucracy*. London: Routledge and Kegan Paul.

Strong, P., and J. Robinson. 1990. *The NHS — Under New Management*. Bristol, Pa.: Open University Press.

Suchman, L. 1987. *Plans and Situated Actions: The Problem of Human-Machine Communication*. Cambridge: Cambridge University Press.

———. 1993. Technologies of Accountability: Of Lizards and Aeroplanes. In *Technology in Working Order: Studies of Work, Interaction, and Technology*, edited by G. Button. London: Routledge.

———. 1994a. Do Categories Have Politics? The Language/Action Perspective Reconsidered. *Computer Supported Cooperative Work* 2:177–90.

———. 1994b. Working Relations of Technology Production and Use. *Computer Supported Cooperative Work* 2:21–39.

Taylor, C. 1989. *Sources of the Self: The Making of the Modern Identity*. Cambridge, Mass.: Harvard University Press.

Terry, J. 1988. The Body Invaded: Medical Surveillance of Women as Reproducers. *Socialist Review* 89 (3): 13–43.

Thomas, S., and G. Rutten. 1993. NHG-Standaarden voor de huisarts. Utrecht: Nederlands Huisartsen Genootschap.

Timmermans, Stefan. 1995. Saving Lives: A Historical and Ethnographic Study of Resuscitation Techniques. Ph.D. diss. University of Illinois.

Timmermans, S., and M. Berg. 1997. Standardization in Action: Achieving Local Universality through Medical Protocols. Social Studies of Science 27:273-305.

Toogood J. H., et al. 1980. Candidiasis and Dysphonia Complicating Beclomethasone Treatment of Asthma. Journal of Allergy and Clinical Immunology 65:143-53.

Traweek, Sharon. 1988. Beamtimes and Lifetimes: The World of High Energy Physicists. Cambridge, Mass.: Harvard University Press.

———. 1993. An Introduction to Cultural and Social Studies of Sciences and Technologies. Culture, Medicine and Psychiatry 17:3-25.

Triechler, Paula. 1990. Feminism, Medicine and the Meaning of Childbirth. In Body/Politics: Women and the Discourses of Science, edited by Mary Jacobus, Evelyn Fox Keller, and Sally Shuttleworth. London: Routledge.

U.S. Department of Health and Human Services. 1991. Guidelines for the Diagnosis and Management of Asthma. Bethesda, Md.: National Asthma Education Program.

Van der Waart, M. A. C., F. W. Dekker, and S. Nijhoff, et al. 1992. NHG-standaard CARA bij volwassenen: Behandeling. Huisarts en Wetenschap 35 (11): 437-43.

Vos, Rein. 1991. Drugs Looking for Diseases: Innovative Drug Research and the Development of the Beta Blockers and the Calcium Antagonists. Dordrecht: Kluwer Academic Publishers.

Wachtel, T., A. W. Moulton, J. Pezzullo, and M. Hamolsky. 1986. Inpatient Management Protocols to Reduce Health Care Costs. Medical Decision Making 6:101-9.

Wagner, Ina. 1993. Women's Voice: The Case of Nursing Information Systems. AI and Society 7:295-310.

Walsh, J. P., and G. R. Ungson. 1991. Organizational Memory. Academy of Management Review 16:57-91.

Warner, John Harley. 1986. The Therapeutic Perspective: Medical Practice, Knowledge and Identity in America, 1820-1885. Cambridge, Mass.: Harvard University Press.

Weber, Max. 1958. The Protestant Ethic and the Spirit of Capitalism. Translated by Talcott Parsons. New York: Charles Scribner's.

Wennberg, J. 1984. Dealing with Medical Practice Variations: A Proposal for Action. Health Affairs 3:6-32.

Werley, H. H., and N. M. Lang. 1988. Identification of the Nursing Minimum Data Set. New York: Springer.

Werley, H. H., N. M. Lang, and S. K. Westlake. 1986. The Nursing Minimum Data Set Conference: Executive Summary. Journal of Professional Nursing 2:217-24.

West, C., and D. H. Zimmerman. 1987. Doing Gender. Gender and Society 1:125-51.

Whalen, J. 1993. Accounting for "Standard" Task Performance in the Execution of 9-1-1 Operations. Paper presented at the annual meeting of the American Sociological Association, Miami.

Willems, Dick. 1992. Susan's Breathlessness: The Construction of Professionals and Lay-persons. In *The Social Construction of Illness: Illness and Medical Knowledge in Past and Present*, edited by Jens Lachmund and Gunnar Stollberg. Stuttgart: Franz Steiner Verlag.

———. 1995. *Tools of Care: Explorations into the Semiotics of Medical Technology*. Ph.D. diss. Amsterdam: Thesis Publishers.

Wittgenstein, L. 1961. *Investigations philosophiques*. Paris: Gallimard.

Wright, Peter, and Andrew Treacher, eds. 1982. *The Problem of Medical Knowledge: Examining the Social Construction of Medicine*. Edinburgh: Edinburgh University Press.

Wulff, H. R. 1981. *Rational Diagnosis and Treatment*. Oxford: Blackwell.

Wulff, Hendrik, Stig Andur Petersen, and Raben Rosenberg. 1986. *Philosophy of Medicine*. Oxford: Blackwell.

Wynne, A. 1988. Accounting for Accounts of the Diagnosis of Multiple Sclerosis. In *Knowledge and Reflexivity: New Frontiers in the Sociology of Knowledge*, edited by S. Woolgar. London: Sage.

Wynne, B. 1987. Uncertainty—Technical and Social. In *Science for Public Policy*, edited by H. Brooks and C. L. Cooper. Oxford: Pergamon Press.

Young, Allan. 1981. The Creation of Medical Knowledge: Some Problems in Interpretation. *Social Science and Medicine* 15B:379–86.

Zuboff, S. 1988. *In the Age of the Smart Machine*. New York: Basic Books.

INDEX

Abbott, Andrew, 220-221
Abortion, 50-51
Actor-network theory, 90, 102, 109
Acupuncture: in pain medicine, 123, 130, 133
Administrative: ethos, 70; individuals, 77. *See also* Frame: administrative
Agency, 166-201; of humans, 26-27; loss of, 177; and selves, 168-169; structured by objectification, 187-192; of things, 26-27
Airway obstruction. *See* Asthma
Airways. *See* Lungs
Akrich, Madeleine, 109, 211
Anesthetic techniques: in pain management, 123-130, 141-142
Angiography, 151-153, 157
Anthropology of medicine, 4-5
Anticipatory socionaturalization, 179-180, 187-188
Asthma, 105-118; differences in, 105-118; drugs in the making of, 105-118
Atherosclerosis, 144-165; clinical, 147-149; pathological, 147-149; performances of, 150, 152, 156, 161; as process over time, 156; as virtual object, 156

Bayesian reasoning, 84
Biomedicine. *See* Medicine
Body: itinerary, 179-186; objectified, 192; ontology of, 3, 6-8, 105-165, 181; performance of, 21, 162-163; pregnant, 28-51;

un-black-boxing of, 180, 187; unity of, 3, 6-8
Body/mind dichotomy, 128-129
Boltanski, Luc, 53-54
Bone marrow transplantation, 244
Bonica, John, 121-122, 126, 128, 132, 136, 140. *See also* Pain
Boundary: object, 120-121, 139-140; theory, 139
Bourdieu, Pierre, 26
Breast cancer: research protocol for, 229-246. *See also* Cancer
Bulechek, Gloria, 206, 216
Bureaucratic ethos. *See* Administrative ethos

Cancer: pain in, 125, 137, 143. *See also* Breast cancer; Cervical Screening Programme
Care: administrative, 215-216; direct, 215-216; indirect, 215-216; plans, 220
CD34: in breast cancer, 232-236, 240-243
Cervical Screening Programme, 86-104; coexistence of formulations of, 102-103; validity and efficacy of, 87-90
Cervical smear samples: analysis of, 93-96, 98; management of, 92-93
Child abuse: creation of category, 203
Classification system, 202-225; as black box, 220; construction of, 240, 211-225
Clinical: decisions, different criteria for, 14-27, 229-246; ethos, 70-72; indi-

Links, 144–165; absent, 145–149; hidden, 153–157; loose, 149–153; making, 144–165; transportable, 157–161, 163
Löwy, Ilana, 120
Lungs: black, 1–2; as constrictable tubes, 112–113, 117; as defense line, 112–113; maps of, 114
Lymph nodes: in breast cancer, 229–243

McCloskey, Joanne, 206, 221
Medical decisions. See Clinical decisions
Medical diagnosis. See Clinical decisions
Medical practice: variations in, 7, 226–227, 237–238
Medical specialties. See Professional groups
Medicine: as institution, 136; logic of traditional, 136; politics inside, 7–8; as unity, 2–8; Western, 4, 11, 144–145, 164

National Association of Cytologists, 99
National Health Service, 86
National Institutes of Health, 44, 108
Negotiated order, 31–32, 47, 50
Neurophysiological techniques: in pain management, 125–135
North American Nursing Diagnosis Association (NANDA), 106, 223
Nursing: activites, 206; autonomy, 220–222; as clinical discipline, 215; community health, 217; diagnoses, 213, 215; intensity, 213; Interventions Classification (NIC), 202–225 (see also Classification system); invisible work of, 210; Minimum Data Set (NMDS), 213; organizations, 206; outcomes, 213; science, 211; social-psychological, 217; specific diagnoses, 206, 210

Objectification, 167–168, 177–180, 182, 184; vs. agency, 189–190; as bureaucratization, 179, 188, 190; cycles of, 187–192; dehumanizing effects of, 190; as epistemically disciplined subject, 188–190; as medical operationalization, 187, 190; as naturalization, 187, 190; nature of, 177; vs. subjectivity, 167

Objects: nature of, 31; multiplicity of, 161–163; social, 30–31; vs. subject, 168; virtual, 150–151, 154–157, 159, 162; work (see Work objects)
Obstetricians, 32–36, 38–51
Obstructive lung disease. See Asthma
Occupational medicine, 53–82; mechanisms, 57; visit, 57–60
Oncology: and breast cancer, 229–246
Ontological choreography, 166–201

Pain: chronic, 121–139; clinic, 120–139; cure vs. management of, 131, 139; definition of, 122, 133; gate control theory of, 121–133, 136–137; management, 129–135; medicine, 119–139; physicians, 119–139; specificity theory of, 122, 140
Pathologists: and atherosclerosis, 147–149; in cervical screening, 89, 96–100, 104
Patient: bureaucratization of, 188 (see also Objectification); different criteria for selection (see Clinical decisions); as disciplined subjects, 169; fetus as, 37–41, 43, 46, 48; generic, 188; as instrument, 176; mother as, 38–40; naturalization of, 187 (see also Objectification); as object, 177–179; as object of study, 176, 178, 240–244; as subject, 177, 188; transsexual as, 17; unity of, 6; women, 28–52, 166–201 (see also Women)
Pelvic exam, 179–182, 187
Peripheral stem cell transplantation, 229–245
Philosophy: empirical, 172; of medicine, 6–7
Politics: of differences between professional groups, 47–49; of identity, 13–14; inside medicine, 7–8; of reproduction, 31, 48
Practice policies. See Protocol
Professional groups: differences between, 4, 36–49; divisions of labor between, 124–139 (see also Work: cooperation in); emergence of, 29–30, 119–139; legitimacy of, 137–139
Professionalization, 220–222

CONTRIBUTORS

ISABELLE BASZANGER is Research Director at the CNRS (Centre National de la Recherche Scientifique) in Paris. Her recent publications include *Douleur et Médecine: La fin d'un oubli* (1995; English translation 1998).

MARC BERG is Postdoctoral Researcher at the Research Group Care, Technology and Culture of the School of Health Sciences, Maastricht University, the Netherlands. He is the author of *Rationalizing Medical Work: Decision Support Techniques and Medical Practices* (1997).

GEOFFREY C. BOWKER is Associate Professor in the Graduate School of Library and Information Science, University of Illinois at Urbana-Champaign. He is author of *Science on the Run: Information Management and Industrial Geophysics at Schlumberger* (1994) and coeditor of *Social Science, Technical Systems and Cooperative Work: Beyond the Great Divide* (1997). His forthcoming book is on the history and sociology of classification systems, written with Leigh Star.

MONICA J. CASPER is Assistant Professor of Sociology at the University of California, Santa Cruz. She is also affiliated with the Stanford University Center for Biomedical Ethics and has served as a consultant for a variety of women's health groups. She is the author of *The Making of the Unborn Patient: A Social Anatomy of Fetal Surgery* (1998).

CHARIS CUSSINS is Visiting Assistant Professor in the Department of Science and Technology Studies at Cornell University. She has written on human reproductive technologies and the politics of conservation.

NICOLAS DODIER is Sociologist at the Institut National de la Santé et de la Recherche Médicale (INSERM), Paris. He is the author of *L'expertise médicale: Essai de sociologie sur l'exercice du jugement* (1993) and *Les hommes et les machines: La conscience collective dans les sociétés technicisées* (1995).

STEFAN HIRSCHAUER is Lecturer in Sociology at the University of Bielefeld, Germany. He has published *The Social Construction of Transsexuality* (1993, in German) and *Alienating Culture* (1997, with Klaus Amann).

ANNEMARIE MOL is the Socrates Professor of Political Philosophy at the University of Twente and Research Fellow in the Policy and Ethics program of the Netherlands

Organization for Scientific Research. She is the author of *Ziek is het woord niet* (1989, with Peter van Lieshout) and *The Body Multiple* (forthcoming).

VICKY SINGLETON works as a Lecturer in the Centre for Science Studies and Science Policy at Lancaster University, United Kingdom. Amongst others, she has published on public responses to science and on feminist approaches to science.

LEIGH STAR is Associate Professor in the Graduate School of Library and Information Science, University of Illinois at Urbana-Champaign. She is the author of *Regions of the Mind: Brain Research and the Quest for Scientific Certainty* (1989), editor of *Ecologies of Knowledge* (1995), *The Cultures of Computing* (1995), and co-editor of *Social Science, Technical Systems and Cooperative Work: Beyond the Great Divide* (1997).

STEFAN TIMMERMANS is Lecturer in Medical Sociology at Brandeis University. His book, *The Paradox of CPR*, is forthcoming from Temple University Press.

DICK WILLEMS is a family physician and a philosopher. He works as Postdoctoral Researcher at the Institute for Extramural Medicine of the Free University of Amsterdam. He is the author of *Tools of Care* (1995).

Library of Congress Cataloging-in-Publication Data
Differences in medicine : unraveling practices, techniques,
and bodies / edited by Marc Berg and Annemarie Mol.
p.   cm. — (Body, commodity, text)
Includes index.
ISBN 0-8223-2162-9 (cloth : alk. paper).
— ISBN 0-8223-2174-2 (pbk. : alk. paper)
1. Social medicine.   2. Medicine—Philosophy.   I. Berg, Marc.
II. Mol, Annemarie.   III. Series.
RA418.D5   1998   610—dc21   97-37836 CIP

55668286R00170

Made in the USA
Middletown, DE
11 December 2017